23 Autopsies

A COMPANION FOR THE STUDY OF PATHOLOGY

Mark L. Mitchell, MD

Omar Zahid Chohan, DO

Book Layout ©2017 BookDesignTemplates.com

23 Autopsies. A Companion for the Study of Pathology/ Mark L. Mitchell, Omar Zahid Chohan —2nd ed.
ISBN 978-0-692-04660-9

To our teachers, and to theirs

Contents

Preface to the Second Edition

The second edition of *Nineteen Autopsies* adds four new cases, two new gross pathology images, two new images of historical figures, an index, and, thanks to my new co-author Dr. Chohan, outstanding radiographs to most of the cases. The concentration of the first edition on gross autopsy findings was one of its most important features, since the autopsy has become a much rarer event. But if one of the reasons for the decline of the autopsy has been the coming of modern whole body cross-sectional imaging techniques, then students will need to see them here, at the very least, for comparison with images of gross pathologic findings. The addition of these and other modern radiologic images should expand this text's usefulness for radiology resident physicians and radiology technologists in training and practice.

Preface to the First Edition

In 1983, I was in the last year of my residency in anatomic and clinical pathology at the University of Rochester in Rochester, New York, and I was looking for a fellowship in anatomic pathology. Since my four-year residency had been equally divided between anatomic pathology, the study of the anatomic basis of disease, and clinical pathology, the study of the laboratory diagnosis of disease, and since I intended to be primarily an anatomic pathologist, I felt that I needed additional training before stepping out into the world and making my own diagnoses. The University of North Carolina at Chapel Hill was well known for its fellowship in surgical pathology and they had a program that would also let me do six months additional training in cytopathology. I flew down to the Raleigh-Durham airport and took a shuttle to Chapel Hill where I met Fred Askin, the program director and head of surgical pathology, for breakfast. I liked Dr. Askin immediately. He was well acquainted with every pathologist I knew or had heard of, and he was delightfully sarcastic about them. He inquired about one of the staff at Rochester, "What was their problem?" followed by a turn of his head and a closed mouth smile.

My tour of the facility included the morning gross pathology conference that Dr. Askin ran. Anatomic pathology is the examination of tissue, and it can be divided into gross pathology, the examination of a surgical or autopsy specimen with one's eyes, and histopathology, the examination of the specimen under the microscope. The residents at UNC who were rotating on surgical pathology service brought interesting unlabeled gross specimens to the conference and they were placed on a laboratory bench. The residents, Dr. Askin, and I stood around the bench. Dr. Askin chose a specimen and started the conference that, he explained to me, was a game called the surgeon's game. It had this name because the participants were permitted to make statements, but to ask no questions. The goal was to identify the specimen. Once an incorrect statement was made, the participant was eliminated from competition and the opportunity to make more statements passed to the next chosen resident. The best strategy, I learned later, was to start with general statements that were likely to be true and then to gradually narrow the specificity of the statements. A sample case might be an esophago-gastrectomy specimen from a patient with gastro-esophageal carcinoma. This tumor has increased in frequency in the last 45 years and is associated with Barrett's esophagus, a metaplastic abnormality of the lower esophagus thought to be caused by reflux of acidic gastric contents into the esophagus, a structure that has not evolved to deal with increased acidity of any chronicity. The resident had already examined and dissected the specimen, selecting pieces for examination under the microscope. He or she had also already fixed the specimen in formalin so that the tissue was somewhat discolored and stiff like a piece of rubber. So, we were looking at a piece of an esophagus and stomach, not the whole thing. Since at this point in our training, we were likely to know that a specimen of this type had a limited number of possible origins, a good starting statement for our permitted statement might be, "This specimen is from below the diaphragm". The statement has the advantage of being quite broad and only excluding about half of the body. Unfortunately, in this case, the specimen comes from both sides of the diaphragm and Dr. Askin would take away the specimen and hand it to someone else. But, since our question was wrong in an unusual way, one of the other residents might make a face or say, "mmmm" when we failed, giving the next resident in line a clue.

I decided to accept a fellowship position at Chapel Hill and spent a great year there in 1983-1984. Now it was my turn to play the surgeon's game, and I was expected to know more than the residents, since I was a fellow and had completed my residency. When faced with an unknown specimen that might come from any organ of the body and might represent any of many different diseases, there can be a tendency to panic. A technique that I used when approaching these specimens was to use a mnemonic, a memory device, to try to summarize all disease types succinctly. At the time, I was using "CIT-N-VIT" that I had learned in Rochester. CIT-N-VIT stands for congenital, infectious, traumatic, neoplastic (a tumor), vascular, idiopathic (of unknown cause) and toxic. Some letters had to do double or triple duty. So toxic had to include both drug related and endocrinologic diseases. The best mnemonic that I've found to date, comes from the radiologists and was told to me by radiology residents in Delaware. VINDICATE has the advantage of being an actual English word and covers more possibilities: vascular, infectious and iatrogenic (caused by the physician), neoplastic, drug related, idiopathic (of unknown cause), congenital (literally present at birth, but used to mean inherited or genetic), allergic or autoimmune, traumatic and endocrinologic (figure 0.1). Obviously, some diseases won't fit (Where does pancreatitis go?), many patients have more than one disease, and some diseases might fit in more than one category (e.g. Diabetes mellitus is endocrinologic, but it might be autoimmune or post-operative, and there is some evidence that some cases are post-infectious.).

I've recently retired from a career as an anatomic pathologist. I was fortunate to be the section chief of autopsy pathology at Christiana Care Health Services (previously The Medical Center of Delaware) in Christiana, Delaware for 28.5 years. Among the places I worked and studied, I performed 971 autopsies. Each autopsy is a fascinating look at a person's life, one of the best ways to learn medicine, a great resource for medical quality assurance, and many other things.

I was sometimes able to teach when I was performing an autopsy, and when I was asked to teach in the classroom, I frequently would choose an autopsy to discuss with findings that were relevant to the students' area of study. In a similar way, I have chosen nineteen of these autopsies to share with you in this book. They have been chosen so that they represent either classical or just interesting examples of the disease categories in the mnemonic VINDICATE. The book is intended as a companion for the study of pathology and pathophysiology at the undergraduate or graduate level. The biggest obstacle to its use by interested students without much exposure to the health sciences is the terminology, so I have attempted to define as much as possible without limiting readability. Each case has five study questions. Some questions are easily answered just from reading the case, but others may require additional research or formulation of an opinion.

My autopsies were usually not forensic in nature. That is, they were usually of no interest to the state and were of patients who had died of natural causes.

Consequently, the results of these autopsies are a private matter, and they are presented completely anonymously. I have sometimes included figures from other similar cases and I have withheld or slightly modified some mostly clinical features to further obscure the decedent's identity.

Lastly, the reader is reminded that disease therapies and diagnostic tests may change rapidly, and this textbook is a snapshot in time of these techniques, many and perhaps all of which will become obsolete at some time in the future (see the quote from Marcel Proust at the beginning of chapter 14). If you have the responsibility for choosing therapy or a diagnostic test for a patient, you should evaluate the most comprehensive and recent references available.

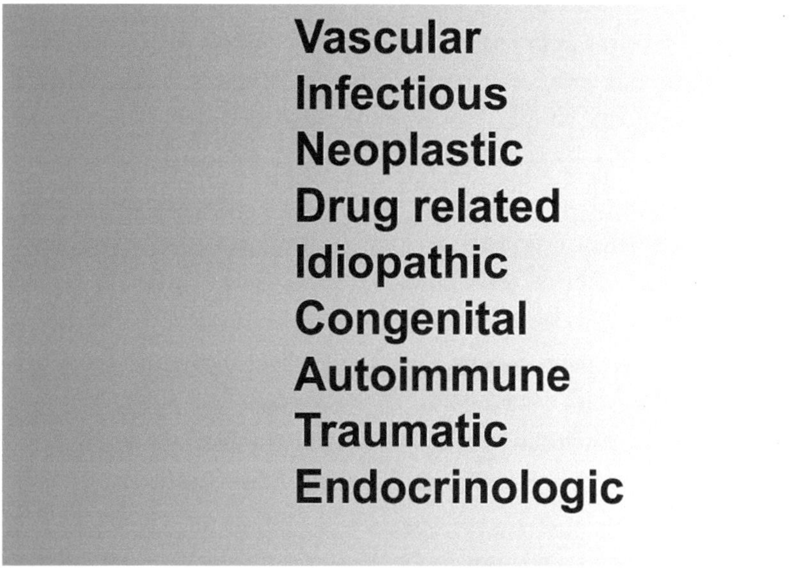

Figure 0.1. VINDICATE, a mnemonic tool to remember the major categories of disease.

Acknowledgments

Figure 2.2 is courtesy of Dr. Perry Habecker at the New Bolton Center Hospital in New Bolton, Pennsylvania.

Figures 6.6 and 6.7 are courtesy of Dr. David Saul at the Nemours Alfred I. duPont Hospital for Children in Wilmington, Delaware.

Figures 20.4, 20.5 and 20.6 are courtesy of Dr. Michael Kanzer at the Christiana Hospital in Newark, Delaware.

Figures 2.6, 4.7, 5.8, 8.5, 10.7, 14.6, 16.4, 17.4, 17.5, 18.5, 19.8, 20.7, 21.6, 21.7, 22.4, 23.7, and 24.7 are public domain images reproduced from Images in the History of Medicine in the National Library of Medicine database and are courtesy of the National Library of Medicine.

Figure 11.3 is a public domain image from https://commons.wikimedia.org/wiki/File:Friedrich_Schatz.png.

Figure 15.4 is courtesy of the Wellcome Library Collection and its use is permitted by the Creative commons BY 4.0 license (http://creativecommons.org/licenses/by/4.0/).

Many thanks to Karen J. Mitchell and to Dr. Andrew J. Mitchell for their critical evaluation of the manuscripts, and to Aaron S. Mitchell for the photographs of Dr. Chohan.

CHAPTER 1

An Introduction to the autopsy

"I believe it is only a matter of time before physicians as well as hospitals will be rated by percentage of autopsies they do or see in their practices." Roscoe C. Giles, 1932. J National Medical Association (Roscoe Giles, 1890 – 1970, was the first African-American admitted to Cornell's medical school and the first to be certified by the American Board of Surgery)

1.1 What is an autopsy?

An autopsy is the postmortem examination of the human body. The body is examined by a trained prosector after the decedent's history or medical record is examined and with the permission of the decedent's next of kin. It is examined using the five senses in a methodical way, and it can be further examined using other techniques commonly including light microscopy of cytologic and histologic specimens, plain radiography, toxicology, microbiological culture, and cytogenetics. The results are recorded in a detailed report that becomes part of the decedent's medical record. A review of the history of the autopsy and a detailed account of how an autopsy is performed in the hospital will give a better understanding of the procedure.

1.2 Medical history of the autopsy

The nature of the first postmortem human examination is lost in antiquity. Our ancestors hunted and so had some familiarity with internal structures in animals, and there is evidence that they sometimes hunted each other. They also performed acts of divination using the internal parts of various domestic animals. Examination of the body to determine the cause of death is documented, but was a rare event, in the dark ages. Autopsies started to become more common as the Renaissance approached. The great Italian polymath, Leonardo da Vinci (1452 – 1519) performed one in the 15th century on an old man in the hospital Santa Maria Nuova in Florence: "without another movement of any sign of accident, he passed away from this life. And I did an autopsy on him to see the cause of such a quiet death" [1]. Theophilus Bonetus of Geneva (1620 – 1689) published a review of the literature describing 3000 autopsy reports in 1689. The great physician and prosector Giovanni Battista Morgagni (1682 – 1771) published a series of letters in 1751 that contained what we would today call clinicopathological case studies. In these 700 cases, the author summarized his career and was the first to systematically correlate clinical with postmortem findings. The work is still considered one of the great achievements in the history of medicine. Morgagni was the first to clearly describe many important anatomical features and pathologies including the anorectal crypts, which are still called the crypts of Morgagni, hepatic cirrhosis, hepatization of the lung and aortic aneurysms.

Other great figures who used the autopsy and clinicopathological correlation to further the development of the science of medicine include René Théophile Hyacinthe Laennec (1781–1826) the inventor of the stethoscope. Laennec performed autopsies on hundreds of patients with pneumonia. He described bronchiectasis, pneumothorax, pulmonary infarct, and emphysema and coined the term cirrhosis of the liver. He discussed the significance of tubercles of the lung and died of tuberculosis himself at age 45. The significance of the autopsy reached new heights in the 19th century with improvements made to the microscope and the coming of the great pathologists Carl von Rokitansky

(1804 – 1878) from Bohemia and Rudolph Virchow (1821 – 1902) from Prussia.

The autopsy contributed to new knowledge on anatomy and helped to define new diseases that could now be separated from the previously poorly distinguishable categories defined by signs and symptoms alone.

In the middle of the 20th century, the number of autopsies performed at a hospital was considered a measure of its quality, since it showed intellectual and academic purpose including teaching and research and suggested an interest in quality assurance using the correlation of antemortem and postmortem findings. This was reflected in the 1953 recommendation by the Joint Commission for the Accreditation of Hospitals that 25% of deaths in teaching hospitals and 20% of deaths in non-teaching hospitals have an autopsy. During the last 50 years of the 20th- century, the rate of non-forensic postmortem examinations declined in the United States. In the 1960s the autopsy rate was 30 to 40% and by 2010 it was less than 5% for adult decedents. A recent report from the United Kingdom found an autopsy rate less than 1%. [2,3]. The beginning of the decline is sometimes linked to a 1956 editorial in the Journal of the American Medical Association by the internist Isaac Starr [4]. Dr. Starr said that an era of medical experimentation had come and that the gathering of routine information at autopsy was a waste of time. Responses from many pathologists defended the value of the autopsy, pointing out its value in the elucidation of many diseases, its use in quality assurance, and the value of the application of new techniques to the autopsy, just as they were used elsewhere in Medicine. I think, however, that complaints about and difficulty with the autopsy stretch back to antiquity, and one need not look far for such evidence. Handling and caring for the dead has always been a special societal task that many have found distasteful. Dissection of a loved one who has recently died is something often not desired by the next-of-kin. Physicians might be concerned that autopsy would show their diagnostic mistakes and might lead to legal action against them. Searching for references to the adage that 'a physician buries his mistakes' will show, in addition to the famous quote from the architect Frank Lloyd Wright, many moldy examples, including the old Ukrainian proverb, "The earth will cover the doctor's mistakes" and "Doctor cures, if the sun sees it; but if he kills, the earth hides it." variously attributed

[5]. Interested physicians have combated these underlying problems with programs to educate resident physicians on ways to request an autopsy sensitively and arguments to use to "sell" the autopsy to the next-of-kin, e.g. an infectious or inherited disease might be discovered that would be of immediate interest to the decedent's relatives. In the latter years of the century, the decline in the autopsy rate was sometimes attributed to the availability of the CT (computerized tomography) scan and the MRI (magnetic resonance imaging), both supposedly making autopsy obsolete. All agree that these fantastic inventions have permitted an amazing look into the body that was never possible before, but the rate of discrepancies between antemortem diagnoses and postmortem diagnoses has been the same before and after the coming of these techniques in many of these studies. Furthermore, the rate of adult autopsies has declined, but the rate of stillborn autopsies has remained high, and whereas the findings at adult autopsy are imagined as potentially damning by clinicians, the findings at stillborn autopsy are imagined as potentially exculpatory [6-8].

1.3 How an autopsy is performed today

An autopsy is the postmortem examination of a deceased person. There are various standard approaches to the examination, but there are different kinds of autopsies and different techniques may be used. Forensic autopsies are performed by physicians with special training in cases that meet certain statutory requirements indicating that they are of special interest to the state. Forensic cases are usually those where it is suspected that the patient did not die of natural causes. Well-known examples are homicides and accidents. Autopsies that are performed in a hospital usually do not meet these statutory requirements, and these patients usually have died of natural causes. Non-forensic autopsies legally require the permission of the next of kin or some similar authoritative person to be performed. Forensic autopsies, of course, do not have this requirement.

There are various ways to perform an autopsy, and the methods carry the names of the 19th century pathologists who described them. In my career, a typical non-forensic hospital autopsy was performed using a technique usually attributed to Anton Ghon (1866 – 1936). The patient's medical record and the autopsy request form were reviewed. I occasionally spoke with the next of kin, but almost never with the clinicians, mostly because the patient had many clinicians and they were usually not aware of or interested in the autopsy. Exceptions included certain autopsies on stillborn infants, cases that had an interested associated physician in training (a so-called resident physician) and cases that were thought to have a chance to lead to litigation. Other interested parties included the hospital Department of Risk Management, some of my colleagues, e.g. the neuropathologist, and my assistant at the autopsy, one of two men or women traditionally called dieners (from the German word for servant). The diener and I put on scrub suits, like surgeons wear during surgery, a water-resistant gown, a waterproof apron, a surgical face mask, and a plastic face mask and shoe covers. In certain cases, e.g. patients with tuberculosis or the acquired immunodeficiency disease, a special respirator called a PAPR (Powered air purifying respirator) respirator is worn in which the prosector's head is covered and air is pumped in through a HEPA filter (high efficiency particulate arrestance) that excludes micro-organisms. The device resembles an old-fashioned hair dryer. Gloves are worn that are slightly thicker than the usual gloves worn at surgery. The body is opened with a Y-shaped incision extending from the shoulders to the epigastrium and then down the midline of the abdomen to the symphysis pubis. The thoracic cavity is opened with a hand-held vibrating saw that cuts through the ribs. The saw is the same kind that is used to remove a plaster cast after a bone fracture has healed. In all cases, the organs are examined in situ and any accumulated fluids in body cavities are measured and described. Some pathologists have dictation equipment available during an autopsy and dictate their findings as they go. At my institutions, we made written notes and dictated the case after it was completed. The heart and lungs are removed separately. The neck organs are dissected free from the body. The pathologist then examines the heart and lungs in detail and weighs them at a slightly separate work area, while the diener removes the neck organs, mediastinum, abdominal and pelvic organs en bloc. Often, the diener ties off and removes the bowel from the ligament of Treitz to the rectum prior to removing the other organs together. In some cases, e.g. aortic dissection or patients who have had a coronary artery bypass graft procedure, the heart is left attached, to be removed with the other organs. The abdominal block is placed with the anterior surface facing down and is then dissected. During this part of the dissection, the abdominal aorta, the inferior vena cava, the adrenal glands, the kidneys, the spleen, the ureters and bladder, the internal genitalia and rectum are examined. Next, the neck organs are examined. The esophagus is opened and the stomach, duodenum, gallbladder, porta hepatis and pancreas are examined. The liver is then examined. In all cases, the organs are examined on their exterior aspect and then on cut section. Relatively small portions of the organs are placed in 10% neutral buffered formalin to fix overnight and to be sampled the next day for histologic examination (under the microscope). Fixation is a physical or chemical process that sterilizes, preserves, hardens, and mechanically stabilizes tissue. Fixation permits tissue to be further processed so that it can be thinly sectioned, stained, and examined under the light microscope. The most common method of fixation in the histology laboratory today is immersion in buffered formalin, an aqueous solution made from formaldehyde. The fixative properties of formalin were discovered in the late 19th century. Prior to that time, many tissue sections were performed on frozen tissue; a method that is still used today when quick results are necessary. The discovery story associated with formalin is that it was being investigated as a disinfectant when, for some reason, a dead mouse was left in it overnight. The next morning the mouse had become stiff and the rest, although probably not exactly as reported, is history. In certain special circumstances, cases of possible poisoning, research protocols, and cases requiring various exotic studies, portions of appropriate tissue are taken and preserved by refrigeration or freezing (usually at -70° Celsius). In cases where infection is suspected, and antemortem cultures were not obtained or were unsatisfactory, tissue is taken for culture. I typically took portions of both lower lung lobes and spleen in cases of suspected sepsis (systemic infection). Tissue might also be taken from a wound or the kidneys in cases where these were suspected to be the source of sepsis. Many clinicians and some pathologists consider postmortem cultures to be of little use and likely to be contaminated, but in patients who have died relatively recently and whose body was refrigerated in the usual fashion, cultures are very useful and virtually never contaminated. If the lung lobes and spleen are sampled with separate sterile culture kits, then the finding of a bacteria or fungal species in more than one location is good evidence for sepsis with that organism. Many pathologists take postmortem blood cultures from the heart, but in my experience, these are insensitive for the detection of sepsis. At the end of the autopsy, the decedent's scalp is reflected, the skull is opened with a circular to somewhat V-shaped cut made with the vibrating saw, and the brain is removed. The brain is a relatively soft organ and it must fix in formalin for some time before the neuropathologist examines it. In those cases without neurologic findings, I often cut the brain in the fresh state and fix representative pieces of it - at the Universities where I have studied and worked, brains were usually fixed for at least 1 week in all cases. Lastly, the bowel is flushed clean, it is opened longitudinally and its lining is examined. Lesions of interest may then be photographed in their fresh state. Following the completion of the initial gross examination part of the autopsy, the results are dictated and an initial report is issued called the Provisional Anatomic Diagnoses with the Provisional Cause of Death. The small pieces of tissue fixed in formalin are examined the day after the autopsy and even smaller representative pieces are submitted for histologic examination. Some tissue, e.g. calcified coronary arteries and a portion of a vertebral body taken for its bone marrow, are first decalcified in a weakly acidic solution. In most adult autopsies 20 - 30 sections are examined histologically. The histologic sections are seen on day 3. At this point, the pathologist must begin his mental synthesis of the case. He or she may need to see some special stains beyond the typical hematoxylin and eosin. Hematoxylin is a basic blue stain derived from the logwood tree that is grown in the Yucatan and in Jamaica. Eosin is a synthetic acidic red aniline dye. The discovery of the aniline dyes in the mid-19th century in Germany revolutionized the textile industry and several of these dyes have been used in histopathology. (The A in the chemical companies BASF and AGFA stands for aniline.) He may need to return to any retained tissue to check for various findings that occurred to him later. He may need to consult with his colleagues or with experts at other institutions. When all is ready, the final report is dictated and distributed. The final report consists of the original provisional diagnoses (PAD), the new final diagnoses (FAD), an abstract of the patient's medical history, a description of the gross findings by organ system, a list of all special studies done and tissue examined histologically, a description of the histologic findings, a list of postmortem culture results and a final correlative summary of the case. For most of my career, the College of American Pathologists required that all autopsies be completed in 30 days unless there were extenuating circumstances, e.g. special studies pending at another institution. Autopsies are considered a private procedure and there are no observers, photographs, or tissue taken for research without the permission of the next-of-kin. If permission is given, medical personnel in training may observe an autopsy. I never encountered a medical educational opportunity that was superior to autopsy.

1.4 References

1. Foster WD. A Short History of Clinical Pathology. London: E&S Livingstone Ltd.; 1961

2. Council on Scientific Affairs. Autopsy. A comprehensive review of current issues. JAMA. 1987;258:364-369.

3. Turnbull A, Osborn M, Nicholas N. Hospital autopsy: Endangered or extinct? J Clin Pathol. 2015;68:601-604.

4. Starr I. Potential values of the autopsy today. J Am Med Assoc. 1956;160:1144- 1145.

5. Anonymous. Ukrainian proverbs. http://www.inspirational-stories.com/proverbs/ukranian-the-earth-will-cover-the-doctors-mistakes/. Accessed March 1, 2015.

6. King LS, Meehan MC. A history of the autopsy. A review. Am J Pathol. 1973;73:514-544.

7. Landefeld CS, Goldman L. The autopsy in clinical medicine. Mayo Clin Proc. 1989;64:1185-1189.

8. Shojania KG, Burton EC, McDonald KM, Goldman L. Changes in rates of autopsy-detected diagnostic errors over time: a systematic review. JAMA. 2003;289:2849-2856.

CHAPTER 2

A middle-aged man with a history of ethanol abuse who fell down stairs. (vinDicaTe, drug, trauma)

"Open up a few corpses: you will dissipate at once the darkness that observation alone could not dissipate." Xavier Bichat (1771 – 1802, Bichat died after falling down a flight of stairs)

2.1 The Autopsy

2.1.1 Case history

A 40-year-old man with a history of ethanol abuse was found unresponsive at the bottom of a flight of concrete steps out of doors. Very little historical information was available. A witness said that the patient had coughed up or vomited blood prior to falling. The patient was brought to the Emergency department and intubated. A CT scan of the head showed an acute left subdural hematoma on top of a chronic subdural hematoma. The midline of the brain was shifted to the right side by 13 mm. There were multiple fractures in the skull including the nasal septum, the right zygomatic arch, the clivus, the body of the sphenoid bone, and the basal occiput. The patient died on the second hospital day.

2.1.2 Postmortem findings

At autopsy, the presence of basilar skull fractures was confirmed (figure 2.1). The patient had a markedly fatty liver and no atherosclerosis, both signs compatible with alcoholism (figures 2.2, 2.3). No cirrhosis or esophageal varices, additional but more severe features of alcoholism, were seen. There was a 3-mm area of red discoloration at the esophagogastric junction associated with a small area of intraepithelial hemorrhage under the microscope. The patient had no coronary artery disease or evidence of a new or old myocardial infarct. There were aspirated gastric contents in large bronchi without any histologic evidence of an inflammatory reaction. The patient had early acute bronchopneumonia in three lung lobes (figures 2.4, 2.5). Histologic sections of lung showed respiratory bronchiolitis, a change seen in patients who smoke cigarettes. The brain was examined by Michael Kanzer, the neuropathologist, and showed focal brain contusions and anoxic encephalopathy.

2.1.3 Case summary

It is common for patients to come to autopsy who were unconscious at the time of admission, came through the Emergency department, and have little or no medical history available. It's important to remember that the patient might have an important discoverable medical history. The best person to talk to is the patient's next of kin; usually, the person who signed permission for the autopsy.

The patient had fatty liver, a common pathological change in liver cells. Various pathological stresses can cause this change, but the most common is the use of ethanol.

A witness had seen the patient cough or vomit blood prior to falling. There are many causes of hemoptysis (coughing up blood) or hematemesis (vomiting up blood) even just within the population or patients who are alcoholics. One cause of special concern is rupture of an esophageal varix (the medical term for a varicose vein). Patients who drink ethanol to excess may develop a chronic fibrosing (scarring) disorder of the liver called cirrhosis (see chapter 10). One of the consequences of cirrhosis is obstruction of the portal blood flow. When the patient has portal hypertension, the blood crosses through anastomotic sites into the systemic blood circulation. One of the sites of anastomosis are veins at the gastro-esophageal junction. These veins dilate and if they rupture, the patient may exsanguinate. This patient had a small area at his gastro-esophageal junction that may have been the source of some bleeding, but he did not have cirrhosis or esophageal varices.

The brain is a relatively soft organ that is protected by the skull. Changes in the brain, such as hemorrhage or edema, that might be consequential but temporary and resolvable in, for example, a skeletal muscle in your arm, are often disastrous in the brain. There is no place for the brain to go, and while the patient can tolerate a non-functional muscle for a while, many functions of the brain are necessary for life. A midline shift in the brain, as seen in this case from hemorrhage and edema on one side, is an ominous finding. Fractures of the basal skull have a relatively poor prognosis for the same reason. A broken finger can be tolerated relatively easily, but changes in the brain next to a basal skull fracture or having a basal skull fracture line that crosses the path of major blood vessels is a much more serious injury. Patients with a basal skull fracture may present with CSF otorrhea (leakage of cerebrospinal fluid from the nose), loss of hearing due to damage of cranial nerve VIII, bruising around the eyes (so-called Raccoon eye appearance) and bruising on the mastoid process (Battle's sign).

There were gastric contents (i.e. food) in the large bronchi of the lungs. Aspiration of gastric contents or vomitus may be a cause of death. If the emergency medical technicians sweep or clean the upper airway before intubating the patient, evidence of the cause of death may be lost. This is an occasional problem at autopsy. It is possible in this case that the patient aspirated vomitus before falling down the steps and striking his head. I commented in the report that there was no inflammatory reaction to the aspirated material indicating that the patient didn't have a more subacute or chronic problem with aspiration pneumonia.

The patient did have pneumonia (inflammation of the lung) in three lung lobes. Based on the appearance of sections of the lung under the microscope, I favored that the patient's pneumonia was a typical bacterial one (alcoholics are at increased risk to get pneumonia). It is likely that the patient was unwell from his pneumonia and that he was more likely to fall when drinking.

2.2 Discussion

2.2.1 Falls

Falls are the second leading cause of death from an accidental injury worldwide. About 420,000 deaths can be attributed to falls each year [1]. Children, the elderly, and the inebriated are at increased risk of falling. Fatal falls from a height are most often a suicide; accidents are less common and homicides of this type are rare. Injuries from a more moderate fall may include scalp laceration, skull fracture, and intracranial injuries as was seen in the case presented here. Many of these cases that come to the attention of the forensic pathologist are associated with alcohol intoxication. Other possible sequelae include fractures of the upper femur, especially in the elderly, and subdural hematomas, which may develop over time [2,3].

2.2.2 Ethanol

Ethanol is in the sedative-hypnotic class of drugs. It is a byproduct of fermentation, and fermented beverages have been drunk in many societies throughout human history. It is the most common drug of abuse and the most commonly encountered toxic substance in forensic medicine. Half of all patients admitted to level 1 trauma centers for motor vehicle accidents are intoxicated and 23 to 32% of decedents in cases of non-motor vehicle fatal injuries are intoxicated [4-6]. About 50% of adults in the Western world drink alcohol and 5 – 10% have chronic alcoholism. There are about 100,000 deaths each year in the US from the effects of alcohol. More than half of these are from motor vehicle accidents, homicides, and suicides and about 15,000 of them are from cirrhosis [7].

Ethanol is absorbed unchanged and is distributed throughout the body. Less than 10% is excreted unchanged in the urine, sweat, and breath, and this is the basis for the use of breath analyzer tests by law enforcement to detect inebriated automobile drivers. The ratio of ethanol in blood to that in the breath is 2200:1 [5]. Most ingested ethanol is oxidized in the liver to acetaldehyde, which is further converted to acetate and enters the Krebs cycle to become carbon dioxide and water. In most states in the US, a driver is considered legally intoxicated with a blood alcohol level of 80 mg/dL. This level can be achieved with the consumption of three standard drinks in a typical man [7]. Some signs of CNS impairment can be detected at a blood level as low as 30 mg/dL and coma and death may result at a level of 300 mg/dL [5]. Tolerance to ethanol develops in chronic alcoholics, and unusually high blood levels may occur in patients who do not seem markedly impaired.

Although ethanol may cause death acutely when consumed in sufficient quantities, most of the medical consequences encountered are due to chronic alcoholism. These include cirrhosis of the liver with portal hypertension and its side effects (e.g. splenomegaly, ascites, esophageal varices, and hemorrhoids), dementia and encephalopathy (Wernicke-Korsakoff encephalopathy), gastric ulcers, fetal alcohol syndrome, and cancer. In addition to hepatoma arising in a background of cirrhosis, alcoholics have an increased risk of carcinoma of the oral cavity, pharynx, esophagus, colon, and breast [8].

2.3 Medical History

2.3.1 Alcoholism

Alcoholism was first considered to be a disease and not a moral failing by Drs. Benjamin Rush (1746 – 1813, figure 2.6) and Thomas Trotter (1760 – 1832) in the late 18th century [9]. Benjamin Rush was a signer of the

Declaration of Independence, an abolitionist and the founder of Dickinson College. He served as surgeon general in the Continental army. Dr. Rush did recommend that chronic alcoholics be incarcerated against their will in hospitals specially designed for the purpose. Thomas Trotter was a Scottish naval physician who, interestingly, was also an abolitionist. One hundred years later, the great William Osler commented in his textbook that treatment for chronic alcoholism was very difficult and that it was best to institutionalize these patients to prevent contact with alcohol [10]. More modern methods have included 12 step programs that teach the patient that their addiction is beyond their personal control and many alternative psychological, behavioral, and pharmaceutical approaches. Unfortunately, if measured by the proportion of patients who relapse, the effectiveness of all therapies is low and Dr. Osler's discussion seems more modern than one would hope from a textbook from 1892.

2.4 Laboratory medicine

2.4.1 Blood alcohol

Blood specimens for the determination of alcohol should have the venipuncture site cleaned using a non-alcohol swab. The specimen should remain sealed, since alcohol is volatile, and non-sterile specimens should be stored with sodium fluoride to prevent contamination by fermentation [11]. Colorimetric methods for the measurement of alcohol have been used for many years. A commonly used current technique is an enzymatic method in which the patient's serum is incubated with a non-human alcohol dehydrogenase. As NAD (nicotinamide adenine dinucleotide) is converted to NADH, the serum is monitored at 340 nm and the amount of alcohol present can be determined [4]. The reference method for ethanol is gas chromatography. This technique has the advantage of being able to separate and quantify all the types of alcohol present, not just ethanol.

2.5 Study questions

1. Alcoholics are sometimes unable to get alcohol. In their desperation, they may ingest non-ethanol alcohols, such as isopropanol (rubbing alcohol) or methanol (wood alcohol). What are the effects of these toxic substances?

2. How is blood ethanol measured in your local hospital?

3. What substances may interfere with the accurate measurement of ethanol?

4. Is any ethanol normally produced in the body?

5. Is the measurement of urine ethanol medically or legally useful?

2.6 References

1. World Health Organization. Falls fact sheet #3244. 2012. http://www.who.int/mediacentre/factsheets/fs344/en/. Accessed 2015.
2. Gonzales T, Vance M, Helpern M, Umberger CJ. Legal Medicine. Pathology and Toxicology. New York:Appleton-Century-Crofts, Inc.; 1954
3. Wetli CV. Practical forensic pathology. New York: Igaku-Shoin; 1988: 150.
4. Pincus MR, Abraham NZ. Toxicology and therapeutic drug monitoring. In: Henry JB, editor. Clinical diagnosis and management by laboratory methods. Philadelphia: W.B.Saunders; 2001
5. Jacobs DS, Oxley DK, DeMott WR. Laboratory test handbook. Hudson (Cleveland), Ohio: Lexi-Comp Inc.; 2001
6. Smith GS, Branas CC, Miller TR. Fatal non-traffic injuries involving alcohol: A metanalysis. Ann Emerg Med 1999;33(6):659 – 668
7. Kumar V, Abbas AK, Aster JC. Robbins and Cotran Pathologic basis of disease. Philadelphia: Elsevier Saunders: 2015

8. Center for disease control and prevention. Alcohol and public health fact sheet. 2014.
http://www.cdc.gov/alcohol/fact-sheet/alcohol-use.htm. Accessed 2015.
9. Talbott JH. A biographical history of medicine: excerpts and essays on the men and their work. New York: Grune & Stratton; 1970:1211
10. Osler W. The principles and practice of medicine. New York: D. Appleton and Company; 1892:1079
11. Thorne DP. Toxicology. In: Bishop ML, Duben-Engelkirk JL, Fody EP, editors. Clinical chemistry. Principles, procedures and correlations. Philadelphia: Lippincott Williams and Wilkins; 2000: 508-510

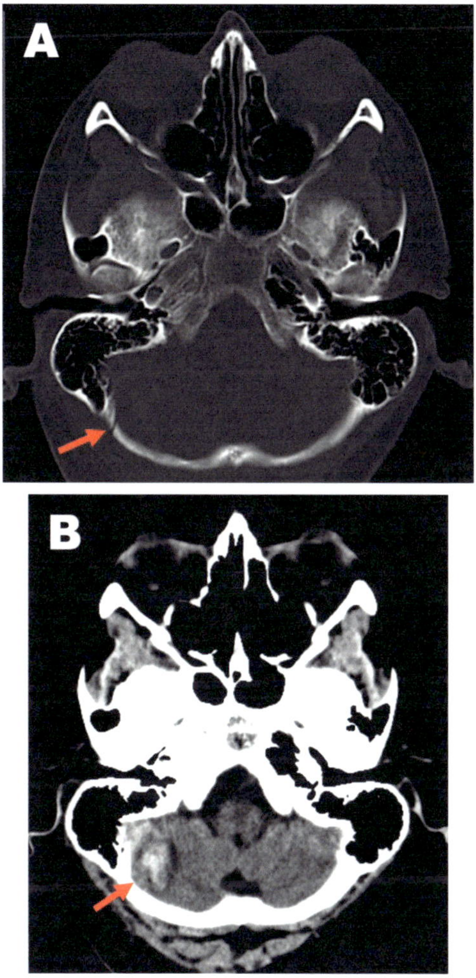

Figure 2.1.A. There is a non-displaced and non-depressed right occipital bone fracture in this image from a different case with basilar skull fracture (red arrow).

Figure 2.1.B. This is the same CT level as figure 2.1.A, but with brain windowing, showing a right inferior cerebellar hemorrhagic contusion (red arrow) adjacent to the right occipital bone fracture.

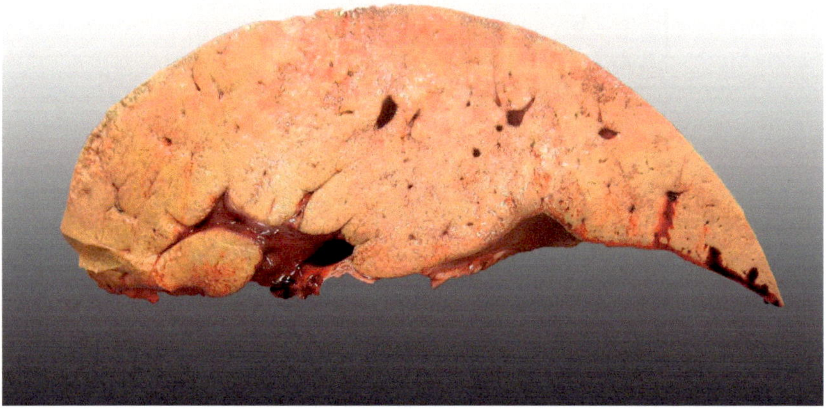

Figure 2.2. Fatty liver also called hepatocellular steatosis. The liver is usually brown, as you know from the kitchen, but a fatty liver is yellow. Fatty liver also has a greasy feel to it on cut section. This image is of a fatty liver from a gravid mare. It is courtesy of Dr. Perry Habecker at the New Bolton Center Hospital in New Bolton, Pennsylvania.

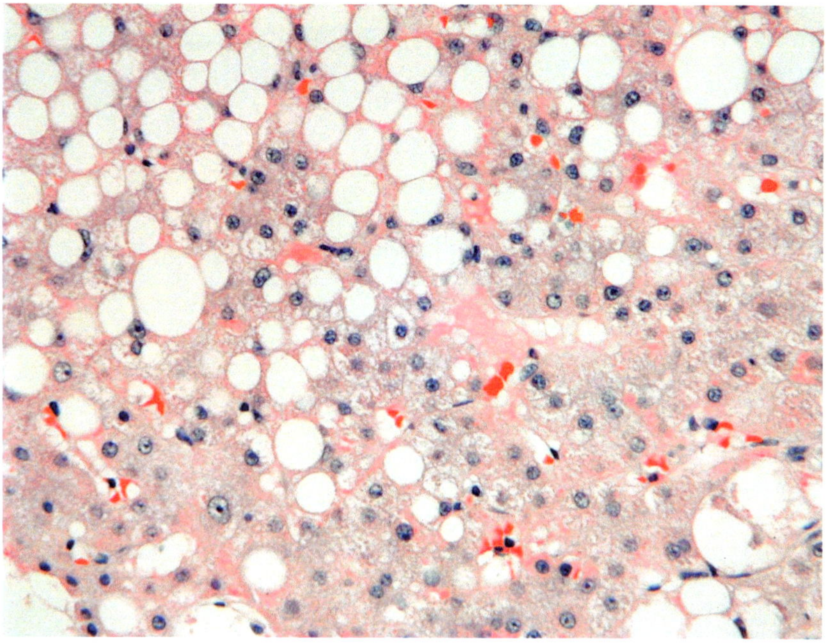

Figure 2.3. A photomicrograph of fatty liver in a case of alcoholic hepatitis. Normal liver cells have pink granular cytoplasm. When they are under assault from a variety of toxins (ethanol in this case) and in several other abnormalities they may accumulate fat. The large intracytoplasmic droplets that are mostly in the left upper part of this image are the typical histologic picture of fatty liver. Tissue for microscopic examination is fixed in formalin, then dehydrated in graded alcohols and finally it is cleared in the organic solvent xylene. Xylene dissolves out fat so that the tissue can be infiltrated with paraffin and cut. The vacuoles seen in this figure are where the dissolved fat used to be. (Original magnification, x200. H&E stain)

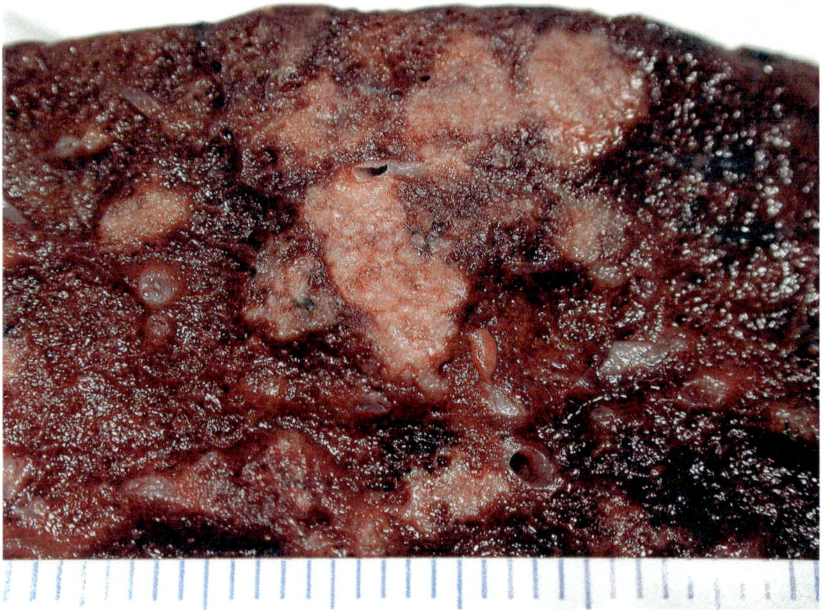

Figure 2.4. Acute bronchopneumonia. The lung is composed of many small air sacs, the alveoli, with capillaries in the alveolar walls since the lung serves to oxygenate the blood. The lung in a living person is usually pink and sponge-like with areas of punctate black discoloration. The alveoli contain some histiocytes and those cells ingest carbon particles that we inhale (bus exhaust, campfires, coal powered electrical power plants, cigarettes etc.) and they give the lung its areas of black discoloration. The blood no longer circulates after death, and since most people die lying down on their backs, the posterior parts of the lung are dark red in color. In this image, we see the normal postmortem dark red appearance in the background. The white elevated areas are pneumonia. The small divisions on the ruler at the bottom of this image are millimeters.

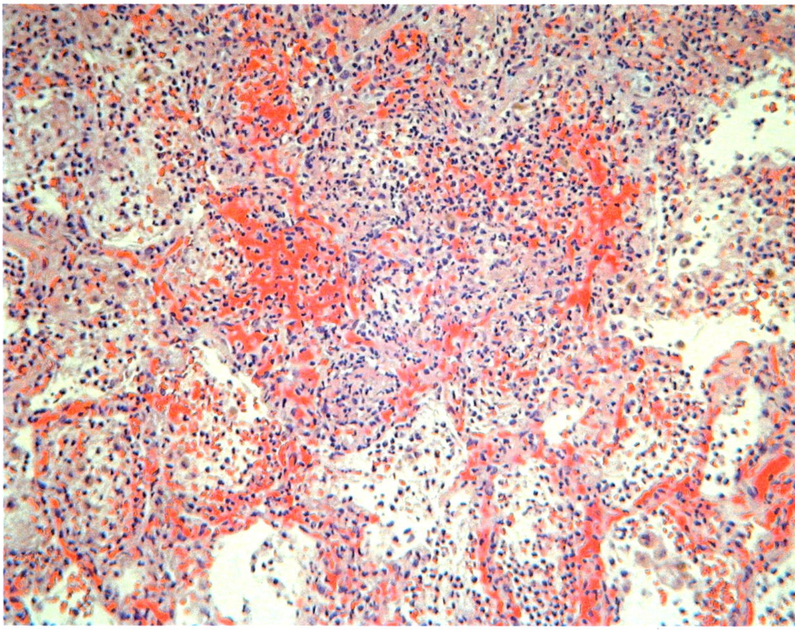

Figure 2.5. Acute bronchopneumonia. The white areas in figure 2.4 are present because the alveoli (the hexagonal shaped spaces in this picture) in pneumonia fill up with an inflammatory exudate containing red blood cells, white blood cells and fibrin. Many of the small dark spots in this picture are the nuclei or nuclear fragments of polymorphonuclear neutrophils (PMNs or just neutrophils). Neutrophils are the main acute reacting white blood cells in the body and the principal cellular component of pus. They often respond to bacterial infection. (Original magnification x100-200. H&E stain)

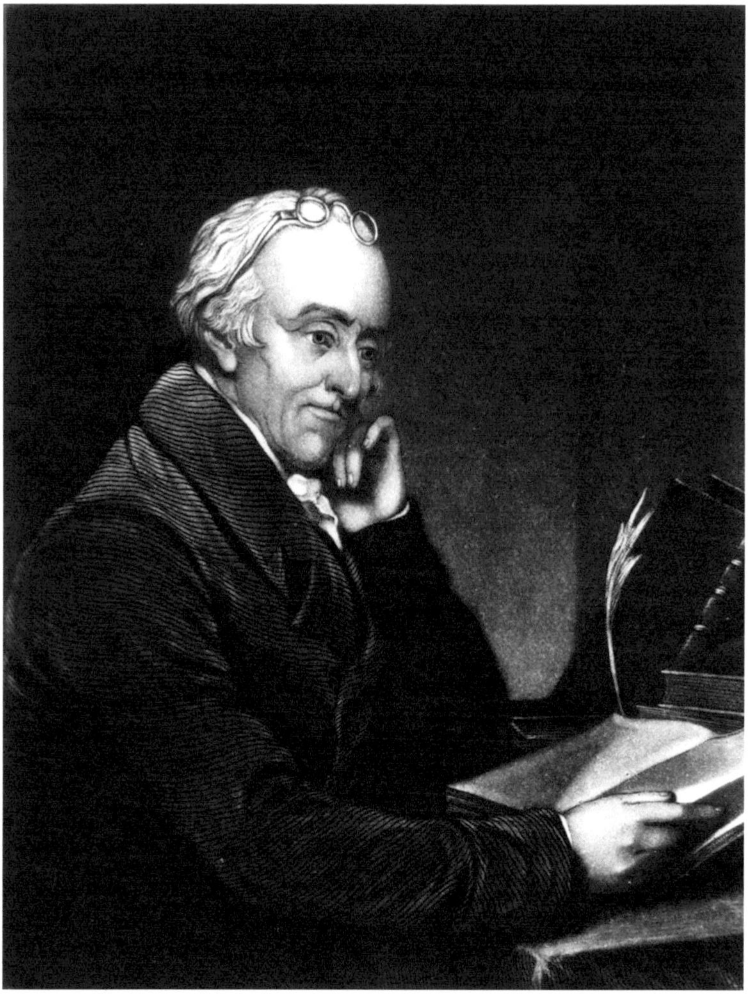

Figure 2.6. Benjamin Rush (1746 – 1813). Courtesy of the National Library of Medicine.

CHAPTER 3

A middle-aged man with sickle cell anemia and pneumonia. (vIndiCate, infectious, congenital)

"I must begin with a good body of facts, and not from principles, in which I always suspect some fallacy." Charles Darwin (1809 – 1882)

3.1 The Autopsy

3.1.1 Case history

A 45-year-old African-American man with sickle cell anemia had a history of multiple complications including stroke, liver disease, diabetes mellitus, pulmonary hypertension, cardiomyopathy, secondary hemosiderosis, coagulopathy, thrombocytopenia, and hepatitis C. He was admitted to the hospital with diarrhea and abdominal pain. He had been recently admitted elsewhere for an hepatic veno-occlusive crisis. The patient's medications were hydromorphone, deferoxamine mesylate, insulin, folate, sertraline, lansoprazole, promethazine, and digoxin. He had a hemoglobin of 9 (normal = 14 – 17 g/dL), and a glucose of 38 (normal = 70 – 105 mg/dL fasting). His glucose varied dramatically during the hospitalization ranging from 38 to 294. The patient's pain was in the right upper quadrant of the abdomen and was thought to be due to his liver disease. The patient became progressively more lethargic and died on the 12th hospital day.

3.1.2 Postmortem findings

At postmortem examination, there was gray - blue discoloration of several organs, including the pancreas and liver. The patient's lungs had areas of firmness and white discoloration in the right middle, right lower and left lower lung lobes. The liver was cirrhotic (figure 3.1). There was prominent thickening of both cardiac ventricles. Examination of tissue sections under the microscope showed extensive hemosiderosis involving the heart, liver, pancreas, adrenal cortex and medulla, testicular interstitium and thyroid gland (figure 3.2). The firm white areas in the lung were confirmed as acute bronchopneumonia. Bacilli of one morphotype were seen in his lungs and the sinusoids of an abdominal lymph node. There was mural thickening of pulmonary arterioles, a feature of pulmonary hypertension. Some sections of lung had deformed erythrocytes in them compatible with sickle cell disease (figure 3.3). Only a small amount of possible splenic tissue was identified. Sections of liver showed both micronodular cirrhosis and extensive hepatocellular and bile duct iron deposition. There was mild to moderate portal chronic inflammation. Postmortem cultures of the lungs grew numerous Klebsiella pneumoniae (figure 3.4).

3.1.3 Case summary

The patient was a middle-aged African-American man with known sickle cell disease; he had so-called auto-splenectomy due to years of splenic infarcts. Sickle cell patients who have lost their spleen are at increased risk for infection by bacteria that are encapsulated, and the patient had Klebsiella pneumoniae pneumonia. There were other features compatible with late stage sickle cell anemia including chronic hepatitis and cirrhosis with hemosiderosis from years of hemolysis and blood transfusions (figure 3.5). I attributed the patient's death to acute bronchopneumonia and probable sepsis in a background of late stage sickle cell anemia.

3.2 Discussion

3.2.1 Sickle cell disease

Red blood cells carry oxygen throughout the body because they contain the protein hemoglobin that binds reversibly with oxygen. The most abundant form of adult hemoglobin is called hemoglobin A and is composed of two alpha protein chains and two beta protein chains. Each chain has an associated non-protein heme group in which a molecule of ferrous iron binds with oxygen as blood passes through the lungs.

About two million African-Americans carry a single copy of a gene mutation that replaces the amino acid glutamic acid with a valine at one point in the beta-globin chain in hemoglobin. These people are said to have sickle trait and are often asymptomatic, but a couple who are each heterozygous for this mutation have a one in four chance of having a child with two copies of the abnormal gene. Patient's affected in this way have sickle cell disease. There are about 50,000 - 70,000 people with sickle cell disease in the United States [1]. Some parts of Africa have a much higher proportion of people with the disease. The disease has many deleterious effects and, at least historically, a marked decrease in lifespan, such that one would expect the incidence to decline over time, but there is evidence that heterozygous patients with sickle trait are resistant to Plasmodium falciparum malaria, and hence actually at increased fitness relative to the general population. In this situation, the presence of homozygotes with sickle cell disease is maintained. Unfortunately, in modern times African-Americans in the US who are heterozygous for HbS will not benefit, but the risk of having children with sickle cell disease persists.

The abnormal hemoglobin in sickle cell disease has an abnormal physical structure when deoxygenated and causes distortion of the patient's red blood cells. Eventually, these cells become sickle-shaped, acquire membrane damage and hemolyze. The degree of sickling is made worse by dehydration, acidosis and with increased capillary transit time, as occurs in the spleen. The patients have a chronic hemolytic anemia, so they have erythroid hyperplasia in the bone marrow, hyperbilirubinemia, secondary hemosiderosis and they develop changes in bone, giving characteristic new bone formation resembling a "crew-cut" on radiographs of the skull. The course of the disease is punctuated by crises in which there are painful episodes of vascular occlusion. These crises may be triggered by dehydration, acidosis, or infection.

The history of vaso-occlusive crises and the chronic micro-ischemia leads to end organ damage including retinopathy, damage to the renal medulla, and destruction of the spleen. Patients without a spleen are at increased risk for infection by encapsulated bacteria. Half of the adults with sickle cell disease have a dilated cardiomyopathy and 30% have pulmonary hypertension. The course and severity of sickle cell disease is quite variable. Symptoms usually develop when hemoglobin is down to 8 – 9 grams and become more severe as the hemoglobin drops to a level of 5 or 6 [2,3].

3.2.2 Klebsiella pneumoniae

Klebsiella is a genus of short Gram-negative rods of the family Enterobacteriaceae. It occurs normally in the gastrointestinal flora and is present in water and on inanimate objects. K. pneumoniae may cause pneumonia, lung abscess, endocarditis, wound infections, urinary tract infections, salpingitis, osteomyelitis, and sepsis. K. pneumoniae may form a capsule. It is most common in immunosuppressed patients and can cause a necrotizing pneumonia with a characteristic red jelly-like sputum. The organism's capsule inhibits the action of neutrophils and the pulmonary exudates in early cases may be free of neutrophils histologically. Klebsiella pneumoniae may be resistant to penicillin and cephalosporin antibiotics [4–6].

3.3 Medical History

3.3.1 Sickle cell disease

In 1910, James B. Herrick (1861–1954) reported the case of a 20-year-old African-American man who had a one-year history of palpitations and shortness of breath and was admitted to the hospital with a two-day history of cough and fever. The patient had scleral icterus, an enlarged heart, a soft systolic heart murmur, and a hemoglobin of 40% (Dare's technique, normal value = 100%). His peripheral smear showed many sickle-shaped red blood cells. The patient was treated with oral iron and his hemoglobin measurement increased to 58%. The author suspected syphilis, but this is the first reported case of sickle cell anemia. For many years sickle cell disease was called Herrick's syndrome [7].

Note: Dare's hemoglobinometer permitted the color of a sample of pipetted blood to be compared to a graduated color scale made with the pigment or dye called golden purple of Cassius that had been calibrated with solutions containing a known quantity of hemoglobin in 100 mL of serum. The light source was a wax candle. At that time blood specimens were usually obtained from a finger or earlobe stick and had to be handled very quickly before they clotted [8].

3.3.2 Klebsiella pneumoniae

The notion that disease could be caused by microorganisms developed over the course of the 19th century. This "germ theory" met with extensive resistance, since many physicians, including some of the greatest of them, found it ludicrous to suppose that an organism so small could cause such extensive disease in an organism as large and complex as a human. The ultimate success of the idea was largely due to the work of Louis Pasteur (1822 – 1895), Robert Koch (1843 – 1910), and their colleagues along with the development of new techniques of culture and identification of microorganisms. Edwin Klebs (1834 – 1913), a student of Rudolph Virchow, had seen bacteria in the bronchi of patients who had died of pneumonia in 1875, but in 1882 Carl Friedländer (1847 – 1887) published a description of a bacteria, at least some of which were probably Klebsiella pneumoniae, that he claimed was nearly always observable in patients dying from pneumonia. It is now thought that some of his cases were likely due to Streptococcus pneumoniae. Freidländer also noted that it was necessary to use the new Gram stain to see the bacteria. A fairly acrimonious debate was touched off by this publication. Like other similar scientific debates from then until now, the history of the debate is quite entertaining, but ultimately there was much more heat than light shed by the arguments made. Carl Friedländer died of pneumonia at age 40, perhaps due to the organism he had studied. For many years, Klebsiella pneumoniae was called Friedländer's bacillus [9].

3.4 Laboratory medicine

3.4.1 Sickle cell disease

Screening tests can be done for Sickle cell disease on whole blood (EDTA, lavender top) with 2% sodium metabisulfite. Sickling is identified under the microscope in the presence of the reducing agent when hemoglobin is deoxygenated. There are also commercial tests in which one looks for turbidity due to decreased solubility of reduced hemoglobin S in a concentrated phosphate buffer solution. More definitive tests are hemoglobin electrophoresis and, more recently, gene sequencing. In hemoglobin electrophoresis, a specimen made from lysed red blood cells is placed on a plate of cellulose acetate in an alkaline buffer. The plate is placed between electrodes and an electric current is passed through the buffer. The cellulose acetate is stained and the migration of the patient's hemoglobins is compared to those in an adjacent row with a control specimen. Normal hemoglobin A migrates quickly to the anode, but hemoglobin S lags behind [10].

3.5 Study questions

1. The patient's history states that he was taking the following drugs: hydromorphone, deferoxamine mesylate, insulin, folate, sertraline, lansoprazole, promethazine, and digoxin. What are these drugs for?

2. Pathologists almost never prescribe medication, but it is important to know what all the drugs are in the decedent's history. Why?

3. Are there any drugs in the list of drugs that this patient was taking that could cause death? Which of his drugs were most likely to be toxic?

4. Who developed the Gram stain?

5. There was considerable acrimony between Drs. Pasteur and Koch and among their supporters. Could there have been a non-microbiological reason for their conflict?

3.6 References

1. Kumar V, Abbas AK, Aster JC. Robbins and Cotran Pathologic basis of disease. Philadelphia: Elsevier Saunders; 2015
2. Berkowitz LR. Anemias. In: Runge MS, Greganti MA, editors. Netter's Internal Medicine. Philadelphia: Saunders Elsevier; 2009. p. 514.
3. Sickle Cell Disease. Basic Principles and Clinical Practice. New York: Raven Press; 1994
4. Schneierson SS. Schneierson's atlas of diagnostic microbiology. North Chicago, IL: Abbott Laboratories; 1979
5. Jorgensen JH, Pfaller MA. A clinician's dictionary of pathogenic microorganisms. Washington, D.C: ASM Press; 2004:273.

6. Abbott SL. Klebsiella, Enterobacter, Citrobacter, Serratia, Plesiomonas and other Enterobacteriaceae. In: Murray PR, editor. Manual of Clinical Microbiology. Washington, D.C.: ASM Press; 2007. p. 698-715.
7. Major RH. Classic descriptions of disease. Baltimore: Charles C. Thomas; 1932
8. Simon CE. A manual of clinical diagnosis by means of laboratory methods: For students, hospital physicians and practitioners. Philadelphia: Lea Brothers & Co; 1907:682.
9. Austrian R. The Gram stain and the etiology of lobar pneumonia, an historical note. Bacteriol Rev. 1960;24:261-265.
10. Lawrence LW. Porphyrins and hemoglobin. In: Bishop MLD-E, JL Fody, EP, editor. Clinical chemistry. Principles, procedures, correlations. Philadelphia: Lippincott William & Wilkins; 2000. p. 280 - 291.

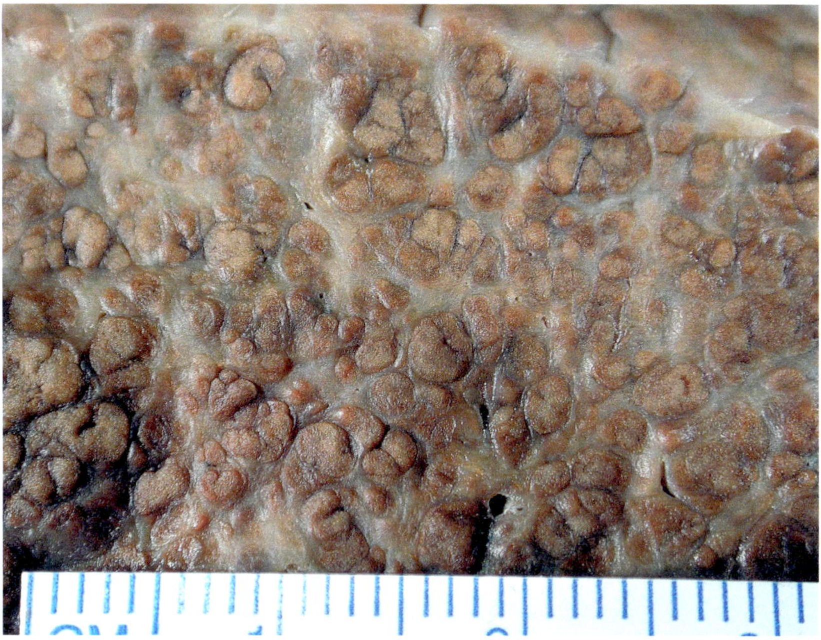

Figure 3.1 Micronodular cirrhosis of the liver comprises many small nodules of architecturally, and sometimes cytologically, abnormal liver surrounded by dense fibrous bands. One occasionally encounters a liver at autopsy that seems somewhat fibrotic but is not clearly cirrhotic. The time-honored test for cirrhosis at the time of gross examination is the finger test. The prosector will find it impossible to press his finger through a piece of cirrhotic liver. The small divisions on the ruler at the bottom of the image are millimeters.

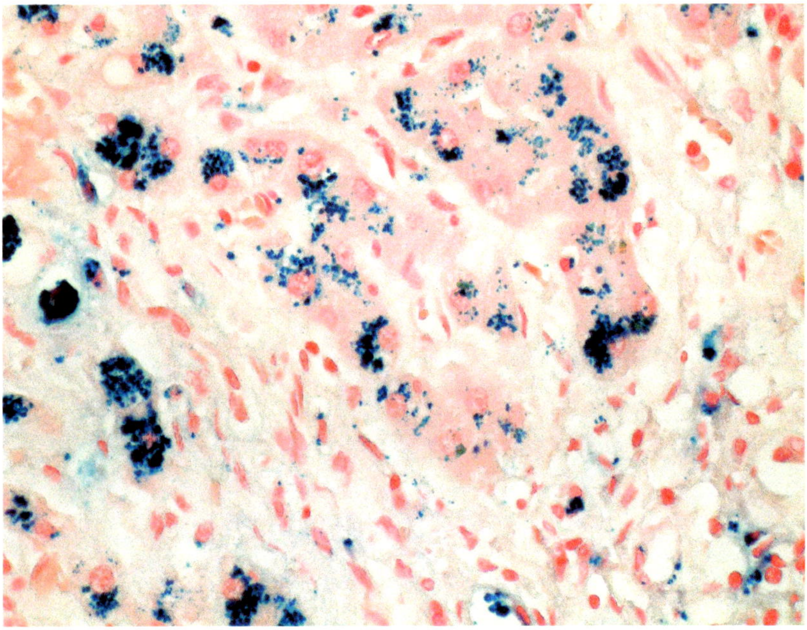

Figure 3.2 Hepatocellular hemosiderosis. Free iron is highly toxic, so in the body, it is bound to the 450,000 Dalton globular protein, ferritin. Ferritin is an ancient molecule and is present in algae and bacteria. In the presence of excess iron, an insoluble pigment comprising ferritin and other substances forms called hemosiderin. Hemosiderin stains blue with the dye Prussian blue. This picture shows the accumulation of intracellular hemosiderin in liver cells. The nuclei have been stained red with a counterstain. (Original magnification 200x. Prussian blue stain)

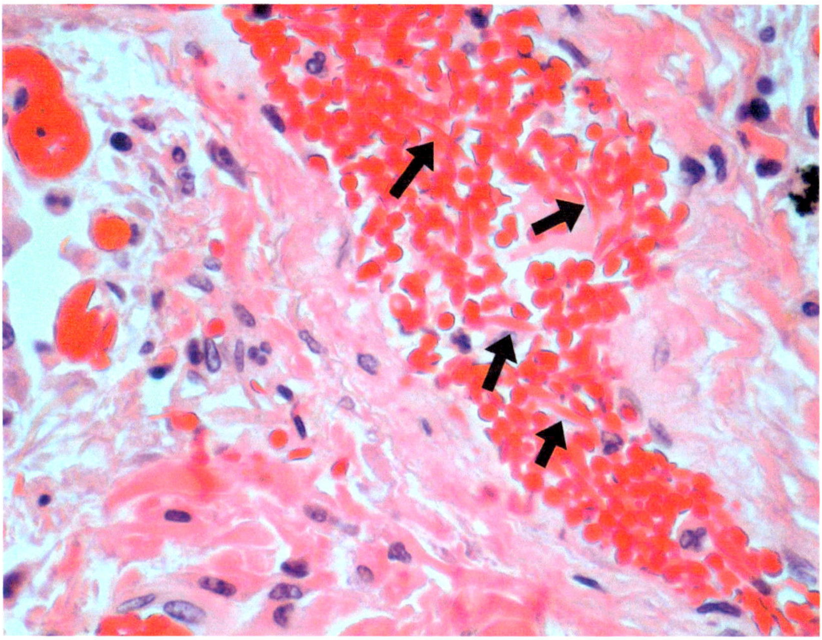

Figure 3.3 This microscopic field of the patient's lung shows many red blood cells. Most are the normal biconcave disc shape, but some are elongated and sickle-shaped. (Original magnification 200x. H&E stain)

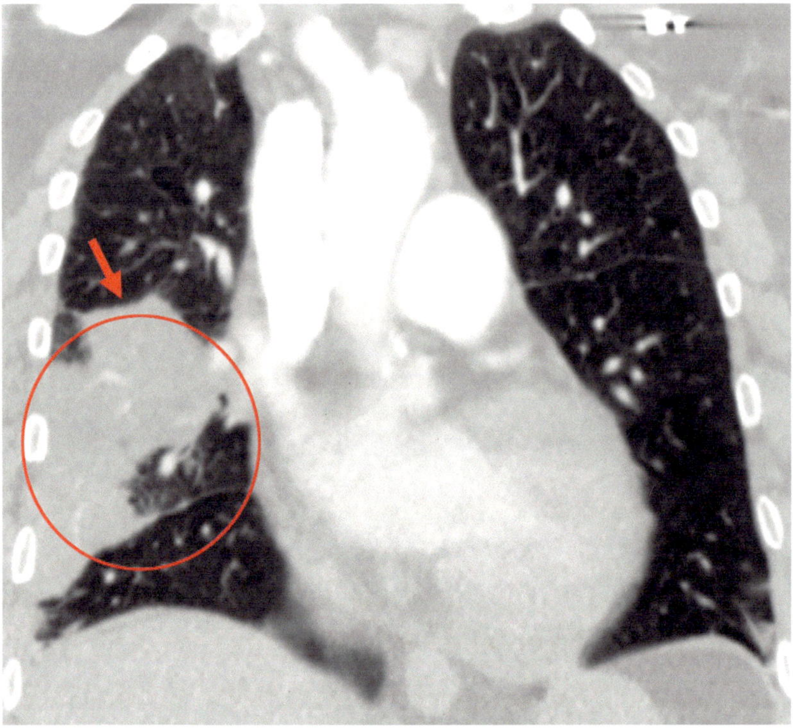

Figure 3.4 A reformatted coronal chest CT from a different case showing dense consolidation in the right middle lung lobe (red circle) with bulging of the minor fissure (red arrow) as a result of accumulated cellular and inflammatory material from pneumonia. Bulging of the minor fissure is characteristic of, but not specific for, Klebsiella pneumonia.

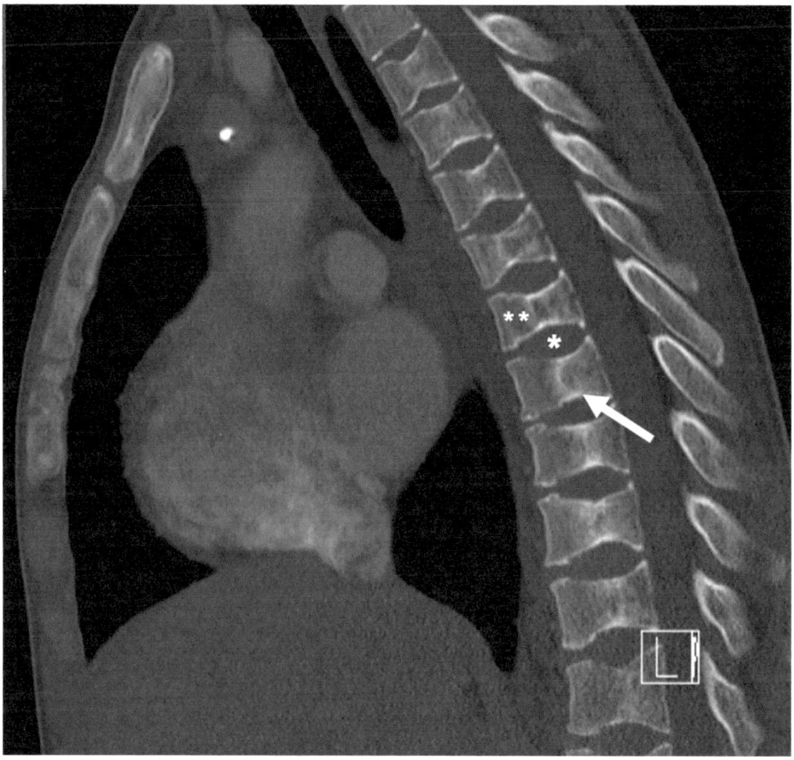

Figure 3.5 A sagittal reformatted chest CT from a different case highlights vertebral body endplate deformities (arrow), producing a fish-mouth appearance of the disc spaces (asterisk) and H-shaped vertebral bodies (two asterisks). This appearance is secondary to vertebral infarcts from microvascular occlusion from abnormally shaped red blood cells occluding small vessels in sickle cell anemia.

CHAPTER 4

A middle-aged woman with dizziness and subsequent sudden death. (Vindicate, vascular)

"For those who have dissected or inspected many [bodies], have at least learn'd to doubt, when the others, who are ignorant of anatomy, and do not take the trouble to attend to it, are in no doubt at all." Giovanni Battista Morgagni (1682 – 1771, Morgagni likely died of a perforated heart).

4.1 The Autopsy

4.1.1 Case history

An 80-year-old woman had a three-day history of dizziness and lethargy. She had recently been treated for an ear infection. She was brought to the Emergency Department by ambulance where she was short of breath. She had a grade 3 systolic heart murmur at the right sternal border and a chest radiograph showed cardiomegaly. Her BNP (brain natriuretic protein) was elevated. CT (computerized tomography) scan of the head showed some basal ganglia lacunae (a type of small, often silent, cerebral infarct sometimes seen in patients with high blood pressure) but was otherwise normal. The patient had no prior history of coronary artery disease. She had smoked one-half pack of cigarettes a day for 43 years (These numbers are commonly multiplied together to give a measure of lifetime exposure to tobacco. This patient had a 26.5 pack-year smoking history.) Her electrocardiogram showed a normal sinus rhythm with some ST segment and T wave changes in inferior leads (i.e. she had EKG evidence of ischemia in the inferior part of her heart). Serum creatine kinase levels on three consecutive specimens were 551, 529 and 499 (normal = 30 – 170 U/L) and serum troponin was 1.11,1.22 and1.32 (normal < 0.1 ng/mL). The MB fraction of her creatine kinase was 13.6 (normal < 4.4 ng/mL). Echocardiogram showed moderate aortic stenosis with a valve area of 0.8 sq cm (normal = 3 – 4 sq cm) and a peak gradient of 32 mm (normal = a few mm). Left ventricular function was said to be normal. Mild to moderate mitral regurgitation and mild tricuspid regurgitation were also present. The patient was thought to have had an acute inferior myocardial infarct and was placed on a low dose beta-blocking drug and aspirin. She developed low systolic blood pressure and ventricular tachycardia on day 2. She also had increased shortness of breath and peripheral oxygen desaturation to 82% (normal = 95 -100%) and was sent to the cardiac catheterization lab emergently. Catheterization showed severe narrowing of the left main coronary artery and significant atherosclerosis of the right and left circumflex coronary arteries with preserved left ventricular function. A coronary artery bypass graft procedure and replacement of her aortic valve was recommended and scheduled, but on hospital day 3, the patient became bradycardic, hypotensive and unresponsive. Resuscitation was unsuccessful and the patient died on the third hospital day.

4.1.2 Postmortem findings

Postmortem examination was limited to the examination of the heart and lungs. A handwritten note on the chart front sheet said to rule out "clot or heart rupture". Very early during the autopsy incision of the pericardium revealed 173 grams of clotted blood and red discoloration of the cardiac surface compatible with cardiac perforation (figure 4.1, 4.2). Examination showed a three-day-old transmural acute myocardial infarct in the posterior left ventricle extending to involve the interventricular septum and right ventricle. The infarct was about 4 cm in circumference and was present in the middle and upper cardiac thirds. There was perforation through the area of infarction into the pericardial space. (figure 4.3 - 4.5) There was severe three-vessel coronary artery disease with total occlusion of the right coronary artery (figure 4.6). The right coronary section showed circumferential necrotic atheroma and a central luminal thrombus. The age of the thrombus was uncertain, but it may have been the cause of the patient's infarct.

4.1.3 Case summary

The patient had perforation of her heart on day three after an acute myocardial infarct and this was the cause of death. Other features of the case including the patient's age and sex, the absence of a prior history of coronary artery disease, the age and histologic appearance of the infarct, the right coronary artery thrombus, and the laboratory findings were all typical for this phenomenon.

4.2 Discussion

4.2.1 Atherosclerosis

Atherosclerosis is the leading cause of death in developed countries. It is a disease characterized by the development of lesions in the lining of arteries that may progress during the patient's lifetime from a relatively subtle fatty intimal elevation to a complex ulcerated calcified plaque with adherent thrombus. Atherosclerotic plaques have pathological consequences because they obstruct the flow of blood and because adherent material may break free and cause various peripheral embolic phenomena. Common pathological effects are myocardial infarct, stroke, claudication (pain or tiredness in leg muscles due to ischemia – from the Latin *claudicare* meaning to limp), and bowel ischemia. Because it is common, atherosclerosis is one of the most studied of diseases. Many risk factors are known, but no single etiology has been found. Risk factors include hyperlipidemia, hypertension, diabetes mellitus, patient gender and age, cigarette smoking and, more controversially, a diet that is high in some kinds of fats. The lipids that circulate in the bloodstream may be associated with a low or high-density lipoprotein (LDL and HDL). LDL carries cholesterol to the cells of the body and to atherosclerotic plaques. HDL carries cholesterol from the periphery including atherosclerotic plaques to the liver where it is excreted in the bile. Consequently, high levels of LDL and low levels of HDL, sometimes called "bad" and "good" cholesterol respectively, may be associated with an increased risk of atherosclerosis. Some adult alcoholic patients may have very little atherosclerosis at autopsy, but most patients have at least some atherosclerotic changes. The most popular model to explain the significance of all the known risk factors is the "response to injury" hypothesis. It states that an initial endothelial injury leads to changes that permit the accumulation of lipoproteins in the arterial wall. Additional changes in the artery involving monocytes, platelets and T lymphocytes lead to progressive development of the complicated atherosclerotic plaque.

At autopsy, the earliest and most benign appearing lesion is the fatty streak. This linear area of yellow discoloration can be seen in children. The next stage is the fibrous plaque that is whiter in color and shows increased thickening. With the infiltration of more inflammatory and smooth muscle cells, the development of areas of necrosis, thrombosis and calcification, the mature and dangerous atherosclerotic plaque can form. If the plaque ruptures or ulcerates leading to hemorrhage into the plaque, the patient may have luminal thrombosis with obstruction or embolization with obstruction at a distant site. Atherosclerosis is most common in certain parts of the arterial tree. The abdominal aorta, the coronary arteries, the popliteal arteries and the internal carotid arteries are common sites of involvement. Atherosclerosis occurs in different places in different patients. Some patients have severe coronary artery disease, but little in the abdominal aorta and so forth [1].

4.2.2 Ischemic heart disease

Ischemic heart disease is a group of cardiac reactions and associated symptoms all due to decreased blood flow to the heart. Ninety-percent of these cases are because of coronary artery atherosclerosis with either acute or chronic decrease in cardiac blood flow. The other 10% are secondary to coronary artery spasm, coronary emboli, or coronary arteritis. The coronary arteries originate above the aortic valve in the root of the aorta. They run around the heart in the groove at the junction of the atria and ventricles, like a crown, and send branches upward and downward to supply the needs of the beating heart. The death rate from ischemia of the heart has fallen by 50% since 1963, but it is still the leading cause of death in the US. The decreased death rate may be attributed to changes in diet, decreased smoking, the use of the medication statins, coronary artery bypass surgery, coronary angioplasty and the use of thrombolytic therapy for acute myocardial infarct. Clinically, cardiac ischemia may present as angina (usually pronounced with the accent on the first syllable) pectoris, classically characterized by crushing chest pain that radiates to the back, jaw or arm and is associated with diaphoresis (sweating), tachycardia (fast heart rate), and shortness of breath [2].

4.2.3 Myocardial Infarct

About 1.5 million people have a myocardial infarct ("heart attack") in the US each year. In most of these patients, the progressive growth of atherosclerotic plaques has gradually decreased the blood flow to their heart. The body responds to this ischemia by developing collateral blood flow through new arterioles, but if there is a sudden non-gradual decrease in blood flow or blood flow oxygenation from sudden blood loss, decreased inhaled oxygen, loss of perfusion of the lungs, coronary artery muscle spasm, a thomboembolus in a coronary artery, or, more likely, rupture of an unstable coronary artery atherosclerotic plaque with formation of a thrombus, then myocardial ischemia may become critical. When the blood flow to part of the heart is acutely inadequate, at least 20 minutes of blood flow that is less than 10% of normal, the myocardial cells begin to die. The dying myofibers release intracellular proteins that we can detect in the patient's blood specimens in the laboratory; the so-called cardiac markers. Myocardial infarcts may develop in different patterns. A transmural infarct is usually due to complete obstruction of an epicardial coronary artery and is associated with ST segment elevation on the patient's EKG. Multifocal small infarcts may be due to small vessel disease in diabetic patients and in patients with hypertensive heart disease, and some patients have infarcts of the subendocardial myocardium only, without elevation of the ST segment on EKG.

Myocardial infarcts usually occur in the left cardiac ventricle. If they are due to disease in a single coronary artery, they occur in the ratio of 3:2:1 corresponding to the left anterior descending artery, the right coronary artery and the left main coronary artery. The infarcts undergo progressive changes over time. At autopsy, they are not usually detectable in the first 24 hours after they occur. The first change is red discoloration due to hemorrhage. After a day or two, a rim of yellow discoloration develops corresponding to necrosis and the infiltration of neutrophils seen histologically. The whole lesion may become yellow or mottled yellow and red. By the end of a week, the neutrophils have disintegrated, some histiocytes are present, there is phagocytosis of cellular debris, and there is ingrowth of new capillaries at the edge of the infarct. In time the lesion is red and depressed appearing, a hemorrhagic scar, and after weeks to months, the lesion is a well-formed white scar. The collagenous scar is only one-third as thick as the myocardium it replaced, and the thinned non-beating scar tissue may bulge outward forming an aneurysm.

Complications of an acute myocardial infarct include loss of normal cardiac contractile function with heart failure, cardiac arrhythmia and, as seen in this case, myocardial rupture.

Myocardial rupture usually occurs in the anterolateral wall of the left ventricle. It can occur between 1 and 10 days after the acute infarct. Some authors have associated rupture with the time of peak neutrophil infiltration or the maximum softness of the necrotic tissue. Female patients, patients over 60 years of age and patients with hypertension are at increased risk for cardiac rupture. The risk also appears to be increased in smaller infarcts and in patients who have had their first infarct, perhaps because they are adjacent to viable beating myocardium and not scar. Perforation of the heart leads to rapid accumulation of blood in the pericardial space, cardiac tamponade, and electromechanical dissociation. Sudden death is common [2–5].

4.3 Medical history

4.3.1 Ischemic heart disease

Angina pectoris was described by William Heberden (1710 – 1801) in 1772 and almost certainly had been recognized for years before then. Matthew Baillie (1761 – 1823) described sclerosis of the coronary arteries in patients with angina at about the same time. Similarly, John Fothergill (1712 – 1780) described an autopsy in 1776 in which "The two coronary arteries, from their origin to many of their ramifications upon the heart, were become one piece of bone.", and the great surgeon John Hunter (1728 – 1793) who died suddenly with angina pectoris was found to have coronaries "in the state of bony tubes" at autopsy. It was not known or commented on at the time, that the important problem in these patients was obstruction of the coronary artery lumen. Despite this gap in the published discussions, it was well known in the 19th century that organs denied their blood flow could infarct and that dogs would die when a coronary artery was tied off (Julius Cohnheim (1839–1884)). Dr. Adam Hammer (1818 – 1878), who had emigrated from Germany to St. Louis, reported a case of sudden death in a 34-year-old man in 1878, in which he had proposed that the patient had an occluded coronary artery at the bedside. At autopsy, the patient had endocarditis with a thrombus in the orifice of the right coronary. In an 1892 case report, Ludvig Hektoen (1863 – 1951) reported a case of sudden death in a 55-year-old man with chest pain with "Embolism of the left coronary artery…" and he mentioned the old saying "a man is only as old as his arteries" and stated that obstruction of a coronary artery was the most common cause of sudden death. George Dock (1860 – 1951) at the University of Michigan published a case in 1896 in which he claimed to be the first in America to make a diagnosis of coronary thrombosis that was confirmed at autopsy. In a series of lectures on angina pectoris published in The Lancet, William Osler (1849 – 1919, figure 4.7), mentioned several interesting questions of the time: Why was angina pectoris more common in the upper classes? Why was it seldom seen in hospital practice? He described a typical patient as a "well 'set' man of from 45 to 55 years of age, with military bearing, iron-grey hair, and a florid complexion". James Herrick (1861 – 1954), the same man mentioned previously for his description of sickle cell disease, published a review of the clinical features of coronary artery obstruction in 1912 in which he stated, "It must be admitted, also, that the reputation of the descending branch of the left coronary as the artery of sudden death is not undeserved." [6,7]

4.4 Laboratory Medicine

4.4.1 Ischemic heart disease

The principle laboratory assays for monitoring acute myocardial ischemia are, in order of decreasing importance, troponin, creatine kinase, and myoglobin. All three are proteins that are released from myocardial cells when they lose their cell membrane integrity at the time of ischemic damage. Troponin is a complex of three proteins that bind to actin in striated muscle and regulate muscle contraction. The three proteins are Troponin C, I, and T. They each have different isoforms depending on their location and the cardiac isoforms of Troponin T (cTnT) and Troponin I (cTnI) are the most widely used markers of cardiac necrosis currently. These troponins are not normally present in the serum and they are specific for heart damage. They begin to rise in the serum of a patient with an acute myocardial infarct in 3 – 4 hours, peak in 10 – 14 hours and may stay elevated for 10 – 14 days. Because of their high sensitivity to heart damage, elevated troponin may be seen in other disorders that are, apparently, associated with small or even minute degrees of myocardial necrosis, e.g. sepsis, aortic dissection and pulmonary embolus [8].

Brain natriuretic protein (BNP) is a hormone that was originally identified in porcine brain. In humans, it is mainly produced by the cardiac ventricles in response to stretching and acts to decrease blood volume and blood vascular resistance. BNP has been used as a marker to help identify patients with heart failure. A typical clinical situation is a patient with evidence of pulmonary edema in whom it is unclear if the fluid in the lungs is due to heart failure or primary lung disease.

4.5 Study questions

1. Myoglobin goes up even faster than troponin in patients with an acute MI. Why don't we use myoglobin instead of troponin as our main marker of a heart attack?

2. William Osler thought that angina pectoris was more common in wealthier patients. Is this true? Why might someone have thought that it was true?

3. There are several theories for the cause of atherosclerosis. How many can you find described on the Internet?

4. Why has the death rate from cardiac ischemia declined recently in the United States?

5. If you make a scatterplot of the incidence of colon cancer versus the incidence of coronary artery disease by patient nationality there is a strong linear relationship. So, for example, people in the United States have a relatively high incidence of both colon cancer and coronary artery disease, but people in Japan have a relatively low incidence for both. Why might this be?

4.6 References

1. Mitchell RN. Blood vessels. In: Kumar V, Abbas AK, Aster JC, editors. Robbins and Cotran Pathologic basis of disease. Philadelphia: Elsevier Saunders; 2015. p. 491 - 500.

2. Schoen FJ, Mitchell RN. The heart. In: Kumar V, Abbas AK, Aster JC, editors. Robbins and Cotran Pathologic basis of disease. Philadelphia: Elsevier Saunders; 2015. p. 523 - 578.

3. Becker AE, Anderson RH. Cardiac pathology. New York: Raven Press; 1982

4. Silver MD, Gotlieb AI, Schoen, FJ. Cardiovascular pathology. New York: Churchill Livingstone; 2001

5. Virmani R, Farb A, Burke A, Atkinson JB. Cardiovascular pathology. Philadelphia: W. B. Saunders; 2001

6. Hill RB, Anderson RE, Narviel MF. The autopsy - medical practice and public policy. Boston, Mass.: Butterworths; 1988:294.

7. Major RH. Classic descriptions of disease. Baltimore: Charles C. Thomas; 1932

8. Schreiber D, Miller SM. Cardiac markers. 2014. http://emedicine.medscape.com/article/811905-overview. Accessed 2015.

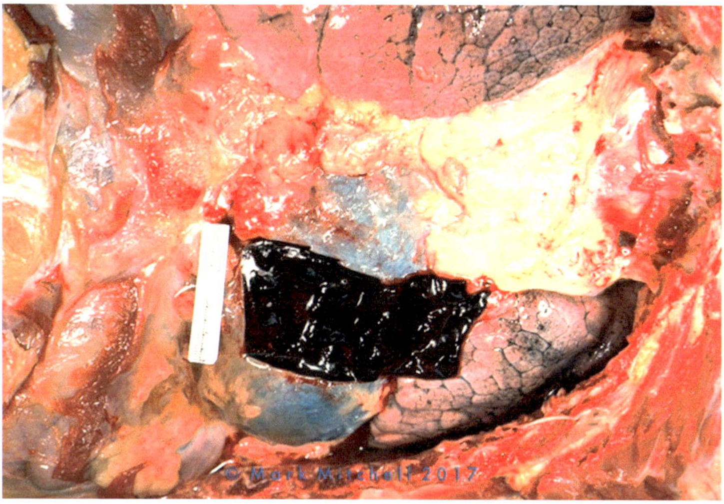

Figure 4.1 The presence of cardiac perforation is plain very early in the performance of the autopsy. Blood clot is present when the pericardial sac is opened to remove the heart from the body. The ruler is 5 cm long.

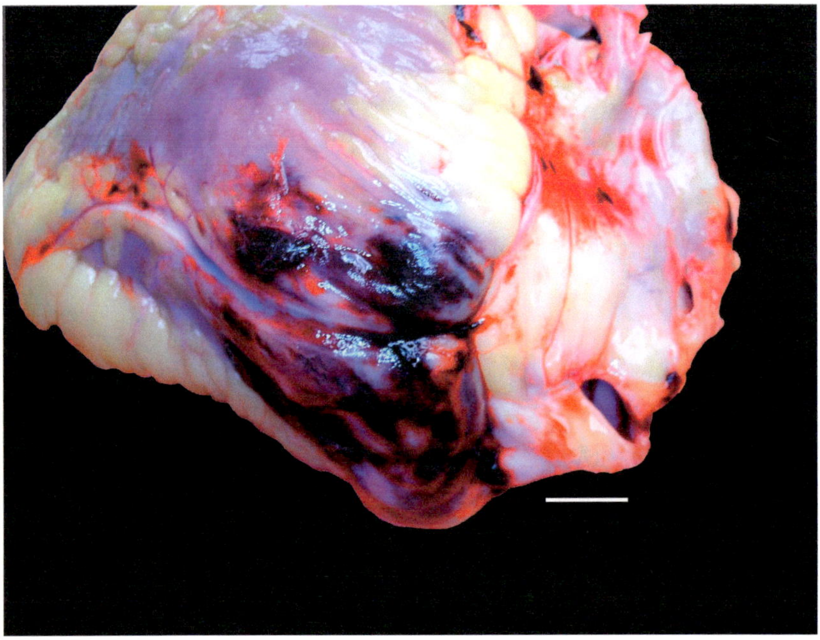

Figure 4.2 The heart was washed off in this case and there was an area of dark red discoloration on the epicardial surface near the point of left ventricular perforation. The white bar is 1 cm long.

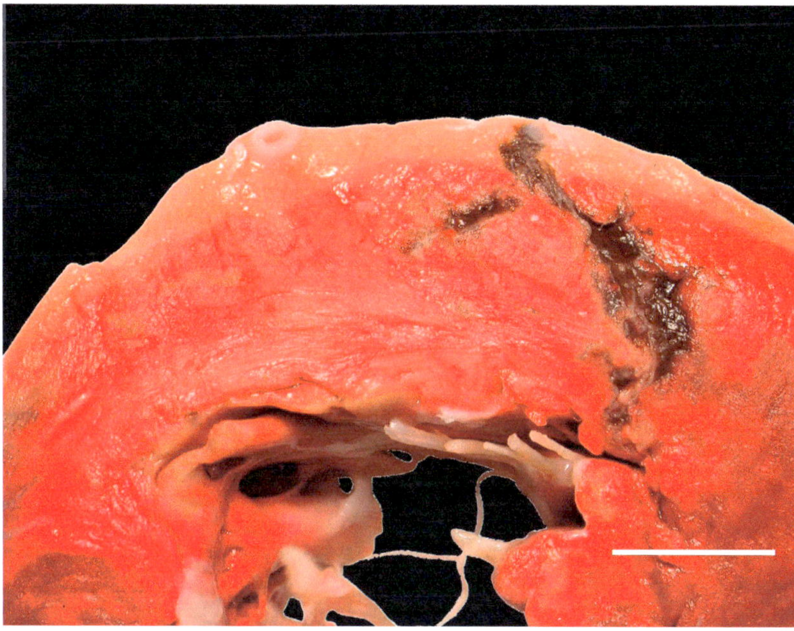

Figure 4.3 This image, from a case similar to the one presented here, shows the dark red track leading from the left ventricular lumen to the epicardial surface of the heart. The track is passing through a transmural acute myocardial infarct. The yellow fatty subepicardial layer is normal. Notice a white epicardial coronary artery at about 11 o'clock. This heart was stained with tetrazolium red giving the cut myocardial surface an intense red color. Tetrazolium red is used to help identify myocardial infarcts that are less than 24 hours old, since the dye stains viable cells red (where NADH has been oxidized to NAD and the stain has been reduced to its red form), but does not stain non-viable cells. The white bar is 1 cm long.

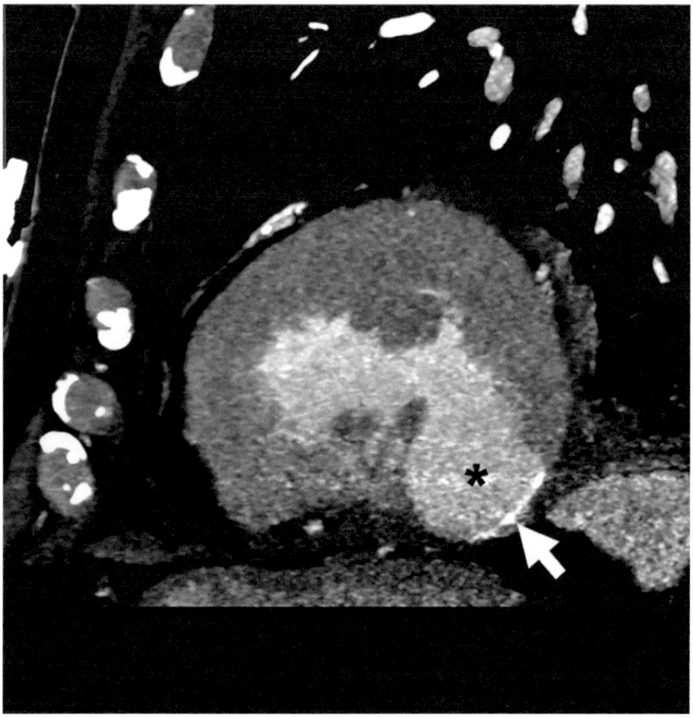

Figure 4.4 An image from a different case showing a short axis view of the left ventricle in a patient with a history of myocardial infarction showing thickening of the left ventricular wall with an area of either absence or thinning of the myocardium with calcification (arrow) and contrast containing blood filling the defect (asterisk), a result of myocardial perforation producing a pseudoaneurysm.

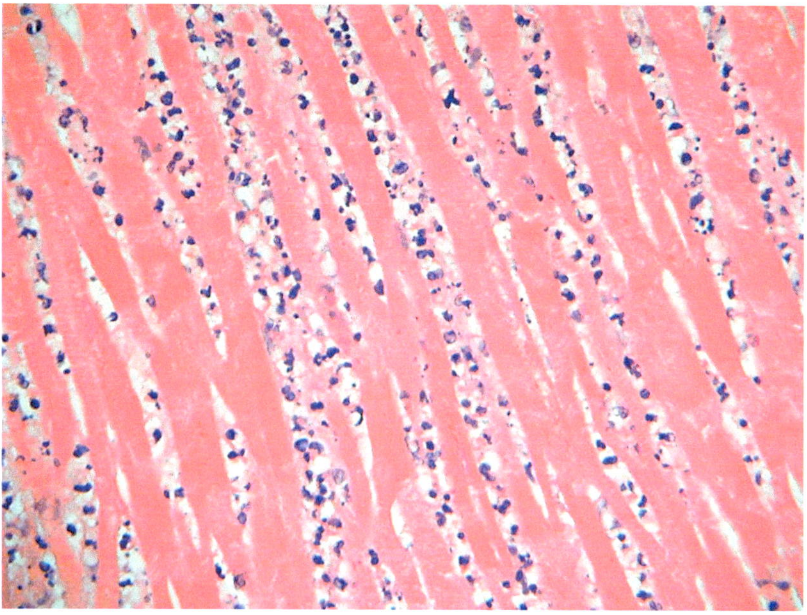

Figure 4.5 An acute myocardial infarct can be dated by its histologic appearance. This microscopic image shows pink myofibers that have lost their nuclei; they are dead or necrotic. The body has responded to the necrosis by sending in neutrophils. Some of the neutrophils have died and their nuclei have broken up into pieces. This appearance is compatible with a myocardial infarct that is about 4 days old. This part of the infarct would look yellow grossly. (Original magnification 200 x, H&E stain)

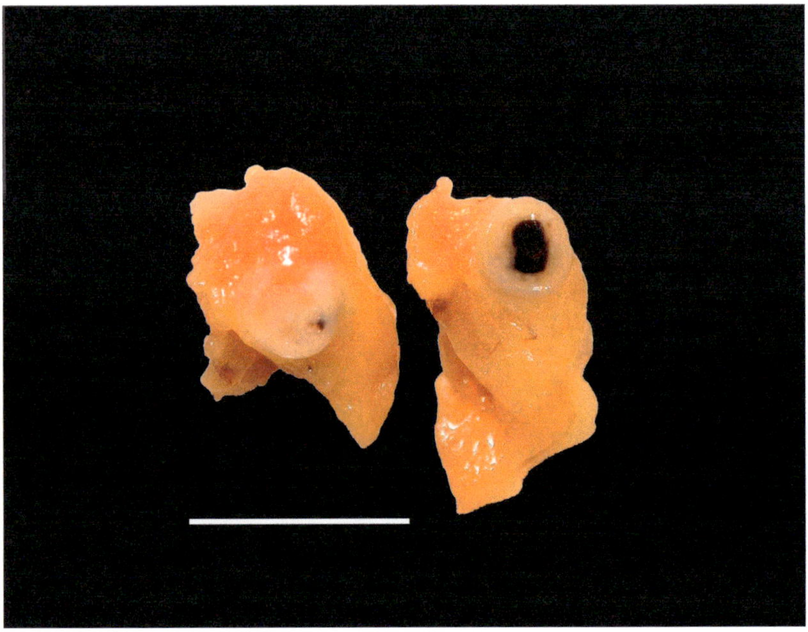

Figure 4.6 Two cross sections of the right coronary artery. A normal coronary artery has a relatively thin wall and a wide-open (or patent) lumen. An example of a relatively normal appearing coronary artery is the one seen in the epicardial fat in figure 4.3. The left cross section above shows near complete loss of the normal lumen by atherosclerotic plaque. The small red dot is the remaining lumen. The right cross section shows obstruction of the lumen by blood clot. Histologic examination confirmed that this clot was probably an antemortem thrombus that formed when the underlying atherosclerotic plaque ruptured. The coronary arteries are dissected free from the heart at autopsy so that they can be carefully examined in cross section. It's usually necessary to decalcify the coronaries in a weakly acidic solution prior to cutting them. The white bar is 1 cm long.

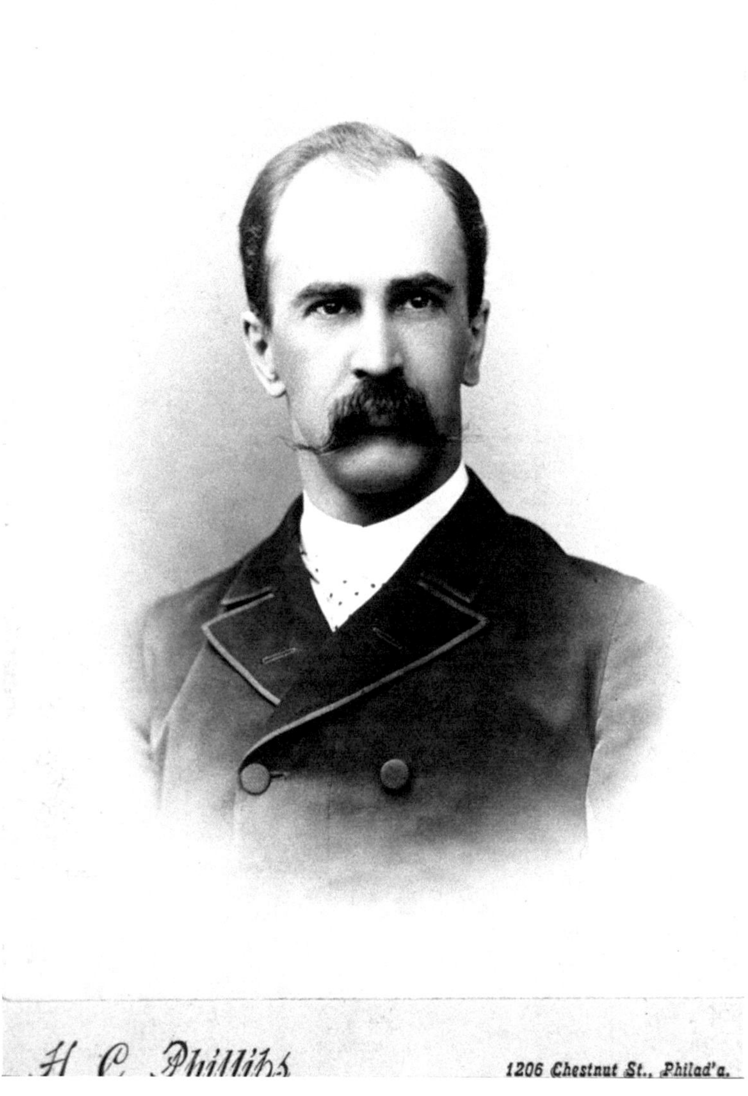

Figure 4.7. William Osler (1849 – 1919). Courtesy of the National Library of Medicine.

CHAPTER 5

A young man with HIV infection and a headache. (uIndicate, infectious)

"If you follow the truth too near the heels, it may happply strike out your teeth."
Walter Raleigh (1554 – 1618)

5.1 The Autopsy

5.1.1 Case history

The patient was a 30-year-old man with a history of IV drug abuse who was diagnosed as HIV (Human Immunodeficiency Virus) positive three years prior to admission. He presented complaining of a posterior headache and a stiff neck for one week. He had diplopia (double vision), nausea, vomiting, and fever. The patient said that he had similar symptoms when he had Cryptococcal meningitis seven months previously. He also had Pneumocystis pneumonia five months earlier. His CD4 level was 83 (normal = 600 - 1500), hemoglobin 11.4 (normal = 14 – 17 g/dL), WBC 7800 (normal = 3900 – 10700 cells/μL and he had 339,000 platelets (normal = 150,000 – 350,000/μL). A lumbar puncture showed CSF (cerebrospinal fluid) with a glucose of 46 (normal = 2/3 of blood glucose), 48 WBCs (normal = 0), 46 RBCs (normal = 0) and a protein of 159 (normal = 15 – 45 mg/dL). A few PMNs were present, but most of the leukocytes were lymphocytes. A test for Cryptococcal antigen was positive in a titer of 1:8. CT scan of the patient's head was unremarkable. His medications were lamivudine (a reverse transcriptase inhibitor (RTI)), nelfinavir (a protease inhibitor), stavudine (RTI), fluconazole (antifungal), azithromycin (antibiotic), and diamino diphenyl sulfone (antibiotic). He was also treated with ceftriaxone (antibiotic), amphotericin B (antifungal), and acyclovir (antiviral). A chest radiograph showed discrete nodules and a 1 cm cavity in the right upper lung lobe. An MRI (magnetic resonance imaging) of the brain on day 3 showed hydrocephalus and extensive leptomeningeal enhancement compatible with meningitis. There was also an area of left basal ganglia enhancement. No abscess or brain shift was seen. On day 4 the patient had hypertension and decreased respiratory effort and was intubated and transferred to the intensive care unit. The patient became unresponsive and died on the 4th hospital day.

5.1.2 Postmortem findings

At autopsy, the patient had an enlarged spleen weighing 530 grams (normal = 150 grams). The leptomeninges on the surface of the brain had a cloudy appearance that was most prominent on the base of the brain (figures 5.1 - 5.3). Histologic examination showed abundant budding yeast with some variability in size (figure 5.4) in the meninges, spleen, left renal cortex, and in a right upper lung lobe cavity (figures 5.5, 5.6). Some of the yeast had capsules that stained with mucicarmine (figure 5.7). The histologic appearance of the yeast was compatible with Cryptococcus neoformans. Sections of the brain also showed granulomatous inflammation and some portions of the cerebellum adjacent to the meningitis had tissue necrosis. Chronic hepatitis with bridging fibrosis was also present.

5.1.3 Case summary

The patient had known HIV infection and a relatively recent history of Cryptococcal meningitis. His CD4 count was 83 (normal = 600 – 1500). Post-mortem findings showed systemic Cryptococcosis with Cryptococcal meningitis, and this was the cause of death.

5.2 Discussion

5.2.1 AIDS and the Medical History of AIDS.

HIV and the acquired immunodeficiency syndrome are a relatively recent story and I've included the history here with the general discussion. A retrovirus is a virus that has RNA as its genetic material instead of DNA. These viruses take over infected cells, just like DNA viruses do, but they use an enzyme called reverse transcriptase to make DNA from their RNA to do so. In 1911 Peyton Rous (1879 – 1970) discovered that a cell-free extract made from a tumor in chickens could cause the development of a sarcoma, a malignant tumor of connective tissue, when injected into another chicken. This extract contained a retrovirus, now called the Rous sarcoma virus or RSV. The first human retrovirus was discovered by Robert Gallo in 1980 (figure 5.8). The virus is associated with malignant tumors of T-lymphocytes and is called HTLV-1 for the human T-cell leukemia virus. Two years later, Gallo's group discovered another retrovirus that they called HTLV-II. In the early 1980's a new disease began to appear in which patients, many of whom were young homosexual men, had the dramatic loss of cell-mediated immunity and died of overwhelming infections and certain malignant tumors. The new disease was called the acquired immunodeficiency syndrome or AIDS and it was widely suspected that it was caused by a viral infection. Since this new disease was associated with decreased numbers of CD4 positive lymphocytes like patients with HTLV infection, some animals with a lymphotropic retrovirus also had an AIDS-like syndrome, HTLV was transmitted similarly to AIDS, and some patients with hemophilia had developed AIDS after receiving only an ultrafiltrate of clotting factors (just as the Rous sarcoma virus had only been passed by an ultrafiltrate), both Robert Gallo at the National Institutes of Health and Luc Montagnier at the Pasteur Institute in Paris thought that AIDS might be caused by a retrovirus. In particular, it was thought that AIDS might by caused by an HTLV type III. In 1984 Montagnier's group and Gallo's group discovered a new virus in AIDS patients that was eventually called the Human immunodeficiency virus or HIV-1. It is now suspected that HIV-1 developed from a similar virus in non-human primates in central Africa in the early 20th century [1,2].

Patients exposed to HIV-1 or HIV-2, usually by sexual intercourse, sharing needles while injecting drugs of abuse, childbirth, breastfeeding, or receiving contaminated therapeutic blood products, may develop an infection that destroys CD4 positive T-lymphocytes. Infected patients may be asymptomatic or they may develop any of various infections or tumors and progress to AIDS. The severity and prognosis of their illness is inversely proportional to their peripheral CD4+ cell count. Most deaths from HIV-related causes occur in patients with a CD4 count less than 50. Tests for the HIV antigen or antibody to the antigen are used for diagnosis, and therapy is based on the use of drug combinations that inhibit retroviral enzymes (HAART, highly active anti-retroviral therapy).

HIV infection has been divided into categories A, B and C, where A includes asymptomatic patients, patients with generalized lymphadenopathy, and patients with symptoms of acute HIV infection. Patients in categories B and C, by definition, have AIDS. Many different infections, tumors and neurological abnormalities are listed in categories B and C, with those in category C being more severe. For example, oropharyngeal Candidiasis (thrush) is in category B and Candidiasis of bronchi or the esophagus is in category C. Extrapulmonary Cryptococcosis, as seen in the autopsy case presented here, is in category C [3].

Most of the infections that AIDS patients get are reactivation of a latent infection that would ordinarily not be a problem for them if their T lymphocytes were present in normal numbers. So, patients who live in central California may develop a severe infection with Coccidiomycosis. In a similar way, homosexual men with type 8 Herpes virus infection may develop Kaposi's sarcoma and patients with Epstein-Barr virus infection may develop Burkitt's lymphoma.

5.2.2 Cryptococcus

We now recognize two Cryptococcus species - C. neoformans is found in bird droppings, especially those of the pigeon, while C. gattii is often associated with certain tree species, e.g. Eucalyptus trees. Most human infections are caused by Cryptococcus neoformans. The inhalation of soil contaminated with the yeast causes pneumonia in susceptible patients, often those with suppressed cellular immunity. Cryptococcus can also cause meningitis and in severe cases, it may disseminate systemically. The pneumonia by itself is not usually fatal, but meningitis and disseminated disease are more often life threatening. Under the microscope, Cryptococcus is a 5 – 10-micron diameter yeast with a thick gelatinous capsule. Involved tissues often contain cystic masses of proliferating yeast that have a grossly gelatinous appearance. Cryptococcus gattii can also cause disease. It is more likely to occur in immunocompetent patients. C. gattii sometimes causes granulomatous masses in infected tissue and it has been reported to cause the formation of masses that may simulate a neoplasm radiographically [4,5].

5.3 Medical History

5.3.1 HIV

See above.

5.3.2 Cryptococcus

In 1894 pathologist Otto Busse (1867 – 1922) and surgeon Abraham Buschke (1868 – 1943) isolated a "Saccharomyces-like" yeast from a bone infection in a young woman. That same year, Francesco Sanfelice (1861 –

1936) reported a similar yeast in fermenting peach juice. He named it Saccharomyces neoformans because of its unusual colony morphology. In 1901, Jean-Paul Vuillemin (1861 – 1932) renamed the organism Cryptococcus neoformans because it had no ascospores (a type of spore that forms inside a fungal structure called an ascus), a defining characteristic of the genus Saccharomyces [6].

5.4 Laboratory Medicine

5.4.1 Cryptococcus

Patients with Cryptococcal meningitis usually have elevated CSF protein, mostly mononuclear cell pleocytosis (an increased cell count in a body fluid) and low glucose. If a drop of the patient's CSF is placed in India ink, the encapsulated yeast may be visible under the microscope by negative staining, i.e. you see them where the ink is displaced by the organism. Some AIDS patients with very low numbers of T lymphocytes may have organisms in their CSF without any inflammatory reaction. Cryptococcus neoformans forms cream to tan colored colonies on Sabouraud dextrose agar at 22° and 37°C. The colonies are usually mucoid appearing.

Cryptococcus neoformans does not ferment sugars, but oxidizes certain sugars and KNO_3, and produces urease. It does not grow on media that contain cycloheximide [7].

Traditional methods for the detection of Cryptococcus are time-consuming and may be insensitive. There is a latex agglutination test for a Cryptococcal antigen that detects more than 90% of patients with Cryptococcal meningitis. Some false positive cases may occur in patients with rheumatoid factor. More modern methods for the detection of Cryptococcus also include enzyme-linked immunoassay and polymerase chain reaction for the detection of Cryptococcal antigens or DNA. In a study of samples from 82 patients in India, latex agglutination, ELISA, and PCR tests showed very high sensitivity and specificity compared to traditional methods. The sensitivity of the tests declined if the patient had been treated with antifungal drugs [8].

5.4.2 HIV

The serious nature of the HIV infection, its prevalence and the fact that 25% of those with HIV are unaware that they have been infected have led to multiple different types of tests, now in multiple technological generations during the last 30 years. Most HIV tests are performed on blood (some point-of-care screening tests can be performed on saliva). The principal screening test is for antibody to HIV-1. HIV-1 is the most common form of the virus in the United States. HIV-2 may occur in some patients here, but it is more prevalent in Africa. More recent screening tests also detect HIV-2 antibody and the p24 antigen. Most of those infected produce antibodies after about 30 days, but some take longer; 97% produce antibody by 90 days. Infected people are most infectious early on when the amount of virus in their blood and body fluids is very high, so the laboratory tests and testing strategies have been designed to detect those infected as early as possible. If patients are given antiretroviral therapy after a known exposure to HIV, antibody formation may take more than 12 months. HIV antibodies are detected using an enzyme-linked immunoassay (ELISA) or a western blot test. Individuals who are ELISA positive must be confirmed by western blot since the ELISA test has high sensitivity, but a higher risk of false positive results. An earlier screening test was for the p24 viral capsid antigen. The capsid antigen is present before antibody is detectable in the so-called seroconversion window, but it is no longer detectable after about 45 days, so it is insensitive as a solitary test and is no longer used this way. Some screening tests have been developed which test for both HIV antibody and p24 together to avoid this problem. Newer tests for nucleic acid are highly sensitive and specific for HIV. A screening test for specific HIV genes is used on pooled blood samples from donated blood for transfusion. When the test is positive, the constituent patient specimens are then tested individually. Tests for viral RNA are used to determine a patient's viral load and monitor the effectiveness of their antiretroviral therapy. Measurement of the number of CD4 positive T lymphocytes is used in HIV-positive patients to monitor their immune status. This test is usually done by flow cytometry. Low

CD4 counts can be found in many other conditions, so they are not, by themselves, diagnostic of HIV infection [9–11].

5.5 Study questions

1. Since many infections in HIV-positive patients are reactivation of common latent infections, patients in what geographic location would be likely to have an increased incidence of Histoplasmosis?

2. What is the difference between Cryptococcus neoformans and Histoplasma capsulatum under the microscope?

3. What is the risk of contracting an infection from the human immunodeficiency virus while performing an autopsy?

4. One-half of the 2008 Nobel Prize in Medicine was awarded to Drs. Barré-Sinoussi and Montagnier for the discovery of HIV. Why do you think Robert Gallo was excluded?

5. HIV is thought to have originated from a similar virus in non-human primates called SIV for the Simian immunodeficiency virus. Can you name any other viral diseases in humans that are thought to have originated in other animals?

5.6 References

1. Gallo RC, Montagnier L. The discovery of HIV as the cause of AIDS. N Engl J Med. 2003;349:2283-2285.
2. Vahlne A. A historical reflection on the discovery of human retroviruses. Retrovirology 2009;6:40.

3. McCutchen JA. Human Immunodeficiency Virus. In: Porter RS, Kaplan JL, editors. The Merck manual of diagnosis and therapy. Whitehouse Station, NJ: Merck Sharpe & Dohme Corp.; 2011. p. 1438 - 1457.
4. Sugar AM. Fungi. In: Porter RS, Kaplan JL, editors. The Merck manual of diagnosis and therapy. Whitehouse Station, NJ: Merck Sharpe & Dohme Corp.; 2011. p. 1329.
5. McAdam AJ, Miller DA, Sharpe AH. Infectious diseases. In: Kumar V, Abbas AK, Aster JC, editors. Robbins and Cotran Pathologic basis of disease. Philadelphia: Elsevier Saunders; 2015. p. 341 - 402.
6. Srikanta D, Santiago-Tirado FH, Doering TL. Cryptococcus neoformans: historical curiosity to modern pathogen. Yeast. 2014;31:47-60.
7. Iwen PC. Mycotic Diseases. In: MacPherson RA, Pincus MR, editors. Henry's Clinical Diagnosis and Management by Laboratory Methods. Philadelphia: Elsevier Saunders; 2011. p. 1169 - 1170.
8. Saha DC, Xess I, Biswas A, Bhowmik DM, Padma MV. Detection of Cryptococcus by conventional, serological and molecular methods. J Med Microbiol. 2009;58:1098-1105.
9. American Association for Clinical Chemistry. Human immunodeficiency virus. Laboratory tests. 2014. https://labtestsonline.org/understanding/conditions/hiv/start/2
10. HIV laboratory diagnosis: New tests and a new algorithm. J Clin Virol. 2013;58 supplement I:e1 - e134.
11. Branson BM OSM, Weselowski LG, Bennett B, Werner BG, Wroblewski KE, Pentella MA. Laboratory testing for the diagnosis of HIV infection: Updated recommendations. 2014. www.cdc.gov/hiv/testing/. Accessed 2015.

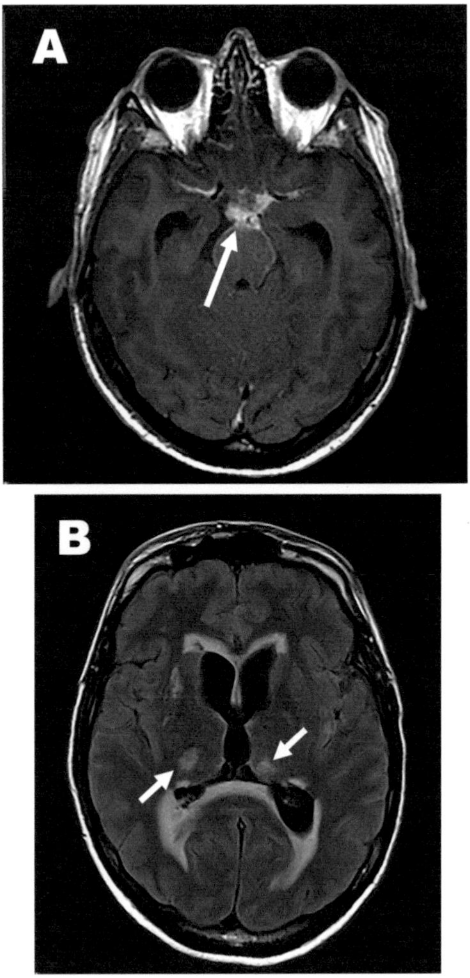

Figure 5.1.A A T1 post-contrast axial MRI of the brain from a different case shows thick nodular enhancement of the leptomeninges in the basilar cistern (arrow) suggesting meningitis.

Figure 5.1.B An Axial Fluid Attenuated Inversion Recovery image shows increased signal in the thalami bilaterally (arrows) suggesting perivascular spread of Cryptococcus resulting in cryptococcomas or gelatinous pseudocysts.

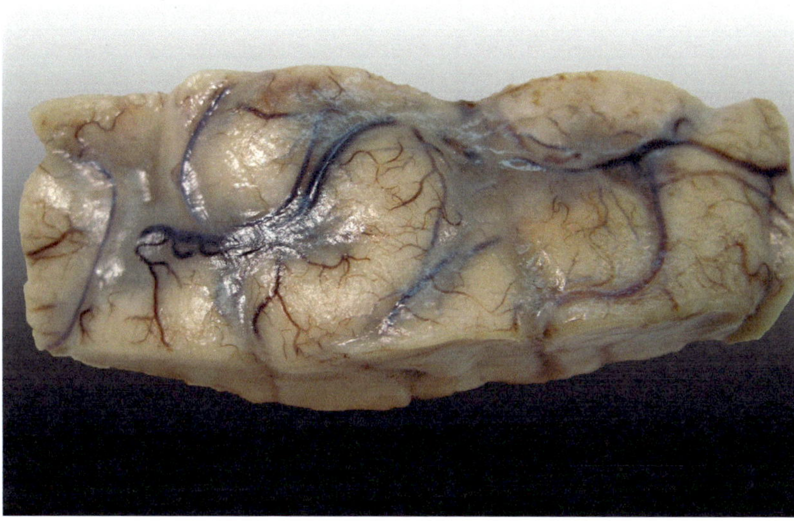

Figure 5.2 A portion of cerebral cortex showing white discoloration or clouding of the surface leptomeninges that is most pronounced along the course of vessels in the sulci (the depressions on the cortical surface); a characteristic feature of meningitis. This image is from a different case with E. coli meningitis.

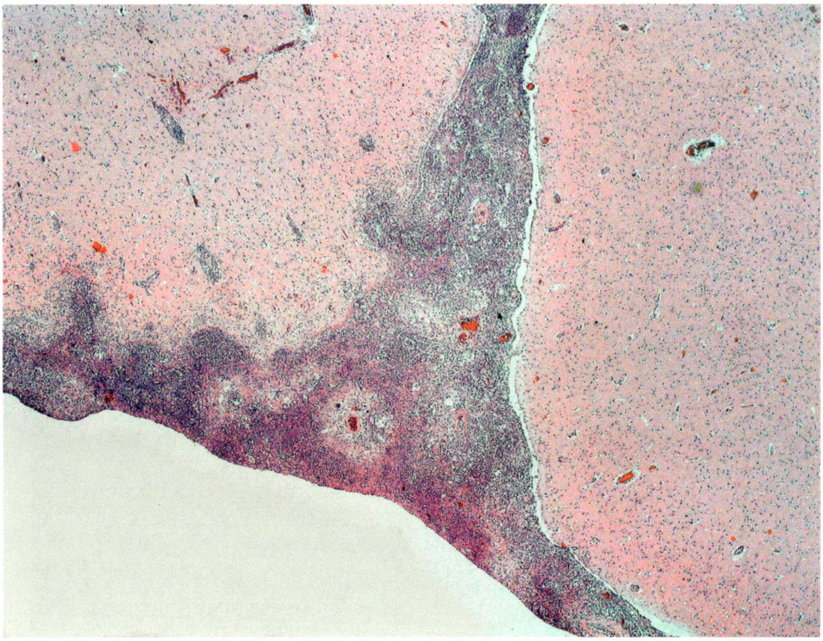

Figure 5.3 This low power microscopic image of the patient's brain shows that the leptomeninges, the membranes that cover the brain surface, have been lifted by an inflammatory exudate. All the small dark spots in the exudate are the nuclei of white blood cells. Meningitis from fungal infections tends to be more prominent on the base of the brain. (Original magnification 40x, H&E stain).

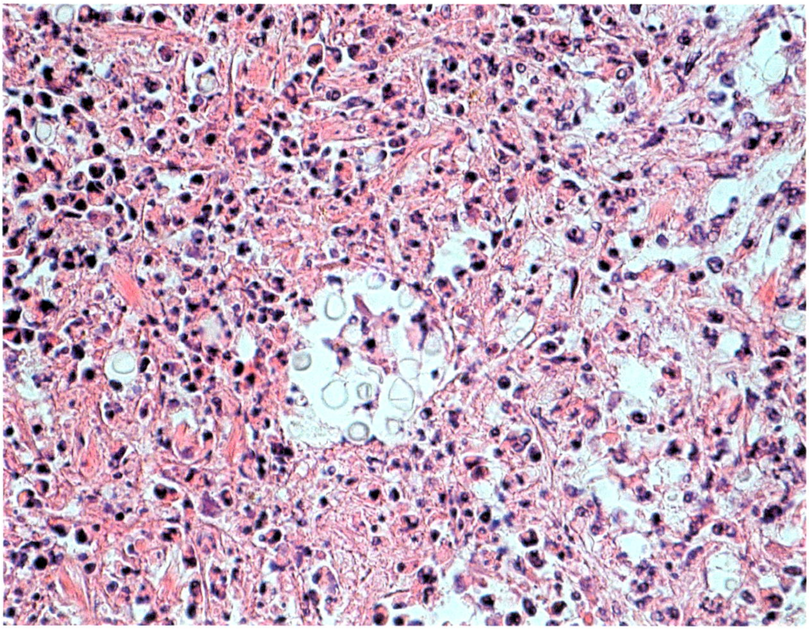

Figure 5.4 This high power microscopic image of the patient's meningeal inflammatory exudate shows many inflammatory cells. In addition, there are some roughly spherical structures that do not stain with either hematoxylin or eosin. The structures have a refractile appearance and many of them seem to have a clear space around them. (Original magnification 200x, H&E stain).

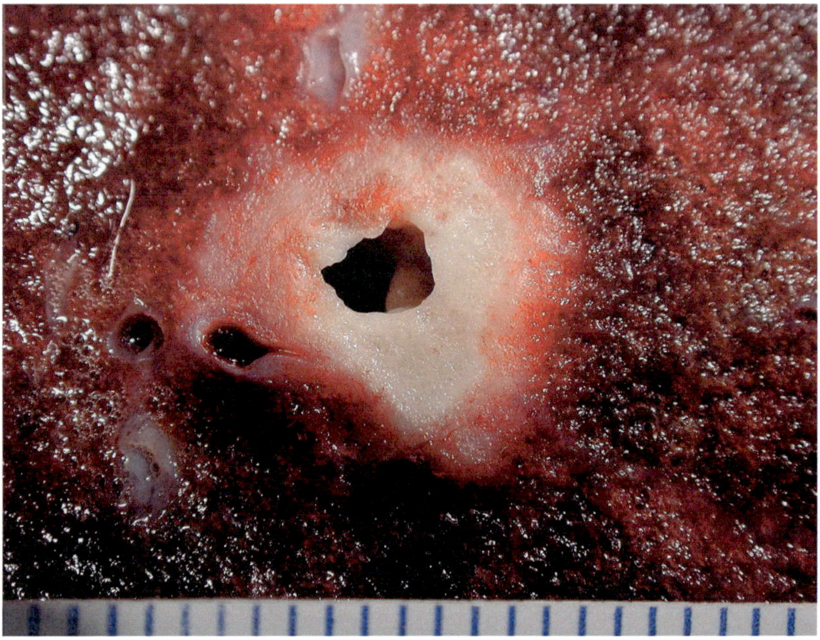

Figure 5.5 A cavity in the lung. The small divisions on the ruler are 1 mm.

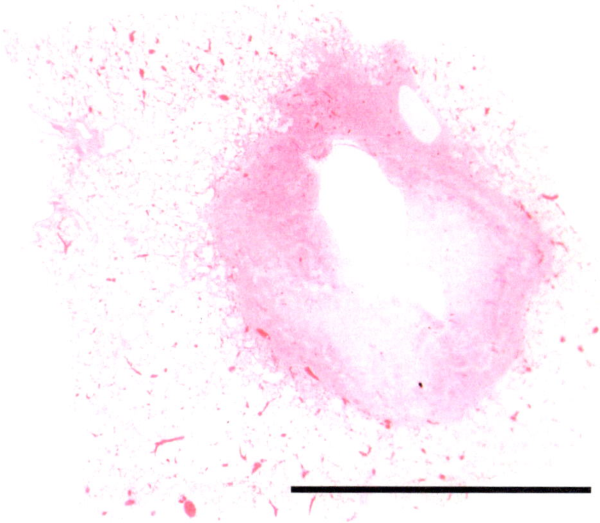

Figure 5.6. A very low power image of the microscopic section of the cavity in the lung. The pulmonary alveoli are visible peripherally. The cavity is surrounded by granulation tissue. The black bar is 1 cm long.

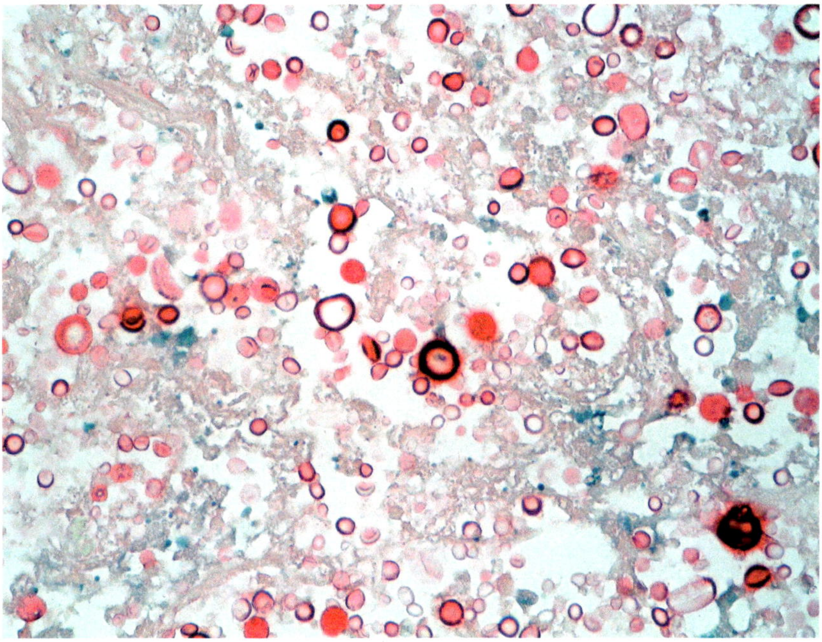

Figure 5.7 An image of the tissue surrounding the lung cavity stained with the Periodic acid – Schiff reagent (PAS). Abundant PAS positive budding yeast are present. The yeast are highly variable in size; a characteristic feature of Cryptococcus.

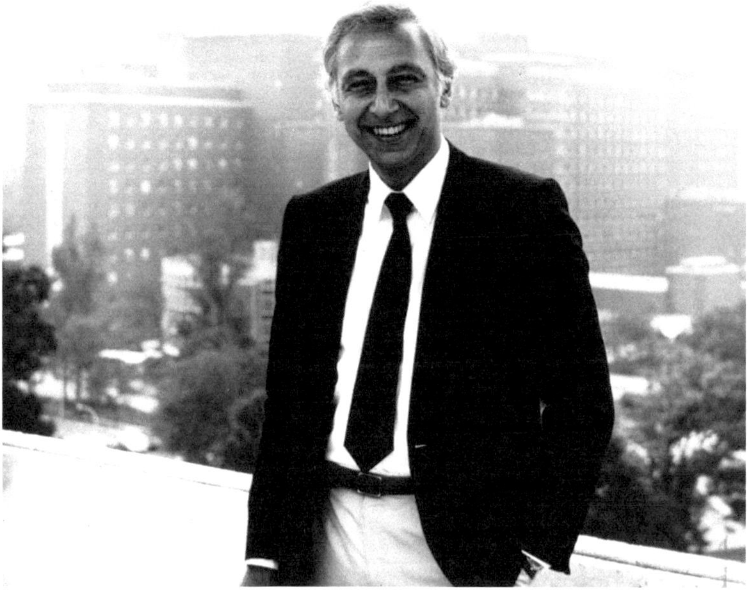

Figure 5.8 Robert Gallo (1937 –). Courtesy of the National Library of Medicine.

Chapter 6

A male fetus at 31 weeks gestation with oligohydramnios and polycystic kidneys. (vindiCate, congenital)

"Classifications are ideal and mutable, observations and experience are solid and unchangeable". Marcello Malpighi (1628 – 1694)

6.1 The Autopsy

6.1.1 Case history

The patient's mother was a G2P1001 woman (i.e. She was pregnant for the second time, had given birth once before after a full-term pregnancy and had one living child. The four digits after the P indicate how many full term pregnancies, how many preterm pregnancies, how many abortions, and how many living children the patient's mother has had. Recall that health care professionals use the term abortion to indicate loss of a fetus from any cause and that in an autopsy report the "patient" is the decedent.) in her mid-twenties who had decreased fetal movement in her late second trimester. An ultrasound showed oligohydramnios (too little amniotic fluid) and bilateral echogenic enlarged kidneys with renal cysts. The previous child had been normal. There were no other significant maternal findings. A 1480-gram stillborn male fetus was delivered early in the third trimester with Apgar scores of 0 at 1 minute and 0 at 5 minutes (Virginia Apgar (1909 – 1974) developed the Apgar scoring system in 1952 to determine how maternal anesthesia had affected newborn infants. The score is used today as an overall indicator of a newborn's health and ranges from 0 to 10. Most normal infants have a score of 7 or higher.)

6.1.2 Postmortem findings

Since a fetus is a developing organism, the pathologist takes many weights and measures during a stillborn autopsy to determine gestational age, whether the fetus was growing normally and to see if there is any unusual pattern of measurements to indicate a particular diagnosis. This fetus had a body weight of 1414 grams, a crown-rump length of 27.7 cm and a heel-toe length of 6.3 cm. Foot length is especially useful since it is easy to measure, it isn't affected much by autolysis and it has been shown to be tightly distributed in study populations. The measurements were compatible with the expected age of 31 weeks. The organ weights were normal for fetal age except that the kidneys weighed 91.3 grams and were expected to weigh about 11.3 grams. The liver was also large at 85.2 grams (expected 46 ± 38 grams).

The fetus was male and had a slightly flattened nose like what is usually seen in the collection of facial features called Potter's facies. There was unusual bilateral deviation of the feet to the right and there was purplish discoloration of the skin along the inner surfaces of the arms and on the chest, both suggesting fetal compression from oligohydramnios (figure 6.1). The placenta weighed 392 grams and was normal. It had a 3-vessel umbilical cord. The left and right kidneys were symmetrically enlarged. The left kidney weighed 44.9 grams and the right kidney weighed 46.4 grams. The kidneys were each about 7 cm long (figures 6.2, 6.3). The ureters and bladder were normal. On cut section, the kidneys had a pattern of many roughly circular areas of whitish discoloration measuring up to about 3 mm in diameter. Some of these areas resembled thin-walled cysts (figures 6.4 – 6.7). No gross cysts were seen in other organs.

Examination under the microscope showed many renal cysts. The cysts were most prominent in the medulla but extended up into the renal cortex. The medullary cysts were mostly round, but toward the cortex, they became elongate and cylindrical. The non-cystic kidney was histologically normal. No glomerular cysts were seen. Sections of the liver showed increased hepatic portal area fibrous tissue. Some portal areas resembled the 'ductal-plate malformation' of congenital hepatic fibrosis with characteristic peripheral bile ductule-like proliferation.

6.1.3 Case summary

This fetus had features of Potter facies and signs of compression, both compatible with oligohydramnios. An important source of amniotic fluid is fetal urine, and one of the causes of oligohydramnios is a renal abnormality. The kidneys in this fetus weighed 8 times normal and the liver was enlarged. Examination under the microscope showed histologic features compatible with the autosomal recessive type of polycystic kidney disease, also called infantile polycystic kidney disease. Cytogenetics was done on a piece of the placenta and it showed a normal 46, XY karyotype. Constitutional comparative genomic hybridization was also done and showed no abnormality.

6.2 Discussion

6.2.1 Renal polycystic kidney disease

Cyst formation is a common morphologic finding in abnormally developed kidneys, so if one looks at all cystic kidneys in stillborn infants, then the group will be quite heterogeneous. There are many causes of multiple renal cysts including, renal dysplasia, glomerulocystic kidney, medullary cystic diseases, and many inherited syndromes that may be associated with renal cystic disease (e.g. Meckel-Grüber syndrome, Tuberous sclerosis, Beckwith-Wiedemann syndrome, and Zellweger's syndrome). Cystic kidneys were classified according to their morphologic features on microdissection by Drs. Osathandondh and Potter in a series of articles in the 1960s. This system, called Potter's classification system, isn't used much today (except perhaps by radiologists) since it doesn't incorporate clinical and genetic information. The term polycystic kidneys is usually used to refer to either of two different diseases, infantile polycystic kidney disease and adult polycystic kidney disease. Infantile PCKD may sometimes present later in life and adult PCKD may sometimes present in an infant, so these diseases are more often called autosomal recessive PCKD and autosomal dominant PCKD respectively. Autosomal recessive polycystic kidney disease (ARPCKD), the diagnosis in the autopsy case presented here, was called type I in the Potter classification and its cysts were shown to develop from the renal collecting tubules. In large series, ARPCKD has occurred in less than 1% of pediatric autopsies. Affected patients usually have very large symmetrical kidneys containing many small cysts. The cysts are often spherical in the medulla but radiate outward into the cortex in cylindrical shapes. Normal glomeruli and tubules are present between the cysts. Patients with ARPCKD have a characteristic histologic change in their livers with portal expansion by increased numbers of peripheral bile ductules associated with loose connective tissue and capillaries. The hepatic appearance was called the ductal plate malformation by Jørgensen. Similar changes occur in some other malformation syndromes. The mortality from ARPCKD in newborn infants is very high. Some reports have had a high survival rate with aggressive treatment. Surviving infants have hypertension and hepatic fibrosis and they will need renal transplantation.

ARPCKD is caused by one of multiple possible mutant alleles in a single gene called PKHD1. The gene is on the short arm of chromosome 6. It makes a large glycoprotein, polycystin, that has some similarities to calcium channel subunits and is probably a cell membrane receptor [1,2].

6.2.2 Potter's sequence

Decreased fetal urine output or chronic leakage of amniotic fluid can lead to oligohydramnios and consequent fetal compression and pulmonary hypoplasia. The findings of fetal compression include a characteristically altered facies with a flattened nose and abnormal positioning of the hands and feet. Breech presentation and increased vernix on the fetal surface of the placenta (amnion nodosum) are also seen in oligohydramnios. Renal function that may seem unnecessary in utero, since waste disposal is handled by the placenta and maternal kidneys, is necessary since urine output supports amniotic fluid volume which is necessary for normal fetal lung development [3].

6.3 Medical history

6.3.1 Renal cysts

Although cysts were known to occur in the kidney for hundreds and perhaps thousands of years, descriptions make it unclear what was being described. Echinococcosis, for example, might simulate autosomal dominant polycystic kidney disease. The first likely description of a case of ADPCK was that of Stefan Bathory a Polish king who defeated Ivan the Terrible in a war lasting from 1576 to 1582. King Bathory died in 1585 and had an autopsy, the results of which were reviewed in 1933 at the time of the 400th anniversary of his death. A group of medical specialists decided that he likely had PCK. Matthew Baillie separated hydatid cysts of the kidney (Echinococcal cysts) from "false hydatids of the kidney" in his 1793 text. A bimodal age distribution of cases was noticed as early as 1902.

Edith Louise Potter (1901 – 1993) was born in Clinton, Iowa and studied Medicine at the University of Minnesota. She came to the Chicago Lying-in Hospital in 1934 and became a professor of pathology there. She performed more than 10,000 perinatal autopsies in her career and worked to create the subspecialty of perinatal pathology. In 1946, she described the findings in 20 autopsies from infants who died in the perinatal period with renal agenesis.

She wrote, "Two anomalies were observed in almost all of these infants which to my knowledge have not previously been recognized as characteristically associated with renal agenesis. These are hypoplasia of the lungs and an abnormal facial expression." [4–6]

6.4 Laboratory Medicine

6.4.1 Evaluation of the fetal genome

Plants, animals, and microorganisms have an outwardly observable physical structure that we call their phenotype. The phenotype is determined by the organism's genetic makeup, its genotype, in interaction with the environment. So, a man might have an unusually shaped head due to his unusual genetic makeup, or due to his typical genetic makeup that interacted with an unusual set of external physical circumstances in utero, or he may merely have been hit in the head in the past. One is more likely to suspect a genetic origin of an abnormality when infants are examined. The patient described here had bilaterally enlarged kidneys containing multiple small cysts with a characteristic histologic appearance, associated hepatic fibrosis with a characteristic histologic appearance, and changes indicating likely oligohydramnios, so we feel confident making the diagnosis of autosomal recessive polycystic kidney disease. The distinction between this disease and others on the differential diagnostic list is important since it helps the parents determine the risk for a similar abnormality occurring in subsequent pregnancies. An autosomal recessive disorder like ARPCKD has a chance of occurring in 1 in 4 pregnancies since each parent is heterozygous for the affected allele, but there is an autosomal dominant form of polycystic kidney disease and there are many other diseases that may have renal cysts but have different patterns of inheritance. The obstetrician in cases like this one usually requests that some laboratory genetic analysis is done. The most common test is called a karyotype in which cells are cultured from fetal tissue. Dividing cells are treated with a drug that stops cell division in metaphase and the cells are stained to highlight different parts of the chromosomes. Photographs of these cells are used to count the number of autosomes and sex chromosomes. This technique can identify if there are too many or too few chromosomes, if there is an abnormality in the sex chromosome number, or if the chromosomes have rearrangements between them. In this case, the karyotype was normal 46, XY, i.e. the right number of normal-appearing autosomes and sex chromosomes were present. Karyotype is a relatively gross way to examine the genotype. Deletions and duplications that are less than 1 or 2 million bases in length cannot be seen in routine karyotype, and other tests may be used to detect abnormalities that might be clinically important. These include DNA probes that detect single nucleotide polymorphisms (SNPs) and fluorescent hybridizing probes for particular DNA abnormalities (FISH). This fetus also had a test called competitive genomic hybridization (CGH) that can detect a few hundred different genetic abnormalities; it was normal. CGH is a fluorescent imaging technique in which the patient's DNA is treated with a green dye and control DNA is treated with a red dye. When these specimens are mixed and hybridized to an array of DNA segments that come from points that are every several thousand bases through the genome, a green fluorescent signal will indicate that an area corresponding to a particular oligonucleotide probe is present in the patient in an amount that is increased relative to the control. Similarly, a red spot indicates an area that is decreased in the patient relative to the control, and areas with equal representation in the patient and the control specimens will appear yellow [7].

6.5 Study questions

1. Why does fetal urine production have any effect on fetal lung development?

2. What is the most common lethal dominantly inherited abnormality in humans?

3. How are autosomal recessive traits inherited? If both parents are heterozygous for an allele associated with a disease, what is the probability that they will have a child with the disease?

4. How is the embryological development of the fetal renal collecting ducts different from the development of the proximal fetal renal tubules?

5. Can you think of an abnormality of the excretory system other than polycystic renal disease that would result in oligohydramnios?

6.6 References

1. Bianchi DW, Crombleholme TM, D'Alton ME, Malone FD. Polycystic kidney disease. Fetology. Diagnosis and management of the fetal patient. New York: McGraw - Hill Medical; 2010. p. 535 - 543.
2. Lacson A, Bernstein J, Risdon RA, Gilbert-Barness E. Renal system. In: Gilbert-Barness E, Kapur RPO, LL Siebert, JR, editors. Potter's pathology of the fetus, infant and child. Philadelphia: Mosby Elsevier; 2007. p. 1304 - 1306.
3. Jones KL, Smith DW. Smith's recognizable patterns of human malformation. Philadelphia: Elsevier Saunders; 2006:954.
4. Dunn PM. Dr Edith Potter (1901–1993) of Chicago: pioneer in perinatal pathology. Arch Dis Child Fetal Neonatal Ed. 2007;92:F419-F420.
5. Rapola J. The kidneys and urinary tract. In: Wigglesworth JS, Singer DB, editors. Textbook of fetal and perinatal pathology. Boston: Blackwell Scientific Publications; 1991. p. 1117 - 1130.
6. Torres VE, Watson ML. Polycystic kidney disease: antiquity to the 20th century. Nephrol Dial Transplant. 1998;13:2690-2696.
7. Nussbaum RL, McInnes RR, Willard HF, Hamosh A. Thompson & Thompson. Genetics in Medicine. Philadelphia: Saunders; 2007
8. R Core Team. R: A language and environment for statistical computing. 2014 http://www.R-project.org/. Accessed 2015
9. Wickham H. ggplot2: elegant graphics for data analysis. New York: Springer; 2009

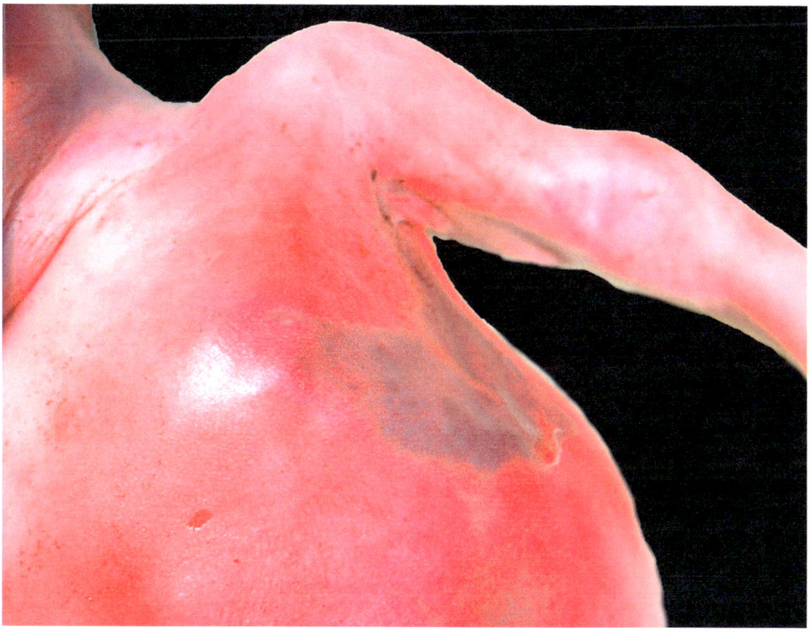

Figure 6.1 An area of purple discoloration on the fetal chest compatible with compression of the arm against the chest, a secondary change from oligohydramnios.

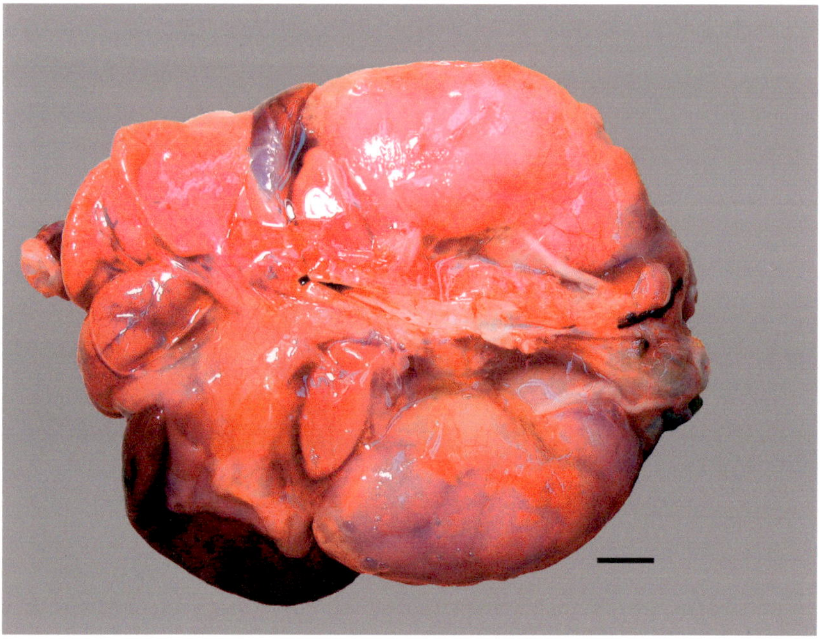

Figure 6.2 A posterior view of the visceral block. There is marked enlargement of the kidneys. The adrenal glands and ureters are visible. The spleen is the dark organ at 11 o'clock. The aorta has been partially opened longitudinally. The black bar is 1 cm long.

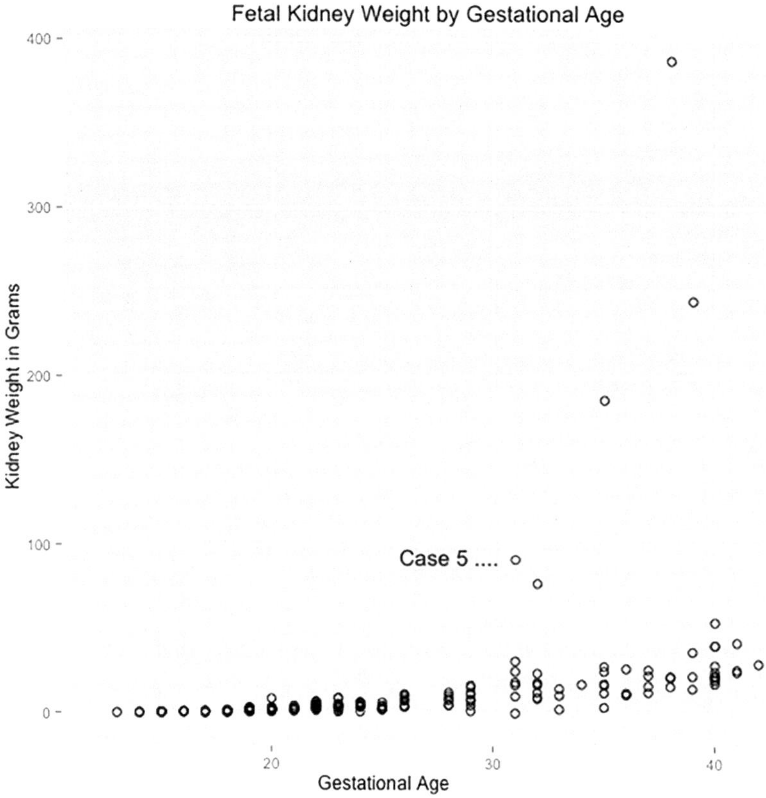

Figure 6.3 A scatterplot of all the fetal decedents in the autopsy database showing the weight of the kidneys in grams by gestational age in weeks. The combined kidney weight is labeled for this case (Case 5). It is a clear outlier. All the outliers in this graph with large kidneys had autosomal recessive polycystic kidney disease except for one case that had Meckel-Grüber syndrome. [8,9]

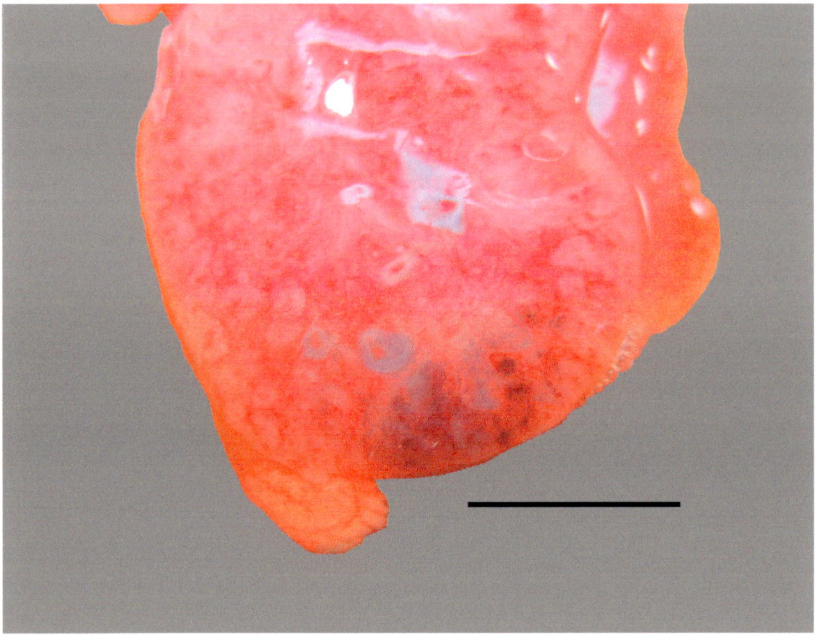

Figure 6.4 Cut section of the lower pole of one kidney. There are multiple cysts ranging up to 3 mm in diameter. The black bar is 1 cm long.

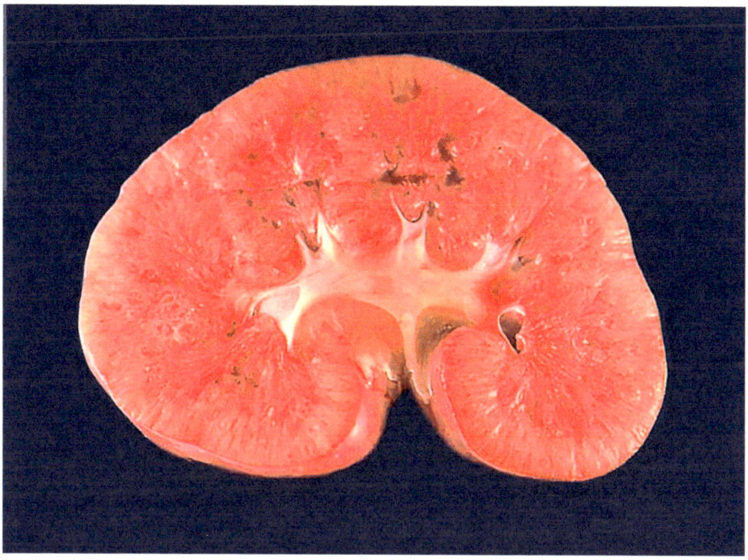

Figure 6.5 A different autopsy case of autosomal recessive polycystic kidney disease. This image was made without a scale; the kidney was about 5 cm long.

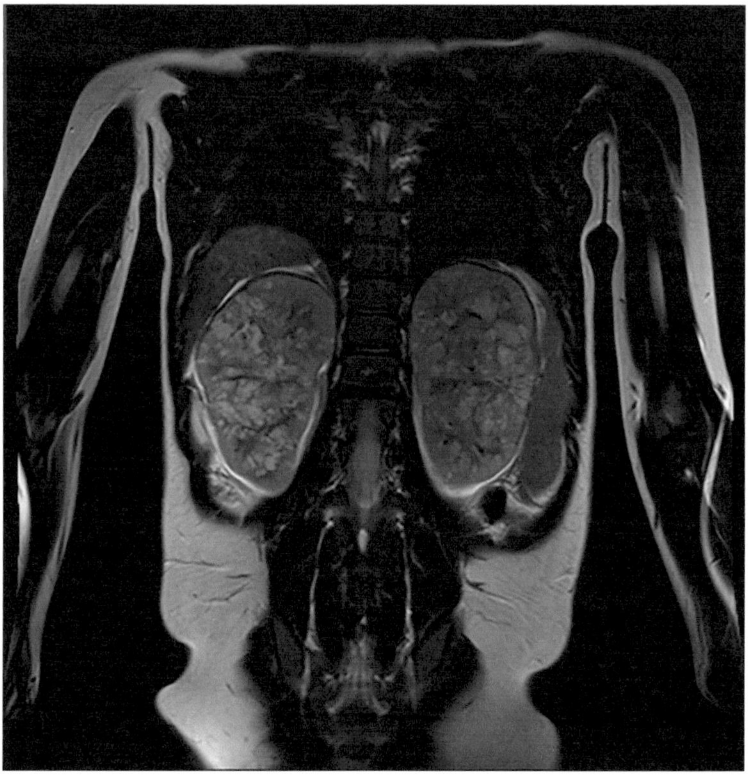

Figure 6.6 A coronal T2 weighted MRI of the kidneys from a different case of ARPCKD demonstrating increased signal and enlargement of the kidneys bilaterally.

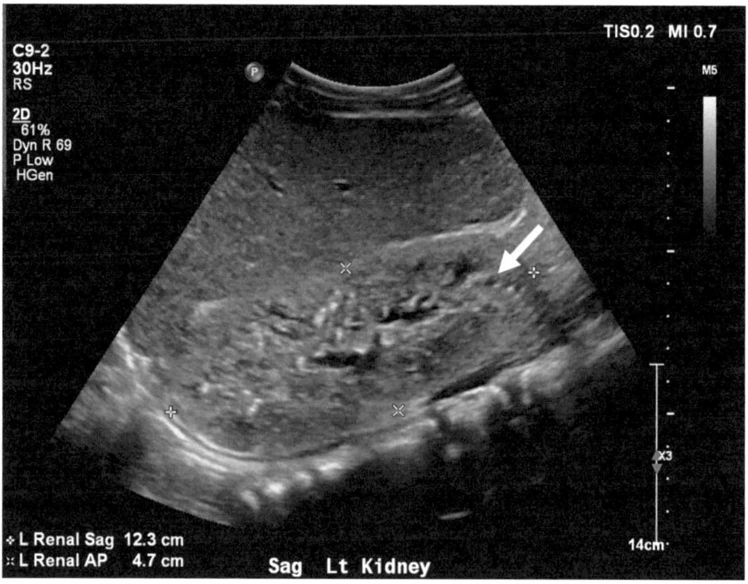

Figure 6.7 A sagittal view gray scale ultrasound of the left kidney from a different case demonstrates enlargement and increased brightness or echogenicity (arrow) as a result of numerous microscopic cysts. Normally the kidneys should be about 1/3 smaller than these enlarged bright kidneys and just slightly darker or equal in signal or greyscale to the adjacent liver. Figures 6.6 and 6.7 are courtesy of Dr. David Saul.

CHAPTER 7

A middle-aged man with systemic hypertension and an adrenal tumor. (ViNdicateE, vascular, neoplastic, endocrinologic)

"There are many things that hinder sure knowledge, the obscurity of the subject and the shortness of human life." Pythagoras (c. 582 BCE – c. 500 BCE)

7.1 The Autopsy

7.1.1 Case history

The patient was a 55-year-old man with a history of hypertension and chronic renal insufficiency. He was found unresponsive at home. He was pronounced dead in the Emergency Department. As is sometimes the case, no other history or information of any kind was available.

7.1.2 Postmortem findings

The patient had only mild to moderate coronary artery atherosclerosis. There was no evidence of a myocardial infarct. He had marked biventricular hypertrophy (the heart weighed 975 grams, about three times normal) with replacement type fibrosis (figure 7.1). There were pulmonary edema and hepatic congestion. There was bilateral arterionephrosclerosis. A 1.8 cm diameter brownish right adrenal tumor was present (figures 7.2 – 7.5). The patient also had a 0.8 cm diameter left thoracic para-radicular tumor and an anterior abdominal brown skin macule resembling a café au lait spot. The patient had gastritis from Helicobacter pylori and diffuse nodular duodenal Brunner gland hyperplasia with focal duodenal pancreatic heterotopia.

7.1.3 Case summary

The tumor in the patient's adrenal gland was centered over the central adrenal medulla and was the characteristic brown-mahogany color of a pheochromocytoma. The tumor next to a left thoracic nerve root had a shiny white appearance and resembled a peripheral nerve sheath tumor. Histologic examination confirmed that the adrenal tumor was a pheochromocytoma (figure 7.6) and that the left thoracic periradicular tumor was a neurofibroma. I attributed the patient's death to cardiac arrhythmia in a background of marked biventricular cardiac hypertrophy from hypertensive heart disease. Since the pheochromocytoma was discovered at autopsy, it was unclear if it had been functional or not. If the pheochromocytoma had been functional and the cause of the patient's hypertensive heart disease, then it was the cause of death. Pheochromocytoma may occur in patients with various other syndromes (von Hippel-Lindau, MEN type 2, Neurofibromatosis type 1). This patient had other abnormalities; a single café au lait spot, a left thoracic nerve root neurofibroma, diffuse duodenal Brunner gland hyperplasia and focal duodenal pancreatic heterotopia (a piece of pancreas located abnormally in the wall of the duodenum). These findings are suspicious for some forme fruste, or incomplete manifestation, of neurofibromatosis, but definitive features of one or more of the syndromes that may be associated with pheochromocytoma were not found.

Of some interest, there is a report in the medical literature of another case with both Brunner gland hyperplasia and pancreatic heterotopia [1]. This case had very little medical history at the time of autopsy, a common problem in patients who die suddenly at home and are brought into the hospital. With the coming of the electronic medical record, it is sometimes possible to find some history if the patient had previously been in my hospital. The absence of medical history might make me fail to do some special examination at autopsy and it might lead me to make some mistaken conclusion when writing the final report. On the other hand, a careful autopsy without any medical history can be exciting and it puts no restrictions on my theorizing. The absence of history when examining surgical specimens, e.g. a surgically resected spleen that comes with the history "spleen", can be more irritating. I once heard a well-known anatomic pathologist from a nearby institution say that he was sometimes tempted to sign out such surgical specimens as, "Diagnosis compatible with history submitted". He was kidding, of course.

7.2 Discussion

7.2.1 Hypertension

Hypertension is the medical term for high blood pressure. Arterial blood pressure is measured as two numbers, the systolic blood pressure or pressure when the cardiac ventricle is contracting and the diastolic blood pressure or pressure when the cardiac ventricle is relaxing. Hypertension is defined as a resting arterial blood pressure that is greater than or equal to 140/90 mm Hg. About 65 million people have hypertension in the United States, but since they are mostly asymptomatic, only about a third of them have their blood pressure adequately controlled and many of them are not aware that they are hypertensive. The incidence of hypertension increases with age and about two-thirds of people over 65 have hypertension. Ninety percent of patients with hypertension have primary hypertension, that is, the cause of their hypertension is unknown. Most of the other 10% of patients with secondary hypertension have kidney disease and only 0.1% of hypertensive patients have a pheochromocytoma.

Over time patients with hypertension have damage to their blood vessels with effects that are most noticeable in their kidneys, brain and heart. So, they are at increased risk for renal failure, cerebrovascular accident (stroke), and myocardial infarct. They often develop hypertensive heart disease characterized by left ventricular hypertrophy and multiple minute areas of myocardial scarring from small vessel ischemia. Patients with hypertensive heart disease are at increased risk of sudden death from cardiac arrhythmia and from aortic dissection.

Patients with high blood pressure are treated with weight loss, restricted sodium diet, and one or more drugs from any of several classes of agents including diuretics, beta blockers, calcium channel blockers, acetylcholinesterase inhibitors, angiotensin type II receptor blockers, adrenergic inhibitors, and vasodilators [2].

7.2.2 Pheochromocytoma

Pheochromocytoma is a tumor of specialized neurosecretory cells in the sympathetic nervous system that arises in the adrenal medulla or in extra-adrenal paraganglia. Outside of the adrenal gland, the tumors are usually called paragangliomas. Some pheochromocytomas are silent, but 90% of them are associated with systemic hypertension from the secretion of catecholamines. The tumor is important to identify, since resecting the tumor can cure the patient's hypertension. Pheochromocytoma has, classically, been referred to as the 10% tumor since it was thought that 10% of the tumors were extra-adrenal, 10% were bilateral, 10% did not have associated hypertension, and 10% were malignant.

Exceptions are that familial cases of pheochromocytoma are bilateral in up to 50% of cases and extra-adrenal cases and some cases associated with inherited mutations have a higher incidence of malignancy. Also, there seem to be more non-functional tumors than the expected 10% that have been found incidentally with the increased use of CT scans, and some studies have found a rate of malignancy higher than 10%, even in solitary tumors of the adrenal gland.

About 2/3 of patients with hypertension from a pheochromocytoma have paroxysmal hypertensive episodes. These episodes may be associated with palpitations, headache, sweating, and chest pain and they may be fatal.

There is increased risk for pheochromocytoma in patients with the Von Hippel-Lindau syndrome, Neurofibromatosis type 1, or Multiple endocrine neoplasia type 2. About a third of patients with pheochromocytoma carry a germline mutation in the RET, VHL, SDHD, or SDHB genes. Screening for these mutations should be considered in patients who are young or who have bilateral or malignant tumors [3,4].

7.2.3 Brief descriptions of syndromes that may be associated with pheochromocytoma:

Von Hippel-Lindau syndrome — An autosomal dominant disease with a mutation in the VHL gene on the short arm of chromosome 3 characterized by an increased risk for various tumors including cerebellar hemangioblastoma, retinal angioma, pheochromocytoma, cysts in the kidneys, liver or pancreas, and renal cell carcinoma. By age 60 the risk of renal cell carcinoma in these patients is 70%.

Neurofibromatosis, type 1 — An autosomal dominant disease described by Friedrich von Recklinghausen (1830 – 1910) in 1882 with a mutation in the gene on chromosome 17 for neurofibromin that is characterized by multiple peripheral neurofibromas, café au lait skin macules, hamartomas of the iris, deformities of bone, and increased risk for various tumors including optic gliomas and pheochromocytomas.

Multiple endocrine neoplasia, type 2 — A hereditary syndrome with a mutation in the RET gene on chromosome 10. Type 2A is characterized by increased risk for various tumors including medullary carcinoma of the thyroid gland, pheochromocytoma and parathyroid adenoma or parathyroid hyperplasia. Type 2B is characterized by increased risk for various tumors including medullary carcinoma of the thyroid gland, pheochromocytoma, multiple mucosal neuromas, and intestinal ganglioneuromas. Type 2B patients may have a Marfanoid appearance with skeletal abnormalities [3,4].

7.3 Medical history

7.3.1 Blood pressure measurement

Physicians have evaluated a patient's heart function by taking the patient's pulse for thousands of years. Works on the evaluation of the pulse were available in China before the Common Era. Four pulsations for each respiration of the physician was described as the natural heart rate. Galen of Pergamon, the great 2nd-century Greek physician, described many qualities of the peripheral arterial pulse in remarkable detail. Pulses were strong or feeble, hard or soft, equal or unequal, decurate (diminishing over time like the tail of a mouse, pulsus myurus), dorcadessans (leaping like a goat, pulsus caprizans, or a gazelle, pulsus gazellans), and so forth, although Galen apparently did not count the heart rate. The pressure at the top of the pulse is called the systolic pressure and the pressure at the lowest point of the pulse is called the diastolic pressure. Since the pulse strength and strength pattern were the principle ways that one could evaluate blood pressure, there was much interest in creating a device that would objectively evaluate or record a trace of the pulse in the mid-19th century. In 1876, Samuel von Basch (1837 – 1905) invented the sphygmomanometer. This device put pressure on the patient's artery until the pulse disappeared and a measure of the pressure required was read from a column of mercury in a graduated glass cylinder. In 1896, Scipione Riva-Rocci (1863 – 1937) modified this device so that a circular rubber bag was placed around the upper arm and inflated with air until the patient's pulse disappeared and in 1905, Nikolai Korotkoff (1874 – 1920) proposed that instead of feeling the pulse, the physician should listen to the brachial artery at the antecubital fossa to obtain an accurate diastolic and systolic blood pressure. Korotkoff's method is used today, although in many instances an electronic device with an LCD screen has replaced the physician, her stethoscope, and column of mercury [5,6].

7.4 Laboratory Medicine

7.4.1 Evaluation of patients with suspected pheochromocytoma

In the past patients with suspected pheochromocytoma were given a drug like histamine to try to induce a hypertensive attack. These tests are now rarely used since they can be dangerous and the results may be difficult to interpret. Testing for pheochromocytoma is usually done by measuring catecholamines and catecholamine metabolites in plasma or urine. The most common screening test is metanephrine in a 24-hour urine specimen using a colorimetric or chromatographic assay. Vanillylmandelic acid (VMA) is also measured, but VMA is more likely to have a problem with interference from vanilla, chocolate, coffee, the drug Carbidopa (used for Parkinson's disease), or propranolol. False negative and positive tests can also occur in the metanephrine assay and certain foods, drugs and smoking should be avoided if possible. Plasma catecholamine tests are more difficult to interpret. Plasma catecholamine can be elevated in patients who do not have pheochromocytoma and it can be normal in patients who have the tumor but are not having a hypertensive episode. Plasma catecholamine is sometimes selectively collected along the course of the inferior vena cava to help make the diagnosis [7,8].

7.5 Study Questions

1. What other tumors occur in the adrenal gland besides pheochromocytoma?

2. This patient had hypertension and died of a cardiac arrhythmia. What other mechanisms of death can be seen in patients with high blood pressure?

3. Why do some patients with hypertension not take their prescribed medication?

4. The study of the patient's pulse has become uncommon. Can you think of anything else that physicians did during the patient's physical examination, that they no longer do? Why did this change happen?

5. Why is it important to consider the possibility of pheochromocytoma in a patient with hypertension?

7.6 References

1. Lee WC, Yang HW, Lee YJ, Jung SH, Choi GY, Go H, Kim A, Cha SW. Brunner's gland hyperplasia: treatment of severe diffuse nodular hyperplasia mimicking a malignancy on pancreatic -duodenal area. J Korean Med Sci. 2008;23:540 - 543.

2. Bakris GL. Arterial hypertension. The Merck Manual of diagnosis and therapy. Whitehouse Station, NJ: Merck Sharp & Dohme Corp.; 2011. p. 2065 - 2076.

3. Miatra A. The endocrine system. In: Kumar V, Abbas AK, Aster JC, editors. Robbins and Cotran Pathologic basis of disease. Philadelphia: Elsevier Saunders; 2015. p. 1134 - 1137.

4. Rosai J. Rosai and Ackerman's surgical pathology. Philadelphia: Mosby Elsevier; 2011

5. Bedford DE. The ancient art of feeling the pulse. Br Heart J. 1951;13:423-437.

6. Reiser SJ. Medicine and the reign of technology. Cambridge: Cambridge University Press; 1988:317.

7. Dons RF, Wians FH Jr. Endocrine and Metabolic Disorders. Clinical Lab Testing Manual. Boca Raton, FL: CRC Press; 2009:310.

8. Jacobs DS, Oxley DK, DeMott WR. Laboratory Test Handbook. Hudson (Cleveland), Ohio: Lexi-Comp, Inc; 2001

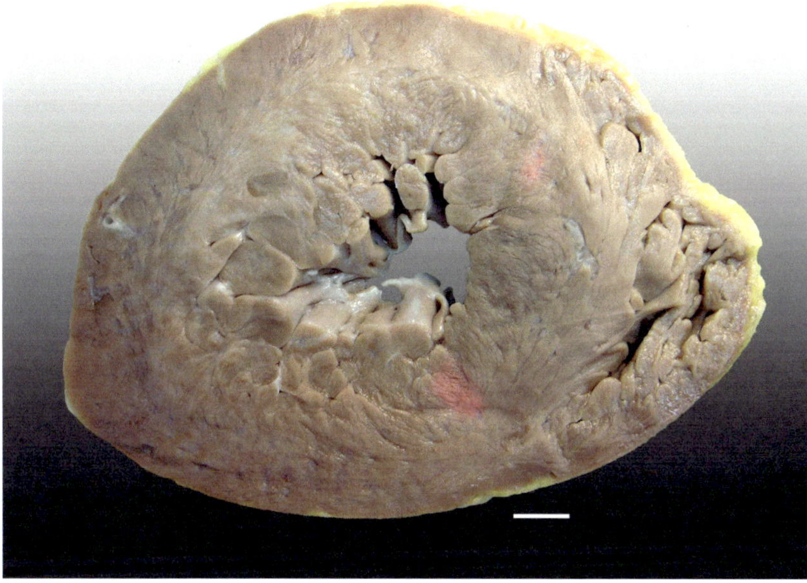

Figure 7.1 A transverse section of the central part of the cardiac ventricles. The left ventricle is on the left side of this picture. The left ventricle pumps your blood into the systemic circulation and must be strong for the task, so it is normally thicker than the right ventricle. The right ventricle is a weaker, bellows-like mechanism since it only pumps blood into the lungs at relatively low pressure. This heart has marked thickening of the left ventricle called left ventricular hypertrophy (LVH). The left ventricle is normally no thicker than 1.5 cm, but it is clearly much thicker than that here. LVH is usually due to systemic hypertension where the left ventricle must pump blood into increased systemic pressure. Patients with LVH are at increased risk for sudden death from cardiac arrhythmia. The pink areas are artifacts of fixation. The white bar is 1 cm long.

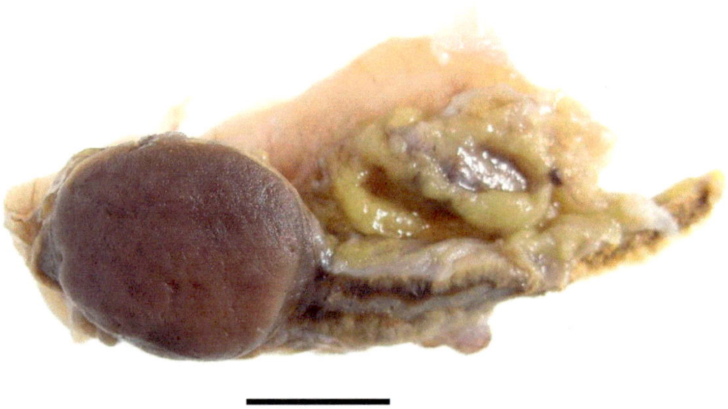

Figure 7.2 The adrenal gland and some surrounding fat. The tumor is the pheochromocytoma. It has a characteristic mahogany color and is centered on the adrenal medulla. The adjacent adrenal gland shows more normal appearing outer yellow and inner brown colored cortex. The central medulla is light gray. The black bar is 1 cm long.

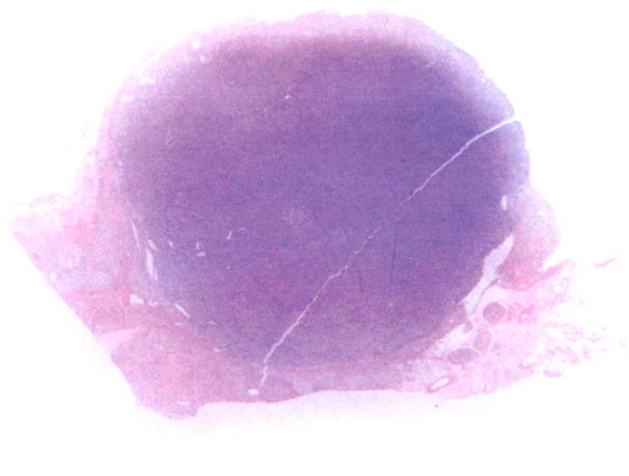

Figure 7.3 A very low power microscopic image of the adrenal tumor. The blue color indicates that the tumor is highly cellular. The black bar is 1 cm long.

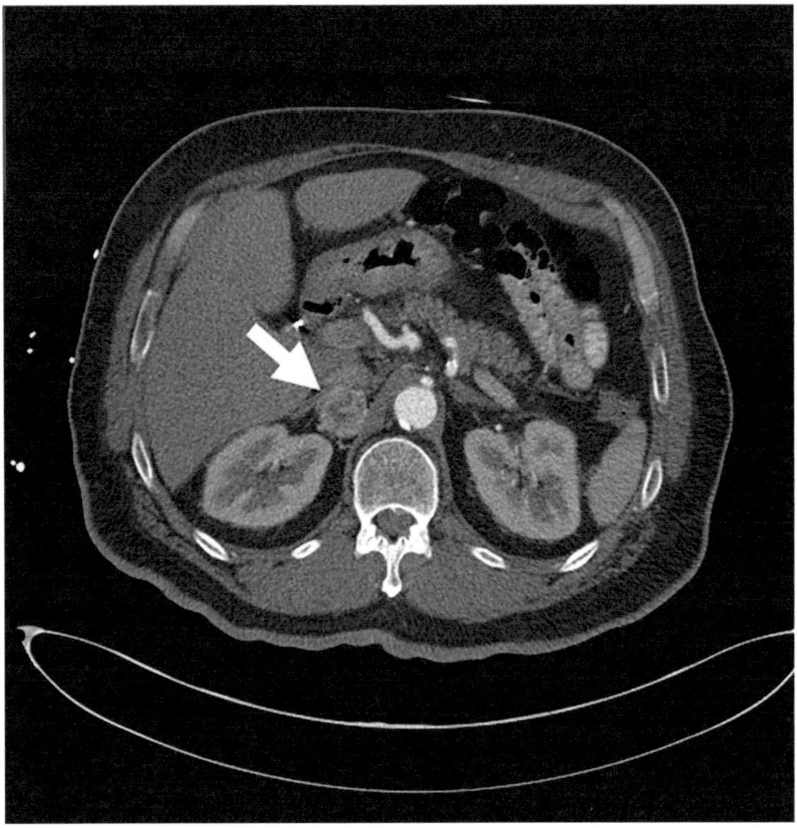

Figure 7.4 An axial CT with contrast through the level of the kidneys from a different case of pheochromocytoma shows a heterogeneously enhancing mass in the region of the right adrenal gland (arrow)

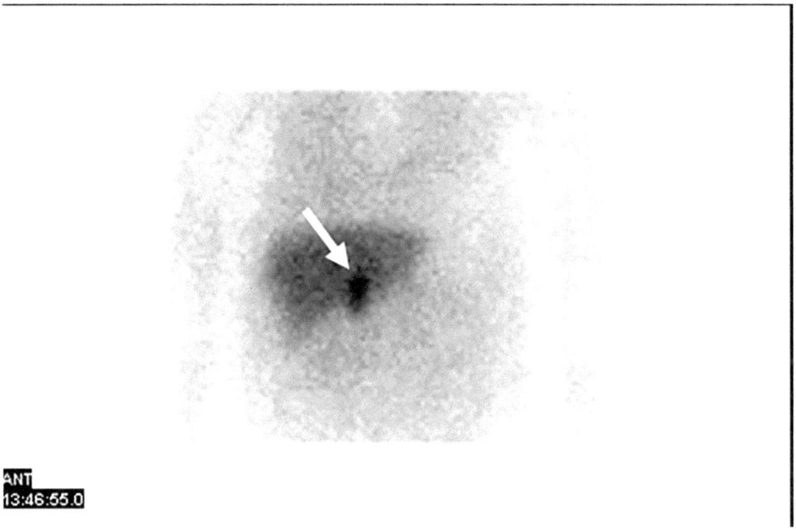

Figure 7.5 A coronal MIBG (metaiodobenzylguanidine) labeled Iodine 123 planar scintiscan image of the abdomen from the same case shown in figure 7.4 demonstrates increased uptake in the region of the right adrenal gland (arrow).

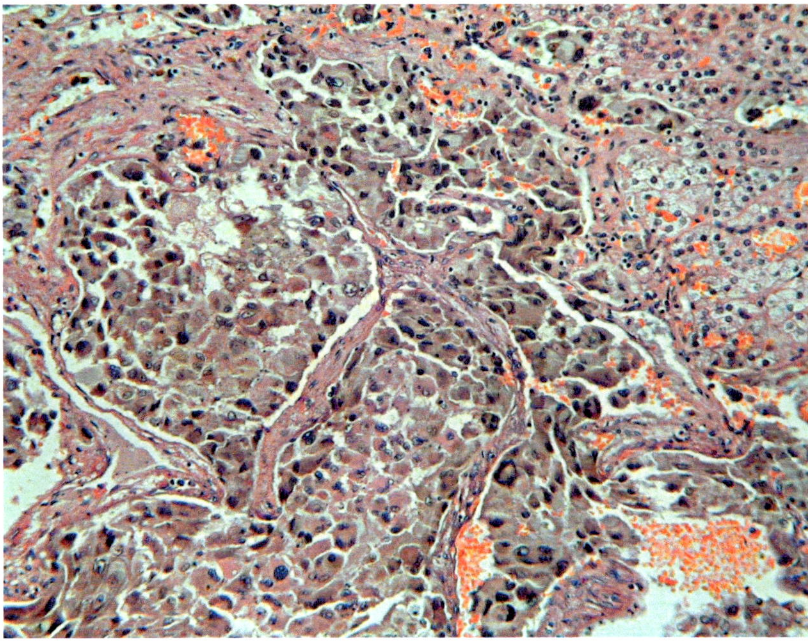

Figure 7.6 A photomicrograph of pheochromocytoma. The tumor cells grow in groups separated by fibrous bands. The tumor sometimes has cell groups that have been called *Zellballen,* or cell balls. Some of the tumor cells have pigmented cytoplasm. (Original magnification, x100. H&E stain)

CHAPTER 8

A young woman with rheumatoid arthritis and systemic lupus erythematosus. (vindicAte, autoimmune)

"If only you ignored everything that refused to come into line, our powers of explanation were unlimited." Alfred North Whitehead (1861 – 1947)

8.1 The Autopsy

8.1.1 Case history

A 35-year-old woman had a history of juvenile onset idiopathic arthritis and systemic lupus erythematosus (SLE). She had a history of hypothyroidism, multinodular goiter, chronic hemolytic anemia, gastroesophageal reflux disease, and pulmonary hypertension. She was admitted with a one-day history of pleuritic chest pain (pleuritic chest pain is usually sharp and associated with breathing), low-grade fever and a cough productive of yellow sputum. In the

Emergency department diagnoses of pneumonia, pleuritis, pericarditis, and acute coronary syndrome were considered. The patient had cardiac arrest with bradycardia and pulseless electrical activity (PEA). She was resuscitated and admitted to the medical intensive care unit. Her EKG showed sinus tachycardia (a normal pattern with increased heart rate) and left posterior fascicular block (a conduction abnormality). Laboratory values included: hemoglobin = 9.2 (normal = 12 – 16 g/dL), creatine kinase (CK) = 30 (normal = 38 – 206 IU/L), CK-MB = 2.8 (normal < 4.4 ng/mL), troponin = 0.6 (normal < 0.6 ng/mL), TSH = 31.19, WBC 37,200 (normal = 4500 – 1000 cells/cubic mm) that was 66% PMNs and 19% band forms. INR = 2.8 (recommended range in patients on warfarin is usually 2 - 3), fibrinogen = 448 (normal = 150 – 448 mg/dL). Her medications included spironolactone (diuretic), prednisone 30 mg per day (anti-inflammatory), warfarin (anticoagulant), lansoprazole (proton pump inhibitor), levothyroxine (thyroid hormone), potassium, furosemide (diuretic), and bosentan (anti-pulmonary hypertension). She was thought to be in septic shock. A chest radiograph was without infiltrate. The patient needed pressor agents to maintain her blood pressure. She developed mild elevation of her transaminases and alkaline phosphatase with a normal total bilirubin. The patient was treated with multiple antibiotics. Her blood and urine cultures were negative. The patient had hypoxia, then bradycardia, then asystole and died on the fourth hospital day.

8.1.2 Postmortem findings

Postmortem examination showed a hemorrhagic pulmonary infarct in the right middle lung lobe, grade 3 pulmonary hypertension with hypertrophy of the right cardiac ventricle, bilateral pleural effusions, adrenal cortical atrophy, hepatomegaly with chronic congestion and erythroid hyperplasia in the bone marrow. A culture from the patient's spleen grew rare Enterococcus species and a culture from the lungs grew yeast.

8.1.3 Case summary

The patient presented with a one-day history of pleuritic chest pain and I attributed that to her right middle lobe pulmonary infarct. The cause of her cardiac arrest was uncertain since she had no significant atherosclerosis and no evidence of a myocardial infarct. She did have postmortem findings indicating pulmonary hypertension, right ventricular hypertrophy due to that, and hepatic congestion due to her right heart failure. It was thought clinically that the patient had sepsis. The diagnosis of sepsis may be difficult to confirm at autopsy. Postmortem cultures showed rare Enterococcus in the splenic specimen. Splenic cultures in a typical autopsy are sterile and Enterococcus should never be in a splenic culture, but with only rare organisms present and no similar bacteria in the lung cultures, I didn't think I could provide conclusive evidence that the patient had been septic. A comment on the patient's chart mentioned some concern that her hypotension was related to a reaction to the dye use in a prior radiographic procedure. It would be difficult or impossible to identify such a reaction at autopsy, but I mention it here to remind us that the patient's medical record comprises only that which was recorded. I happened to notice the comment about the possible dye reaction, but on more than one occasion I have been questioned by a clinician after completion of an autopsy concerning a question of some interest (or even much concern) to them about which there was no mention in the patient's chart. This case is also an example of a situation in which the patient's main underlying autoimmune disease might be difficult or impossible to detect at autopsy since the disease is defined by clinical and laboratory findings.

8.2 Discussion

8.2.1 Autoimmune diseases

The connective tissue diseases, also called collagen vascular diseases, are a diverse collection of disorders characterized by abnormalities of muscle, fat, bone, joints, and blood vessels. Many of these diseases are autoimmune diseases and pathological changes may also be seen in other tissues of the body.

Since we live intimately with thousands of microorganisms and encounter more in our external environment, we have evolved a sophisticated immune system that defends the body from these organisms and their toxins. The body may sometimes attack its own antigens, either by an apparent pathological mistake or as a normal function. When a disorder is characterized by evidence of primary autoimmunity without another primary cause, it is considered an autoimmune disease. The autoimmune diseases can be divided into those mediated by autoantibodies, those mediated by T lymphocytes and others of uncertain etiology. These groups can be further subdivided into those that are organ specific and those that are systemic. These diseases are, in fact, often even more complicated than that. This patient was said to have Still's disease, the name given either to adult cases of rheumatoid arthritis that also have a fever and a characteristic skin rash or to cases of a systemic juvenile onset arthritis. It is likely that these diseases are not the same entity. She also had systemic lupus erythematosus, a prototypical systemic autoimmune disease. Certain autoantibodies are known to be associated with particular autoimmune diseases and they may be used in the laboratory as diagnostic tests.

8.2.2. Systemic lupus erythematosus

The incidence of systemic lupus erythematosus (SLE) is difficult to determine because the diagnosis is difficult to make, the disease has many variable manifestations and the disease, like most autoimmune diseases, is chronic with remissions and relapses.

Patients have many autoantibodies, especially anti-nuclear antibodies and injury is due to antibodies to various tissues and to the deposition of immune complexes. The skin, joints, kidneys and serosal membranes are often affected. Because of the difficulty in making the diagnosis, there are criteria for the diagnosis from the American College of Rheumatology in which a person must have 4 of 11 listed symptoms, signs, or laboratory findings for a diagnosis of SLE to be made with certainty [1]. Classical findings include an erythematous malar rash, photosensitive dermatitis, pleuritis, glomerulonephritis, arthritis, hemolytic anemia and various neuropsychiatric disorders. SLE may sometimes be induced by drug therapy, examples are hydralazine, procainamide and isoniazid. The findings at autopsy are, as expected, quite variable and usually correspond to the patient's signs and symptoms [2].

8.2.3 Rheumatoid Arthritis

Rheumatoid arthritis (RA) occurs in 1% of the population and is the most common autoimmune disease. Most patients with rheumatoid arthritis are women, and the usual age of onset is in the 5th decade. The etiology of RA is unknown. It is associated with a conserved sequence in the hypervariable region of the HLA gene called the shared epitope. RA is characterized by an inflammatory synovitis containing lymphoid follicles (Allison-Gormley bodies) that produce autoantibodies. Much of the synovitis is due to CD4+ T lymphocytes and associated cytokines. Many of the autoantibodies are made to citrullinated peptides (CCPs). About 75% of patients with rheumatoid arthritis eventually produce a serum IgM antibody to the Fc portion of their own IgG antibody. This antibody is called rheumatoid factor, but it is not specific for RA. Clinical criteria for a diagnosis of RA include morning stiffness, symmetrical arthritis especially in the small joints of the hands and feet, rheumatoid nodules (a histologically specific type of necrotizing granuloma most commonly found in the dermis at pressure points), and characteristic radiographs with periarticular bony erosions and ulnar deviation of the hand (figure 8.4). Rheumatoid arthritis may be treated with steroids, methotrexate, and tumor necrosis factor (TNF) antagonists (e.g. infliximab and adalimumab) [3,4].

8.3 Medical History

8.3.1 Systemic lupus erythematosus

Moritz Kaposi (1837 – 1902, figure 8.5) was born in Koposavar, Hungary. He became a student (and son-in-law) of the great dermatologist Ferdinand von Hebra at the University of Vienna. Kaposi described the systemic signs of SLE in 1872. He also described and named discoid lupus of the skin. The name SLE was coined by William Osler (1849 – 1919). Osler was born in Bond Head, Ontario and received his degree from McGill University in Montreal. He was one of the principle founding faculty of the Johns Hopkins Hospital, sometimes called the Hopkins four (William Osler in medicine, William Welch in pathology, Howard Kelly in gynecology and William Halstead in surgery). Osler observed 24 SLE patients from 1894 to 1903. According to Mallavarapu and Grimsley, only two of these patients clearly had SLE and these included a 15- year-old girl with a photosensitive malar rash, joint pain, pleuritis, fever and nephritis. In 1948, Malcolm Hargraves took serum from patients with SLE and added it to bone marrow from normal subjects. This led to the formation of neutrophils that had phagocytized amorphous masses of nuclear material, called LE cells. These cells may be seen in vivo in cytology specimens from body cavity fluid [5,6].

8.3.2 Rheumatoid arthritis

There is evidence of arthritis, inflammation of the joints, in writings from Egypt in 1500 BC. Arthritis is also mentioned in the writings of Hippocrates. Thomas Sydenham (1624 – 1689) commented that "gout attacks women but rarely" and that when you have the symptoms of gout in slender females, they are either the symptoms of hysteria or rheumatism. The latter could be treated with a julep made from water-lily water, purslane water, lettuce water, syrup of lemon, and syrup of violets. Emil Vidal (1825 – 1893) published "Considerations on Chronic Primary Articular Rheumatism" in 1855 in which he described the higher incidence in women, ulnar deviation, fixation in flexion, skin changes, and atrophy of the digits. He termed the disease the atrophic type of chronic articular rheumatism. A. B. Garrod (1819 – 1909) proposed the name rheumatoid arthritis in 1858. The name was proposed to replace arthritis deformans and rheumatic gout, so he was drawing a distinction among forms of arthritis that had not often been made previously [6-8].

8.4 Laboratory Medicine

8.4.1 Serological tests for SLE and Rheumatoid arthritis

The most sensitive test for SLE is the general test for antinuclear antibodies which is found in 95% of SLE patients, but the test is not specific and as many as 15% of normal people older than 65 years are ANA positive. The double-stranded DNA antibody and Sm (Smith) antibody are specific for SLE, but they are only present in 20 - 60% of patients. Other antibodies in SLE patients include U1-RNP, SS-A and SS-B nucleoproteins, and anti-phospholipid.

Rheumatoid factor is present in 60 – 70% of patients with rheumatoid arthritis, but it is non-specific. Examples of other disorders that may have positive rheumatoid factor are SLE, granulomatous inflammation, tuberculosis, viral hepatitis and carcinomas.

Cyclic citrullinated peptides (CCP) are much more specific for RA, but they are also only present in 60 – 80% of patients [3].

8.5 Study questions

1. Since a general antinuclear antibody test is sensitive for the detection of SLE, but not specific, what would be the result of using it as a screening test on normal patients?

2. Moritz Kaposi and his father-in-law Ferdinand von Hebra worked at the Allgemeines Krankenhaus in Vienna. This is one of the most famous hospitals

in the world and in the 19th century its faculty included many great figures in the history of Medicine. Can you name any of them?

3. How would you design an experiment to see if a julep containing water-lily water was an effective treatment for rheumatoid arthritis?

4. Why is the determination of an arthritic patient's rheumatoid factor insufficient to make a diagnosis of rheumatoid arthritis?

5. There are various drugs used to treat rheumatoid arthritis. What are the advantages and disadvantages of steroids, methotrexate, and the anti-tissue necrosis factor agents?

8.6 References

1. American College of Rheumatology. 2010 RA Classification - Tree. 2010. http://www.rheumatology.org/ACR/practice/clinical/classification/ra/ratree_2010.asp. Accessed 2015.
2. Kumar V, Abbas AK, Aster JC. Robbins and Cotran Pathologic basis of disease. Philadelphia: Elsevier Saunders; 2015
3. Jonas BL, Roubey RAS. Rheumatoid Arthritis. In: Runge MS, Greganti MA, editor. Netter's internal medicine. Philadelphia: Saunders Elsevier; 2009. p. 1079 - 1084.
4. Horvai A. Bone, joints, and soft tissue tumors. In: Kumar V, Abbas AK, Aster JC, editors. Robbins and Cotran Pathologic basis of disease. Philadelphia: Elsevier Saunders; 2015. p. 1209 - 1212.
5. Mallavarapu RK, Grimsley EW. The history of lupus erythematosus. South Med J. 2007;100:896 - 898.
6. Talbott JH. A biographical history of medicine: excerpts and essays on the men and their work. New York: Grune & Stratton; 1970:1211.
7. Mandal A. Rheumatoid arthritis history. 2015. http://www.news-medical.net/health/Rheumatoid-Arthritis-History.aspx. Accessed 2015.

8. Sydenham T. A Treatise on Gout and Dropsy. The works of Thomas Sydenham. London: The Sydenham Society; 1848. p. 245.

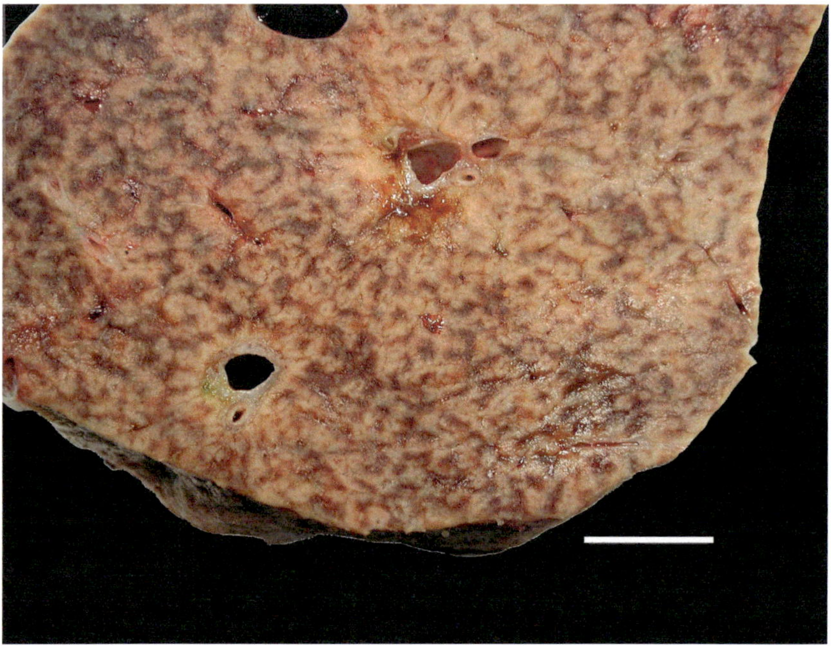

Figure 8.1 Hepatic congestion. The liver is our largest internal organ. It is a highly vascular organ that serves to chemically process our food, store glycogen, manufacture bile, and to detoxify native and foreign toxins (like ethanol). In some circumstances, e.g. right heart failure, the blood can back up into the liver making it congested. Congested liver has a characteristic gross appearance shown here, called nutmeg liver. This image is from a different case than the one described in this chapter's case. The white bar is 1 cm long.

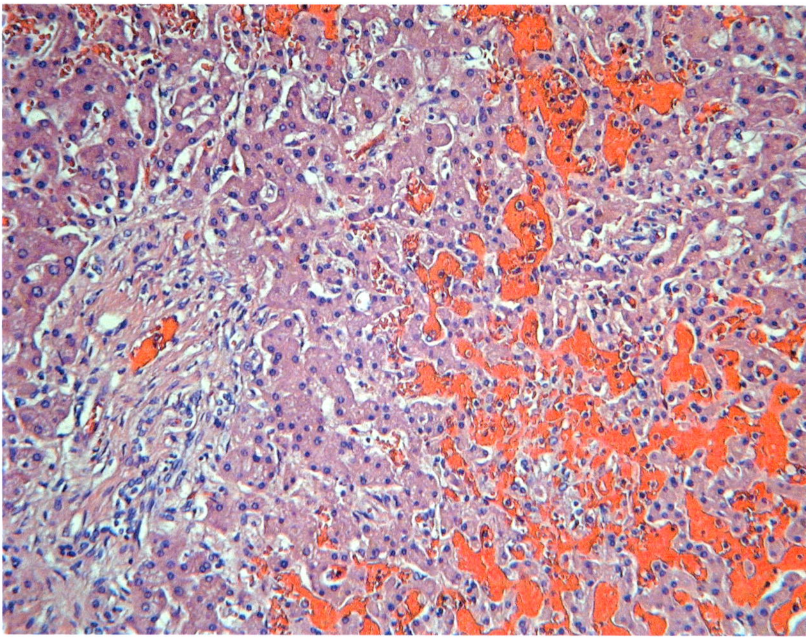

Figure 8.2 Hepatic congestion. This histologic section of the patient's liver shown in figure 7.1 shows that the reddish-brown bands seen grossly are due to red blood cells distending the hepatic sinusoids. (Original magnification x200, H&E stain)

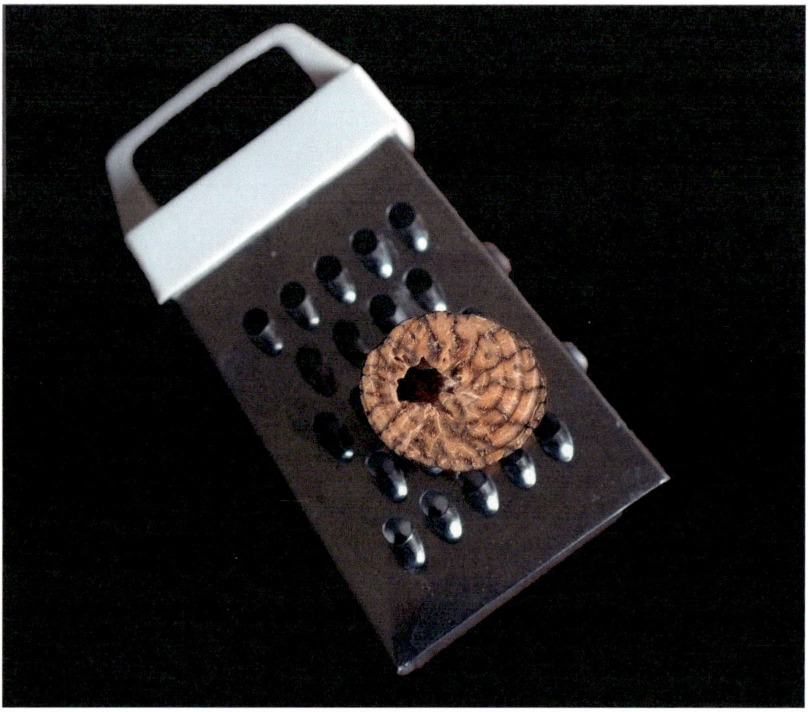

Figure 8.3 When I was in training, I asked why nutmeg liver had its name. I was told that the liver looked as if nutmeg had been sprinkled on it, but if we look at the nutmeg seed itself, we see the striking similarity between it and a congested liver. The nutmeg tree also produces the spice called mace.

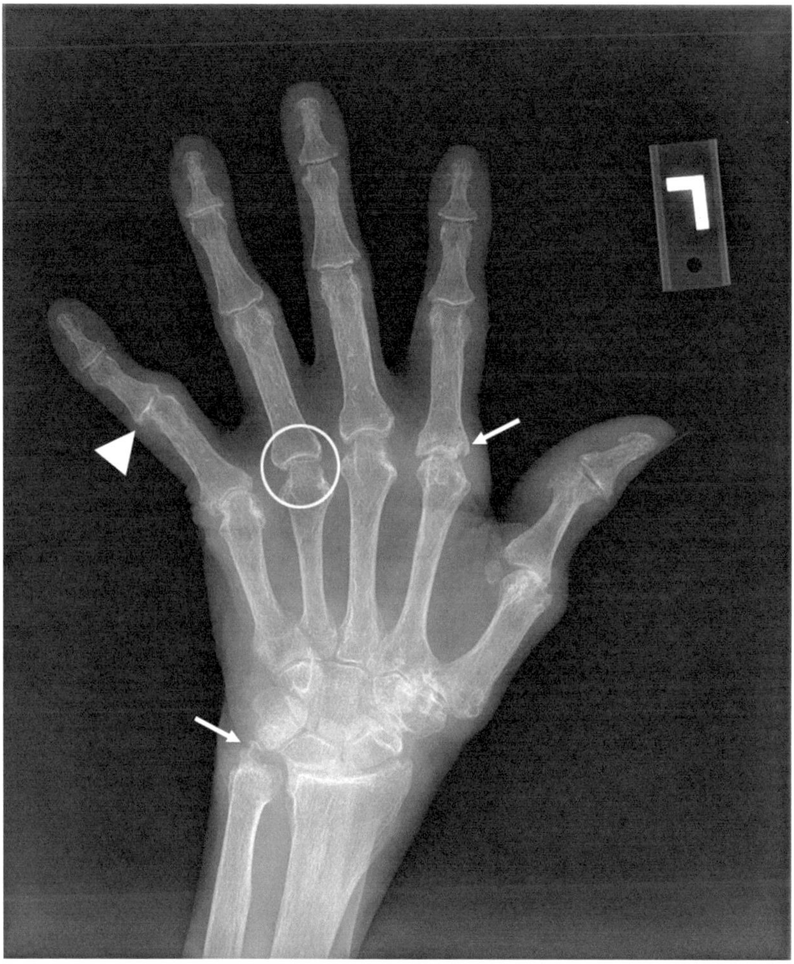

Figure 8.4 A single AP projection of the left hand from a different patient demonstrating multiple marginal erosions at the joint spaces (arrows) compatible with rheumatoid arthritis. The circle surrounds a normal appearing joint. Notice the ulnar subluxation of the interphalangeal joint of the 5th digit, another feature suggestive of rheumatoid arthritis (arrow head).

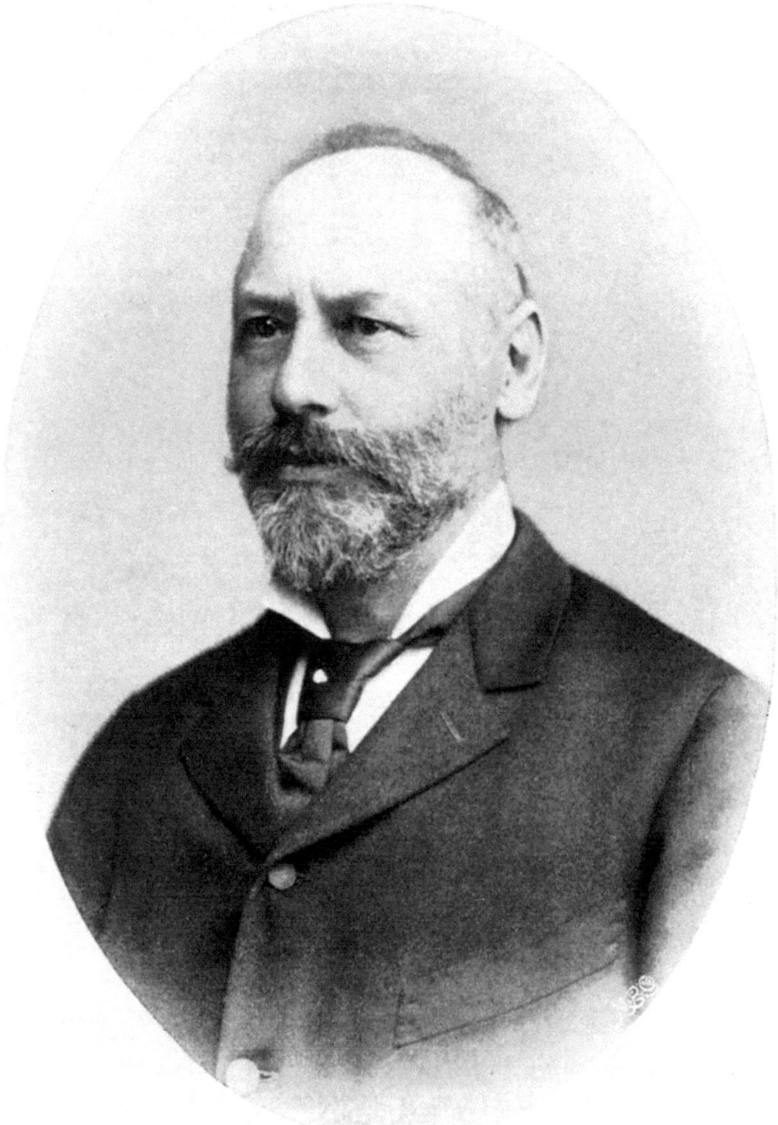

Figure 8.5 Moritz Kaposi (1837 – 1902). Courtesy of the National Library of Medicine.

CHAPTER 9

A middle-aged man with dyspnea on exertion who died suddenly on the second hospital day. (ViNdicate, vascular, neoplastic)

"And generally let every student of nature take this as a rule that whatever his mind seizes and dwells upon with peculiar satisfaction is to be held in suspicion."
Francis Bacon (1561 – 1626)

9.1 The Autopsy

9.1.1 Case history.

The patient was a 65-year-old man with a history of hypertension and hyperlipidemia. He smoked 1 pack of cigarettes a day from age 20 to age 50. He had a recent normal cardiac stress test. The patient had a one-month history of dyspnea on exertion and was admitted to the hospital. He was hypoxic and treated with oxygen by nasal cannulae. He was afebrile but had leukocytosis (16,900 leukocytes/cubic mm). He had a mild anemia and his peripheral smear had features of microangiopathic hemolytic anemia (i.e. the red blood cells looked traumatized as if they had passed through a narrow space with a rough surface) with some nucleated red cells. The patient had thrombocytopenia (69,000 platelets/cubic mm). Cardiac ultrasound showed pulmonary hypertension with tricuspid regurgitation and normal left ventricular systolic function. A CT angiogram showed no pulmonary embolus. There was mild emphysema. Ultrasound of the abdomen showed hepatic steatosis and renal cysts only. The patient had low fibrinogen and was thought to have disseminated intravascular coagulation (DIC). Occult carcinoma, idiopathic thrombocytopenic purpura (ITP) and thrombotic thrombocytopenic purpura (TTP) were considered. The patient became dizzy using the bathroom and had cardiac arrest on hospital day 2.

9.1.2 Postmortem findings

Postmortem examination showed massive para-aortic abdominal lymphadenopathy and no other grossly identifiable primary tumor (figure 9.1). On the patient's provisional anatomic diagnoses, before the use of the microscope, I opined that he had a malignant lymphoma, but histologic sections showed metastatic papillary adenocarcinoma in the enlarged lymph nodes and in pulmonary arterioles and capillaries. The pleural surface of the lung showed lymphangitic tumor (figure 9.2). Some arterioles had an intraluminal desmoplastic response with near total luminal obstruction (figure 9.3). This appearance has been termed pulmonary tumor thrombotic microangiopathy. Some tumor cells had intracellular mucin, a feature of adenocarcinoma (figure 9.4).

9.1.3 Case summary

The previous autopsies that we've discussed were chosen to show relatively common, or if not common, classic examples of disease. This case is different and represents both an unusual disorder and a case in which some basic questions could not be answered after the autopsy.

The big question is, where did the patient's tumor come from? One of the properties of malignant tumors is that they metastasize to other locations in the body. The location that the tumor originates from is called the primary site, and the locations that the tumor metastasizes to are called secondary sites. The tumor's actions on the body may be due to the location to which they have metastasized. In this case, the tumor was filling blood and lymphatic vessels in the lungs. This prevented oxygenation of blood, it increased the blood pressure through the lungs, it altered the function of the right side of the heart, it damaged the patient's red blood cells, and it consumed fibrinogen and platelets in his blood. With this pattern of tumor metastasis, this might happen no matter where the tumor was originally from, but we want to know the primary site for several reasons. Certain tumors are more common in some people than others. Was this tumor a common one or an uncommon one? Was this a tumor that has a known cause? Was this a tumor that has a genetic component and should the patient's living relatives be screened for it?

Malignant tumors can be divided into a few large categories. Sarcomas arise in soft tissue and bone and they often metastasize to the lungs. Carcinomas arise from epithelial cells, the constituent cells of organs and the lining cells of the skin and gastrointestinal tract, and they often metastasize to lymph nodes, the liver, the lungs, and the brain. Leukemias and lymphomas arise from blood cells or lymphocytes. There are some tumors that don't fit into these categories. Examples are malignant melanoma that arises from specialized cells in the skin and the pheochromocytoma discussed in chapter #7. The most common malignant tumors in adults in the United States are carcinomas of the lung, the breast, the colon and the prostate gland. These tumors account for about 700,000 new cancer cases in the US each year [1]. This patient only had tumor in large intra-abdominal para-aortic lymph nodes identifiable grossly at autopsy. Consequently, I originally suspected that he had a malignant lymphoma, but it was clear under the microscope that the patient had a carcinoma. It was a carcinoma that made mucin and that grew in a papillary pattern. The patient was a man, so carcinoma of the breast would be unusual (the incidence of breast cancer in men is 1/100 the incidence in women), but carcinoma of the prostate gland was a consideration. The patient's prostate gland was grossly enlarged, as it is likely to be in an elderly man, but multiple sections showed no tumor. Prostate cancer does not usually metastasize to the lung, it prefers to go to the pleura, and prostate cancer does not usually make mucin like the mucin seen in this case.

The next step was the use of some special diagnostic stains to try to determine the site of origin of this tumor. First, a brief introduction to these immunohistochemical stains.

Vertebrates have evolved the ability for their lymphocytes to produce special proteins as part of their immune system called antibodies. Antibodies are assembled from protein chains that together make a Y-shaped structure. The "top" ends of the Y have highly variable amino acid constituents so that the body is able to produce many kinds of antibodies that bind to many kinds of antigens. In this way as, for example, microorganisms evolve to penetrate our defenses we can produce antibodies that bind to them and permit their destruction. Even before people knew what antibodies were, they were using them for diagnostic purposes as "antisera". Many laboratory tests now use specifically manufactured antibodies using laboratory animals or modified microorganisms in culture. Pathologists began using antibodies linked to a colored reagent to make stains specific for certain cell elements in the 1980s. Today there are thousands of these stains.

The stains that I used when this autopsy was performed included prostate specific antigen (PSA, which preferentially stains prostate gland epithelium), gross cyst disease fluid protein-15 (GCDFP-15 or BRST-2, which stains some breast carcinomas), estrogen receptor (ER, which stains some breast carcinomas), thyroid transcription factor-1(TTF1, which stains some tumors of the lung and thyroid gland), cytokeratin 7 (CK7, which stains some types of carcinoma), cytokeratin 20 (CK20, which stains some types of carcinoma) and CDX-2 (which preferentially stains carcinomas originating in the gastrointestinal tract).

The tumor did not stain for TTF-1 making primary carcinoma of the lung unlikely. It did not stain for estrogen receptor and it did not stain for CDX-2. These antibodies are used to help identify tumors of the breast and the GI tract. The tumor stained for CK7 and was negative for CK20, but this is a common pattern of cytokeratin staining in carcinomas from many different primary sites. The tumor was focally positive for PSA and BRST-2. PSA is relatively specific for prostate cancer, but for the reasons mentioned above, I thought that we had eliminated prostate cancer as a possibility. BRST-2 stains some carcinomas of the breast, and it may stain some unusual tumors such as carcinomas arising from the sweat glands in the skin. Some carcinomas of the breast may be PSA positive. So, I was left with the question whether this patient had a very rare primary carcinoma of the breast that did not make a significant sized tumor and that metastasized in a very rare pattern. By the time that I had the information listed here, the funeral director had already removed the patient's remains, and I could not re-examine the patient's breasts, so this case will remain at least a partial mystery. Since this case was done, an antibody called GATTA3 has become available that preferentially stains carcinomas of the breast; it might be useful if this case is reviewed.

9.2 Discussion

9.2.1 Pulmonary tumor thrombotic microangiopathy

Pulmonary tumor thrombotic microangiopathy (PTTM) is a rare presentation of metastatic carcinoma where the tumor grows in an extensive intravascular pattern in the lungs and incites a reactive fibroplasia in the vessels that further obstructs the pulmonary vascular tree. PTTM is often confused with other diagnoses clinically and the diagnosis is often only made at autopsy. PTTM may mimic pneumonia, a pulmonary thromboembolus, and idiopathic pulmonary hypertension. In a review of 630 consecutive autopsies at the University of Heidelberg 19 cases of PTTM from carcinoma were found [2]. Of these, 11 had metastatic gastric carcinoma. Others have mentioned cases of carcinoma of the breast, choriocarcinoma, and hepatocellular carcinoma [3].

9.2.2 Carcinoma of the breast

Carcinoma of the breast is the leading cause of cancer death in women worldwide. It accounted for 14% of all new cancer cases and 7% of cancer deaths in 2015. About 12% of women will be diagnosed with breast cancer in their lifetime. The incidence is relatively high in the US and northern Europe and low in Asia and Africa. There are multiple known risk factors for the development of carcinoma of the breast. The most important is patient age. Two-thirds of cases occur in postmenopausal women. Other risk factors include family history, nulliparity, and proliferative fibrocystic changes. Familial breast cancer accounts for 5 – 10% of cases. Most familial cases have a mutation in the BRCA1 (chromosome 17q21) or BRCA2 (chromosome 13q12.3) genes. Women with these mutations have a 70 – 80% lifetime risk of carcinoma and an increased risk of premenopausal and bilateral disease. Invasive breast cancer presents as a painless firm mass or as a radiographic abnormality. Only 60% of the tumors detected by mammography are palpable. Mammography permits the detection of very small tumors by the detection of characteristic patterns of calcification, architectural distortion, or asymmetrical density. The incidence of calcification in breast cancer is 50 – 60%, but benign lesions calcify 20% of the time. Only 20% of mammographically suspicious lesions turn out to be malignant and 20% of palpable carcinomas are not detectable by mammography.

Hubert and Wainer point out that, "In the US about 180,000 women are found to have breast cancer each year from among the 33.5 million women who annually have a mammogram. Thus, the probability of [carcinoma] is about 180,000/33,500,000 = .0054. So, given a positive mammogram the probability of carcinoma (predictive value of a positive result) is 0.0049. "[4]

The prognosis of a patient with breast cancer has been related to many different factors. Rosai lists 46 different prognostic indicators! [7] For the purposes of this discussion, I will note hormone receptors and the epidermal growth factor HER-2 (also referred to by its gene's name c-erbB-2). The presence or absence of estrogen receptors (ER) on a patient's tumor cells is the single most important prognostic marker and predictor of response to therapy.

Progesterone receptor is also measured in breast cancer patients, but it is a weaker predictor.

These receptors are currently measured with immunohistochemical stains. About 80% of breast cancers are ER-positive. ER positivity is more common in postmenopausal women and in tumors with a lower grade. The two most popular methods for measuring HER-2 are by immunohistochemistry, which shows the amount of the epidermal growth factor that is present on the tumor cell membranes, or by in-situ hybridization, which shows the number of HER-2 genes on chromosome 17 in the tumor cell nuclei. HER-2 is a weaker overall prognostic indicator than ER, but it is used to help determine if the patient should be treated with trastuzumab, a drug that binds to HER-2. Some patient's tumors do not stain with ER, PR or HER-2 and are often referred to as "triple negative". These tumors are more common in patients with a BRCA1 mutation and often behave in an aggressive fashion.

Starting with work reported in Nature in 2000 it has been possible to categorize breast cancers using a microarray of genetic probes [5]. This technique separates breast carcinomas into categories usually called luminal A, luminal B, HER-2 type, basal-like, and normal breast-like. There has been considerable work on the possible use of these categories for diagnosis and prognosis, perhaps one day obviating histologic examination, but currently, several problems exist. The categories do not account for many of the known types of breast cancer with special behavior, various patented microarray gene collections classify some breast tumors differently, and the categories are heterogeneous using traditional techniques. So, some HER-2 type carcinomas are HER-2 negative and some basal-like carcinomas correspond to tumors with a special histology with a known favorable prognosis, e.g. adenoid cystic carcinoma of the breast.

A technique called the sentinel lymph node became popular in the evaluation of breast cancer beginning in the early 1990s. The patient is injected with a blue dye and a radioactive marker during surgery and an attempt is made to find a single lymph node (or a small number of lymph nodes) that are the first to receive marker material from the injection site from the breast. The identified node(s) are sent to pathology for careful frozen section examination. Studies have shown that if this sentinel lymph node is negative for metastatic carcinoma, it is very likely that all the patient's axillary lymph nodes will be negative for metastases and no further lymph node dissection is necessary. On the other hand, if the sentinel lymph node is positive for metastatic carcinoma, then there is about 1 chance in 3 that additional lymph nodes will be positive, and a more traditional lymph node dissection is done at that time [6,7].

9.3 Medical History

9.3.1 Carcinoma of the breast

Carcinoma of the breast was described in antiquity. E. R. Long has a photograph of an ancient Greek votive statuette that has an apparent ulcerating tumor of the left breast. Archigenes of Apameia (c. 100 AD) described the rare occurrence of carcinoma of the breast in men. He commented on the usual futility of surgery for breast cancer and he described a salve, *medicamentum Archigenis ad cancros ulceratos*, that was still in use in the sixteenth century. "De Recondita Abscessum Natura" by Neapolitan surgeon Marco Aurelio Severino (1580 – 1656) and published in 1632 may be the first illustrated work in surgical pathology. In the chapter on tumors of the breast, Severino separated these into glandular, strumous, scirrhous, and cancerous. From his descriptions, the glandular and strumous tumors are palpable and movable tumors some of which probably correspond to what would be called a fibroadenoma today. The strumous tumors were apparently firmer and their significance was more confusing, both to Severino and the modern reader. Severino said of the strumous tumors, "So they are plainly wrong, and cannot be justified, who think that type of affection in the breast is an incurable cancer, and wish to treat it by painting on some remedy. Furthermore, since it does not adhere to the underlying flesh and is of the same color, and does not become surrounded by turgid veins, no one who is not unlearned would call it a cancer." For this reason, Servino recommended that strumous tumors be excised immediately; recall that the obviously malignant tumors were not considered resectable. Resection of breast cancer, or anything else for that matter, became a viable option in the 19th century with the invention of general anesthesia and antisepsis. A great figure in the treatment of breast cancer was William Stewart Halsted (1852 – 1922) who showed early aptitude as an athlete but was not a great scholar at Yale. Like others who experimented with cocaine at the end of the nineteenth century (e.g. Sigmund Freud), Halsted became an addict. During his recovery, he was persuaded to join the faculty at Johns Hopkins University in Baltimore. Halsted was an introspective man and was said to have spent considerable energy avoiding his patients and students. Some of his students referred to their rounds with Dr. Halsted as "shifting dullness" a pun on the sign for fluid in the abdominal cavity. Halsted's achievements were many. Besides his radical mastectomy, he was the first to introduce the use of rubber gloves during surgery; not for antisepsis, but initially because a nurse had dermatitis from exposure to the carbolic acid that was used for hand washing. Halsted's importance in surgery was so great, that as a medical student I was advised that a safe response to a question asked on rounds about who had originated a surgical procedure was always, "Halsted at the turn of the century". If the correct answer was Dr. Charles Child III (1908 – 1991) at the University of Michigan, then one looked like an idiot, but it is important to remember that questions of that sort are only asked when the attending is confident that no one knows the answer [8 – 10].

9.4 Laboratory Medicine

9.4.1 Disseminated intravascular coagulation

Disseminated intravascular coagulation (DIC) is a serious abnormality that is triggered by any one of many different diseases, which causes the release of the glycoprotein thromboplastin (tissue factor) and activates the hemostasis system. An affected patient has both thrombotic and hemorrhagic complications. Recall that blood clots formed in blood vessels during life are called thrombi and are formed through the activation of a pathway of clotting factors. The pathway is initiated by platelets that are activated and release thromboplastin that leads to the conversion of fibrinogen to fibrin in the presence of thrombin. The fibrin is cross-linked to stabilize the thrombus by factor XIIIa. Thrombi are lysed by plasmin. Fibrinolysis leads to the presence of fibrin degradation products, which are detectable in the patient's serum. Laboratory findings in acute or uncompensated DIC include low platelets, low fibrinogen, microangiopathic hemolytic anemia, decreased factor VIII, prolonged prothrombin time, prolonged partial thromboplastin time, and elevated fibrin split products and D-dimers. Depending on the underlying abnormality, fibrinogen may not be depressed, since it is an acute phase reactant and microangiopathic hemolytic anemia may not be present. Patients with hepatic necrosis may have laboratory findings mimicking DIC, but they do not have decreased factor VIII since it is released into the circulation by necrotic liver. Patients with a chronic or compensated form of DIC have more subtle laboratory findings and a diagnosis may be even more difficult to make. There are diagnostic scoring algorithms for acute and chronic DIC from the International Society of Thrombosis and Haemostasis in 2001. Points are awarded for low platelet count, prolonged PT, low fibrinogen, and elevated fibrin-degradation products. The scoring system was validated prospectively in a 2004 paper in patients in intensive care who had clinical suspicion of acute DIC [11-13].

9.5 Study Questions

1. The patient in this case had decreased fibrinogen and platelets and evidence of red cell destruction that was due to his unusual intrapulmonary metastases and the associated endovascular fibroplasia. What would be more usual causes for these laboratory results?

2. Some surgeons have asked me to perform immunohistochemical stains so that they could classify a patient's tumor into one of the molecular categories of breast cancer. Why might this be a bad idea?

3. Some patients have a sentinel lymph node biopsy that shows scant isolated tumor cells only. There is some evidence that these patients do not have a clinically significantly poorer prognosis than patients with no detectable sentinel lymph node tumor cells. How could this be?

4. What are the arguments for and against routine mammography of women who have no known risk factor for breast cancer?

5. What are the most likely metastatic sites of a typical invasive ductal carcinoma of the breast?

9.6 References

1. National Institutes of Health. Common Cancer Types. 2015. http://www.cancer.gov/cancertopics/types/. Accessed 2015.
2. von Herbay A, Illes A, Waldherr R, Otto HF. Pulmonary tumor thrombotic microangiopathy with pulmonary hypertension. Cancer. 1990;66:587-592.
3. Chakeres DW, Spiegel PK. Fatal pulmonary hypertension secondary to intravascular metastatic tumor emboli. Am J Roentgenol. 1982;139:997-1000.
4. Hubert L, Wainer H. A statistical guide for the ethically perplexed. New York: CRC press; 2013:32.
5. Perou CM, Sørlie T, Eisen MB, van de Rijn M, Jeffre SS, Rees CA, Pollack JR, Ross DT, Johnsen H, Akslen LA, Fluge O, Pergamenschiko VA, Williams C, Zhu SX, Lønning PE, Børresen-Dale AL, Brown PO, Botstein D. Molecular portraits of human breast tumours. Nature. 2000;406:747 - 752.
6. Carey LA. Breast Cancer. In: Runge MS, Greganti, MA, editor. Netter's internal medicine. Philadelphia: Saunders Elsevier; 2011. p. 572 - 577.
7. Rosai J. Rosai and Ackerman's surgical pathology. Philadelphia: Mosby Elsevier; 2011
8. Long ER. Selected readings in pathology. Springfield, Illinois: Charles C. Thomas; 1961
9. Long ER. A history of pathology. New York: Dover; 1965:199.
10. Talbott JH. A biographical history of medicine: excerpts and essays on the men and their work. New York: Grune & Stratton; 1970:1211.
11. Markel H. An Anatomy of Addiction. Sigmund Freud, William Halsted, and the Miracle Drug Cocaine. New York: Pantheon Books; 2011

12. Bakhtiari K, Meijers JC, de Jonge E, Levi M. Prospective validation of the International Society of Thrombosis and Haemostasis scoring system for disseminated intravascular coagulation. Crit Care Med. 2004;32:2416 - 2421.

13. Mammen EF. Disseminated intravascular coagulation (DIC). Clin Lab Sci. 2000;13:239-245.

14. Moll S, Key NS. Disseminated intravascular coagulation. In: Runge MS, Greganti MA, editor. Netter's internal medicine. Philadelphia: Saunders Elsevier; 2009. p. 489 - 494.

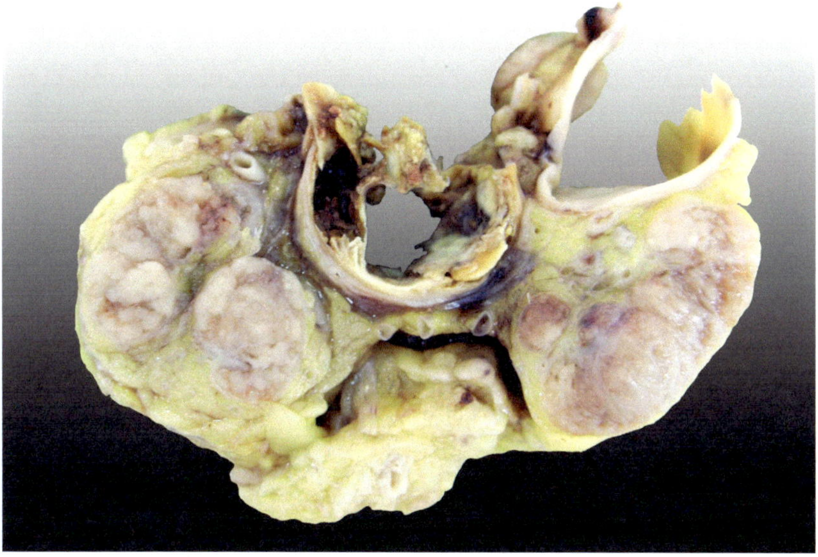

Figure 9.1 Massive para-aortic lymphadenopathy seen in cross-section. The two large vessels are the abdominal aorta and the inferior vena cava. The aorta contains some complex atherosclerotic plaque. The cut surface of a lymph node that contains lymphoma often resembles the cut surface of a scallop and does not have the irregular appearance seen here; a hint that this is not lymphoma. There is no reference scale in this image, but the aorta is about 3 cm in diameter.

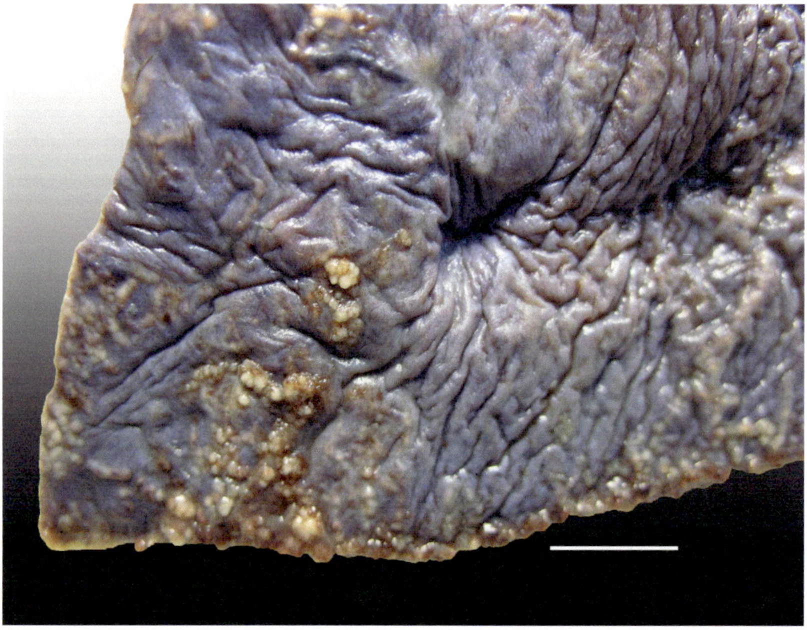

Figure 9.2 Areas of white discoloration and elevation of the pleural surface of the lung resemble worms and represent metastatic carcinoma in lymphatic vessels. The white bar is 1 cm long.

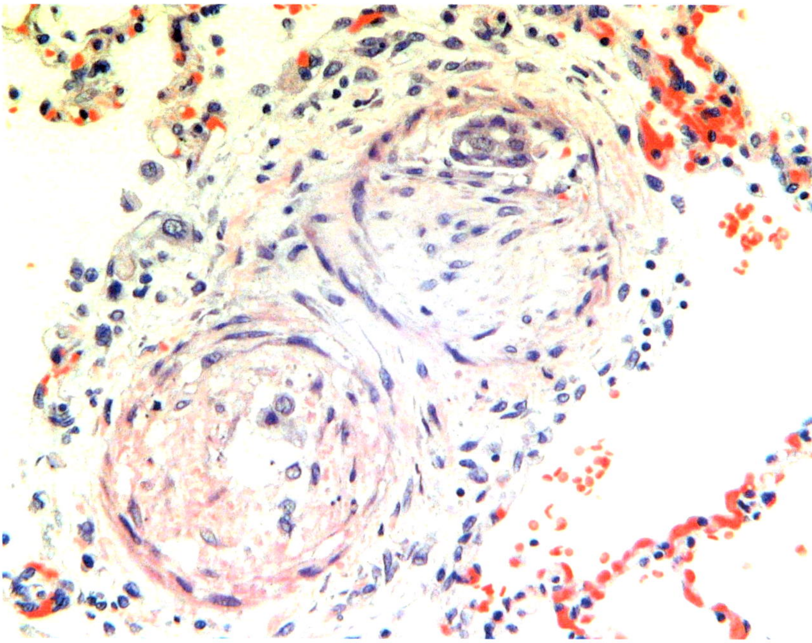

Figure 9.3 Pulmonary blood vessels containing clusters of carcinoma cells and showing intimal fibroplasia with marked narrowing of the lumen. (Original magnification, x200. H&E stain)

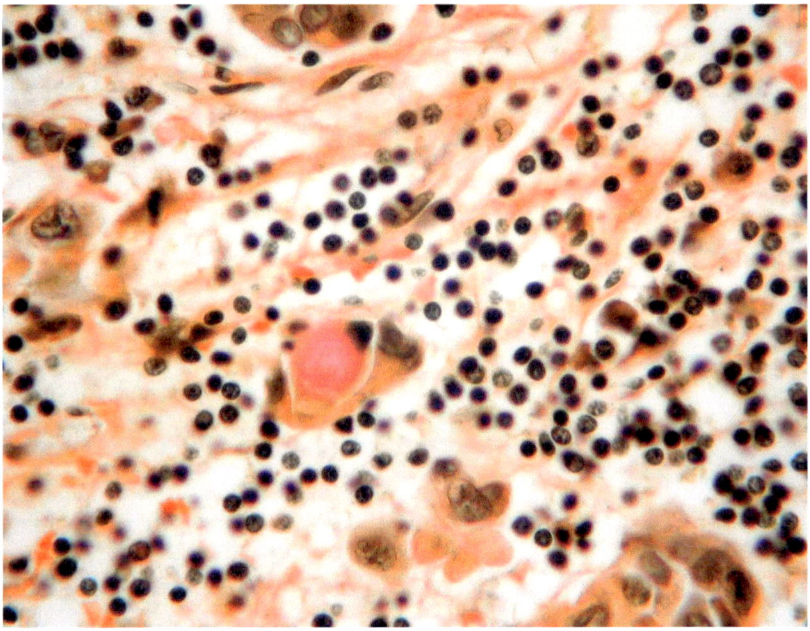

Figure 9.4 An intravascular carcinoma cell in a pulmonary blood vessel. The tumor cell has intracytoplasmic mucin that stains red. (Original magnification, x400. Mucicarmine stain)

CHAPTER 10

A middle-aged woman with hepatic cirrhosis and abdominal pain. (vINDicate, infectious, neoplastic, drug)

"You know my methods. Apply them!" Sherlock Holmes to Dr. Watson (on more than one occasion) Arthur Conan Doyle (1859 – 1930)

10.1 The Autopsy

10.1.1 Case history

The patient was a 40-year-old woman with a past medical history of hepatitis C and diabetes mellitus. She had a history of alcohol and cocaine use. The patient presented with a 3-day history of progressive abdominal pain and lethargy. She had vomiting and diarrhea. Her medications were phenytoin (anticonvulsant), glipizide (treatment for type 2 diabetes), and sertraline (antidepressant). The patient had smoked 1 pack of cigarettes per day for 25 years. She claimed that she had not used crack cocaine or ethanol for 2 months prior to admission. The patient had no fever, headache, chest pain, or dyspnea. Her blood pressure was 94/58 mm Hg. She had an ammonia of 127 (normal $<$ 50 μmol/L), AST = 321 (normal = 10 – 40 U/L), ALT = 131 (normal = 10 – 40 U/L), alkaline phosphatase = 144 (normal = 30 – 115 U/L), bilirubin = 0.8 (normal = 0 – 1.0 mg/dL), lipase = 100 (normal = 0 – 50 U/L), hemoglobin = 4.9 (normal = 12 – 16 g/dL). The patient had a BUN of 11 and creatinine of 1.8. She had an INR of 4.7 (normal = 1) and a PTT of 47 (Normal = 22.1 – 34.1 seconds). She had 45,700 white cells (normal = 4,500 – 11,000 leukocytes/cubic mm) that were 57% PMNs and 9% bands. She had metabolic acidosis with an anion gap of 20 (normal = 8 – 16). The patient was hemodynamically unstable and was admitted to the MICU. A CT scan of the abdomen showed a large intra-abdominal hemorrhage of uncertain origin. The patient was treated with packed red cells (pRBCs), fresh frozen plasma, and intravenous fluids. She was also treated with the antibiotics piperacillin/tazobactam, metronidazole, and vancomycin. She had lactic acidosis with a lactate of 20.1 (normal = 4.5 – 19.8 mg/dL). An emergency laparotomy was performed on hospital day 2. The liver was cirrhotic and an area of bleeding was identified on the inferior right hepatic lobe just medial to the gallbladder fossa. This area was cauterized and biopsied. There were 1.5 liters of blood evacuated. The patient continued to bleed after the procedure and required pressor agents to maintain her blood pressure. She received a total of 16 units of pRBCs and required increasing levels of PEEP (positive end-expiratory pressure ventilation) for ventilation. A "Do not resuscitate" order type 2 was written on hospital day 3. The patient died on the third hospital day.

10.1.2 Postmortem findings

At autopsy, the patient had micronodular cirrhosis and multicentric hepatocellular carcinoma, grade 2 with vascular invasion, and penetration through Glisson's capsule (the membrane covering the surface of the liver) near the cystic duct of the gallbladder (figures 10.1, 10.2). Other findings were moderate atherosclerosis of the middle left anterior descending coronary and splenomegaly.

10.1.3 Case Summary

The patient had hepatitis C and had a history of possible ethanol abuse. She presented with a three-day history of progressive lethargy and abdominal pain and was found to have multiple abnormal serum analytes, some indicating probable liver disease and a hemoglobin of only 4.9 grams. A sudden drop in hemoglobin from the normal range to 4.9 would be incompatible with life, but patients may have very low hemoglobin if it declined slowly over time. A CT scan showed an intra-abdominal hemorrhage and at laparotomy, the patient had cirrhosis and was bleeding from the surface of her liver. The liver biopsy, and her autopsy showed a moderate grade hepatocellular carcinoma (figure 10.5). I attributed the patient's death to intra-abdominal hemorrhage from her hepatocellular carcinoma.

10.2 Discussion

10.2.1 DNR status

Seriously ill patients in the hospital may be assigned to a DNR (do not resuscitate) category based on decisions made by their physicians, the patient's next of kin, and verbal or written instructions left by the patient him or herself in accordance with state law. Some have complained that DNR is an inappropriate name for what is being done since the point is not to deny the patient an effective therapy, but to permit a natural death when no further therapy is useful, and keeping in mind that cardiopulmonary resuscitation is often unsuccessful. There are many possible variations to a DNR order, but in general a lower level (DNR #1 in my hospital) means that the patient will not be resuscitated (i.e. no chest compression, no defibrillation, no intubation, no cardiotonic drugs), but will receive most other therapy including fluids, antibiotics, pain medication, have any bleeding controlled, receive oxygen, and so forth. A DNR #3 order is usually written in a terminally ill and unresponsive patient for whom most care is to be discontinued to allow a natural death. DNR #3 patients usually just receive pain medication and other care to ensure that they are comfortable. DNR #2 orders are complicated and somewhat problematic in reviewing a patient's chart since it usually is not clear what the expression DNR #2 by itself means exactly. These patients or their guardian or next of kin have decided, based on the patient's illness, the therapies available, and the physician's opinion that some selected therapies will be used if necessary, but cardiopulmonary resuscitation will not be done [1,2].

10.2.2 Cirrhosis

Cirrhosis is a reaction pattern in the liver to any of many different noxious stimuli. It is characterized by the formation of fibrous bands that bridge the normal hepatic architecture and the formation of regenerative nodules of liver cells. The most common causes are alcoholism, viral hepatitis, and fatty liver. The patient in the case presented here had chronic hepatitis C and was an alcoholic. The portal system is a system of blood vessels that brings the products of food digestion from capillaries in the bowel mucosa to the portal vein that carries the blood to the liver. Patients with cirrhosis have fibrous destruction of the hepatic end vessels of the portal system, so these patients develop portal hypertension. The blood in the portal system still needs to get back to the right heart and it passes through several areas of anastomosis with the systemic venous system. The most clinically important anastomotic site is in the distal esophagus. Submucosal esophageal varices form there and may rupture and lead to life-threatening gastrointestinal hemorrhage (figure 10.4). Other complications of cirrhosis include splenomegaly, ascites, coagulopathy due to the loss of the ability of the liver to manufacture the coagulation factors, liver failure, and hepatocellular carcinoma. Patients with cirrhosis may be asymptomatic for many years. Their first symptoms are often nonspecific, such as fatigue or weight loss, and patients may have signs and symptoms associated with the cause of their cirrhosis, e.g. alcoholism. As cirrhosis progresses the symptoms of the various complications mentioned above develop. Disease severity and prognosis can be categorized with the Child-Turcotte-Pugh scoring system. The patient is given points for the presence and degree of abnormality of encephalopathy, ascites, prothrombin time, serum albumin, and serum bilirubin. Diagnosis of cirrhosis may require liver biopsy, but some newer techniques are available that use an ultrasound probe on the abdomen to measure the stiffness of the liver called transient elastography, and these have become popular, especially outside the United States, for the diagnosis of cirrhosis without a biopsy. There are some reported cases of reversal of hepatic fibrosis, but, in general cirrhosis of the liver is irreversible and treatment is supportive [3-6].

10.2.3 Hepatocellular carcinoma

Hepatocellular carcinoma, also called hepatoma, is a primary malignancy of the liver. The NIH classifies it as a rare disease since it occurs in less than 1 in 2000 people in the United States, but the incidence has increased in the last few decades because of chronic hepatitis C infection. The disease is more common in sub-Saharan Africa and southeast Asia where there is both a high incidence of chronic hepatitis B infection and the possibility of exposure to aflatoxin, a powerful carcinogen produced by some Aspergillus species of fungus found in maize and sorghum. Less common risk factors are a history of exposure to thorium dioxide, congenital biliary atresia, alpha 1 antitrypsin deficiency, hemochromatosis, and tyrosinemia.

In the United States, hepatoma usually occurs in elderly adult males with hepatic cirrhosis. In Asia and sub-Saharan Africa, hepatoma is more likely to occur in younger patients and is more common in patients without cirrhosis. Patients usually present with weight loss, abdominal pain, and a right upper quadrant abdominal mass, but the signs and symptoms of hepatocellular carcinoma may be obscured by the concomitant liver disease that these patients often have. The diagnosis is usually made by ultrasound, CT scan, MRI scan, and biopsy. Hepatocellular carcinomas may grow as a single mass, as multifocal separate masses, or diffusely. Tumors with a diffuse pattern of growth, especially when infiltrating cirrhosis, may be difficult to identify radiographically. Hepatocellular carcinoma has a propensity to invade the veins in the liver. The tumor may sometimes form a long invasive tail in the portal or hepatic veins. Hepatocellular carcinoma often has characteristic vascular changes on CT scan with evidence of arterio-portal shunts and arterial phase enhancement (figures 10.3, 10.5, 10.6) [7,8].

10.3 Medical history

10.3.1 Cirrhosis

Matthew Baillie (1761 – 1823, figure 10.7) was born in Scotland, a nephew of the great surgeons and anatomists John and William Hunter. He studied Medicine with William Hunter and was bequeathed the Hunterian museum in his will. In 1770 William Hunter had built a house in Great Windmill Street, London with an amphitheater, dissecting room and museum to become his school of anatomy. Baillie worked in the dissecting room, and his careful observations were published in 1796 as "The morbid anatomy of some of the most important parts of the human body", one of the first systematic collections of morbid anatomical findings. Baillie described cirrhosis as

"Common tubercle of the liver.

One of the most common diseases in the liver…is the formation of tubercles in its substance. This disease is hardly ever met with in a young person, but frequently takes place in persons of middle or advanced age; it is likewise more common in men than women. This would seem to depend upon the habit of drinking being more common in the one sex than in the other; for this disease is most frequently found in hard drinkers…. The tubercles which are formed in this disease occupy generally the whole mass of the liver, are placed near each other, and are of a rounded shape. They give the appearance every where of irregularity to its surface. When cut into, they are found to consist of a brownish or yellowish white solid matter…When the liver is thus tuberculated, it feels much harder to the touch than natural, and not uncommonly its lower edge is bent a little forwards. Its size, however, is generally not larger than in a healthy state, and I think it is sometimes smaller.... It very frequently happens that in this state the liver is of a yellow colour, arising from the bile accumulated in its substance; and there is also water in the cavity of the abdomen.... This is the general appearance of what is commonly called a scirrhous liver...." [9]

René Théophile Hyacinthe Laennec (1781 – 1826) was born in Quimper in Brittany and was 5 years old when his mother died of tuberculosis, a disease that he would suffer from himself. He studied medicine in Paris at the Charité and his faculty included Corvisart (physician to Emperor Napoleon), Bichat, and Dupuytren. Laennec became expert in pathological anatomy but is best known for the invention of the stethoscope, which he described in 1816. In a case report that was added to the 1826 edition of his book on diseases of the chest and auscultation, Laennec described a case of cirrhosis and gave the disease its name:

"This structure was similar to a number of conditions which we call scirrhous. I would like to name it cirrhosis because of its color. Its development in the liver is one of the common causes of ascites and when cirrhosis develops, normal liver tissue is reduced and as happened in this patient, it disappears entirely; also in all of the cases, a liver which becomes cirrhotic will lose rather than increase its volume." [10]

10.4 Laboratory Medicine

10.4.1 Alpha-1 fetoprotein

Alpha-1 fetoprotein (AFP) is a glycoprotein found in normal fetal plasma. The name alpha-1 indicates the area where AFP migrates in serum protein electrophoresis. Low levels of AFP are present in normal adults. It is elevated in amniotic fluid, and so also in the plasma of pregnant women. Marked elevation of serum alpha-1 fetoprotein is usually secondary to hepatocellular carcinoma or a germ cell tumor with a yolk sac component. Moderate elevations are common in non-malignant liver diseases. AFP may be elevated in maternal serum in some types of fetal congenital abnormality, especially open neural tube defects, and it may be decreased in the first and second-trimester maternal serum in some cases of trisomy 21. An immunohistochemical stain for AFP is sometimes used in the diagnosis of hepatocellular carcinoma and yolk sac tumor.

10.5 Study Questions

1. This patient had a "DNR #2" order written in her medical record on the day before she died. DNR #2 stands for "do not resuscitate, level 2". What does it mean?

2. What is Stigler's law? Does it apply to the name "Laennec's cirrhosis"?

3. Why is hepatocellular carcinoma more likely to occur in a patient without cirrhosis in Africa than in the United States?

4. How is hepatocellular carcinoma treated?

5. Auscultation of the chest using the stethoscope was a great discovery, but it was not used widely for several years. Why?

10.6 References

1. Chen YY, Youngner SJ. "Allow natural death" is not equivalent to " do not resuscitate": a response. J Med Ethics. 2008;34:887-888.
2. Venneman SS, Narnor-Harris P, Perish M, Hamilton M. "Allow natural death" versus "do not resuscitate": three words that can change a life. J Med Ethics. 2008;34:2-6.
3. Bacon BR. Cirrhosis and its complications. In: Longo DL, Fauci ASL, CA Harrison, TR, editors. Harrison's gastroenterology and hepatology. New York: McGraw-Hill; 2013. p. 431-445.

4. Durand F, Valla D. Assessment of prognosis of cirrhosis. Semin Liver Dis. 2008;28:110-122.
5. Gómez-Domínguez E MJ, Rubio S, Moreno-Monteagudo JA, García-Buey L, Moreno-Otero, R. Transient elastography: A valid alternative to biopsy in patients with chronic liver disease. Aliment Pharmacol Ther. 2006;24:513 - 518.
6. Shaffer EA. Fibrosis and Cirrhosis. The Merck manual of diagnosis and therapy. Whitehouse Station, NJ: Merck Sharp & Dohme Corp; 2011. p. 239 - 246.
7. Theise ND. Liver and gallbladder. In: Kumar V, Abbas AK, Aster JC, editors. Robbins and Cotran Pathologic basis of disease. Philadelphia: Elsevier Saunders; 2015. p. 821 - 881.
8. Rosai J. Rosai and Ackerman's surgical pathology. Philadelphia: Mosby Elsevier; 2011
9. Baillie M. The morbid anatomy of some of the most important parts of the human body. London: J. Johnson & G. Nicol; 1793:314.
10. Talbott JH. A biographical history of medicine: excerpts and essays on the men and their work. New York: Grune & Stratton; 1970:1211.

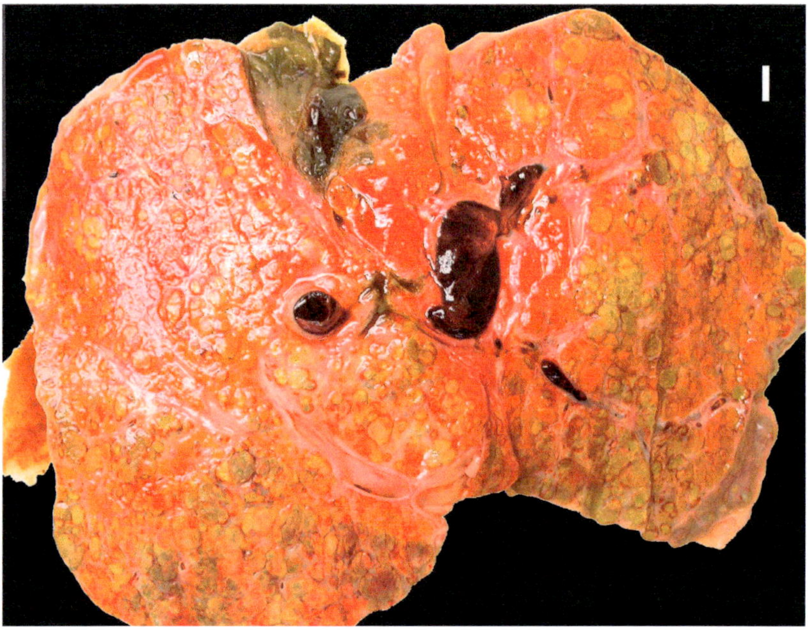

Figure 10.1 The cut surface of the liver shows cirrhosis with nodules of both normal liver and hepatocellular carcinoma, and yellow-green discoloration from bile. The gallbladder is green at the edge of the specimen at about 11 o'clock. Directly beneath the gallbladder in the center of the specimen is a tumor thrombus distending a blood vessel. The white bar is 1 cm long

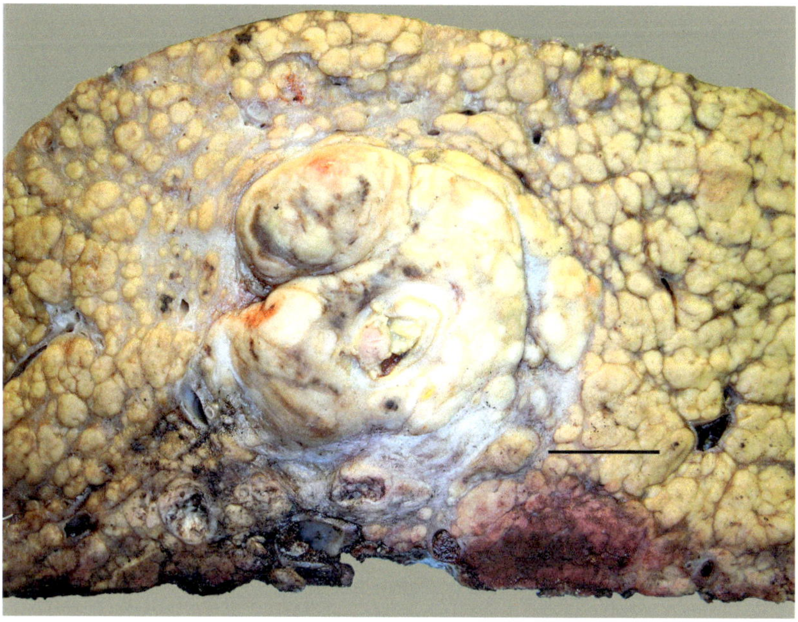

Figure 10.2 A different case of hepatocellular carcinoma arising in cirrhosis of the liver. The white mass in the center of the specimen is the tumor. This specimen has black ink on its lower surface indicating that it was a surgical specimen. The black bar is 1 cm long.

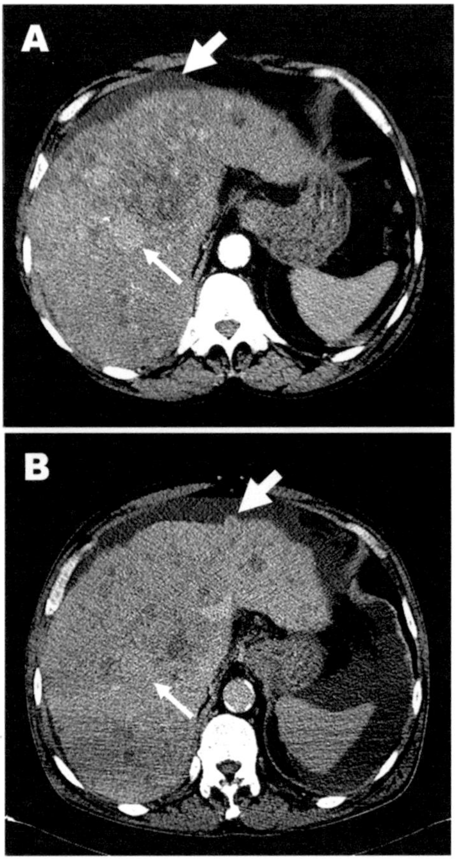

Figure 10.3.A An axial contrast enhanced CT in the arterial phase from a different patient demonstrates heterogeneous enhancement of the liver parenchyma with multiple hyper-enhancing nodular lesions and a dominant round enhancing lesion (small arrow). Additionally, there is ascites surrounding the liver (large arrow).

Figure 10.3.B The axial contrast enhanced CT in the venous phase shows a cirrhotic liver with a nodular liver contour (large arrow) and surrounding ascites. There is decreased enhancement (washout) of the previously enhancing lesions in image 10.3.A (small arrow) that is highly suspicious for hepatocellular carcinoma in the background of cirrhosis.

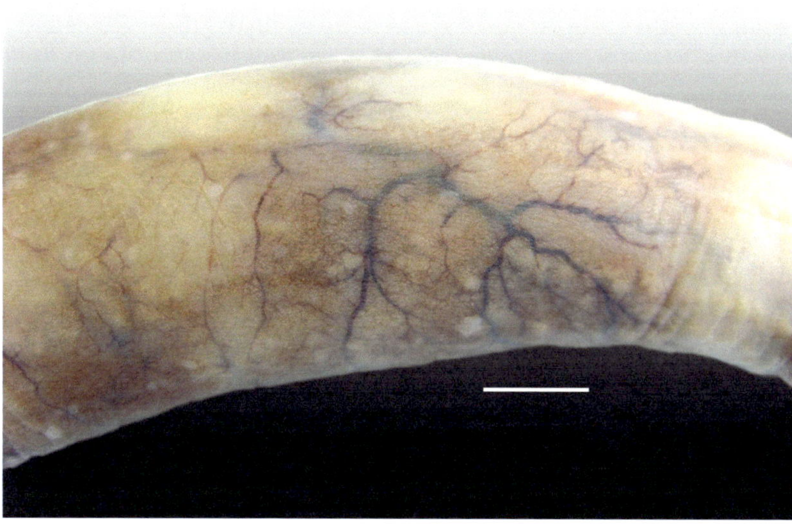

Figure 10.4 Esophageal varices at the gastroesophageal junction may be difficult to detect postmortem when there is no blood pressure distending them. For this reason, the esophagus is sometimes opened inside-out at autopsy through an incision in the stomach trapping blood in the varices. This picture is of such a specimen. The blue varicose veins are now clearly visible. The white bar is 1 cm long.

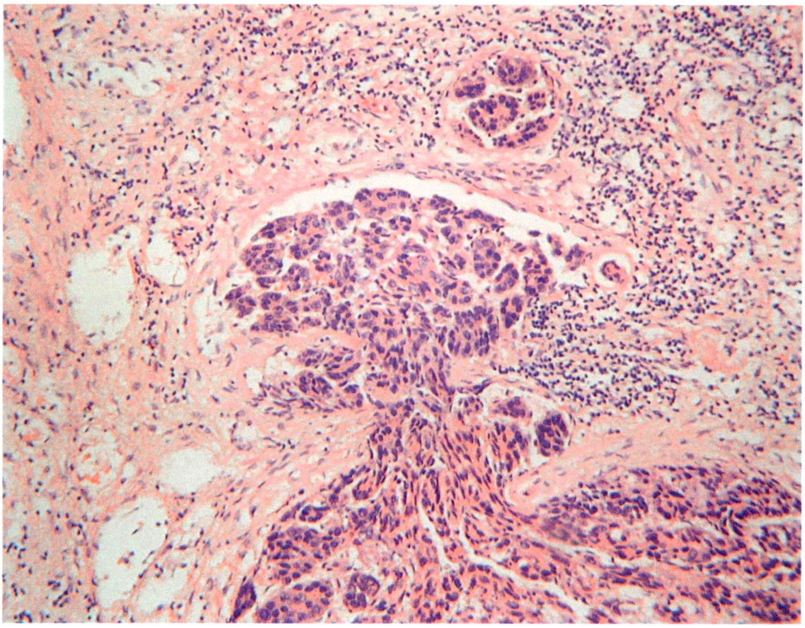

Figure 10.5 Relatively well-differentiated (low grade) hepatocellular carcinoma invading into a blood vessel in the liver. (Original magnification, x100. H&E stain).

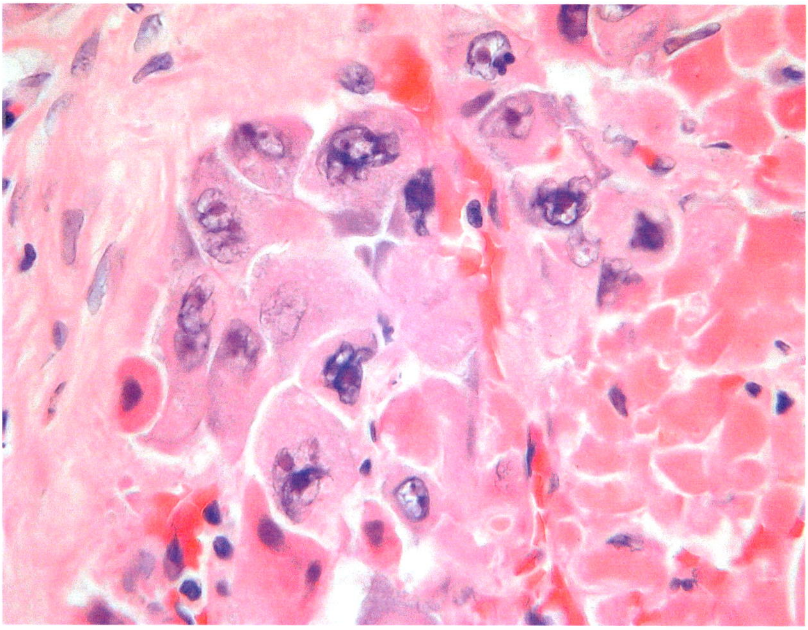

Figure 10.6 An area of poorly differentiated (high grade) hepatocellular carcinoma. The pink cells on the right side of the image are necrotic tumor cells. The tumor cells show increased size, haphazard cell to cell organization, very large purple nucleoli, and some cells have more than one nucleus. (Original magnification, x400. H&E stain).

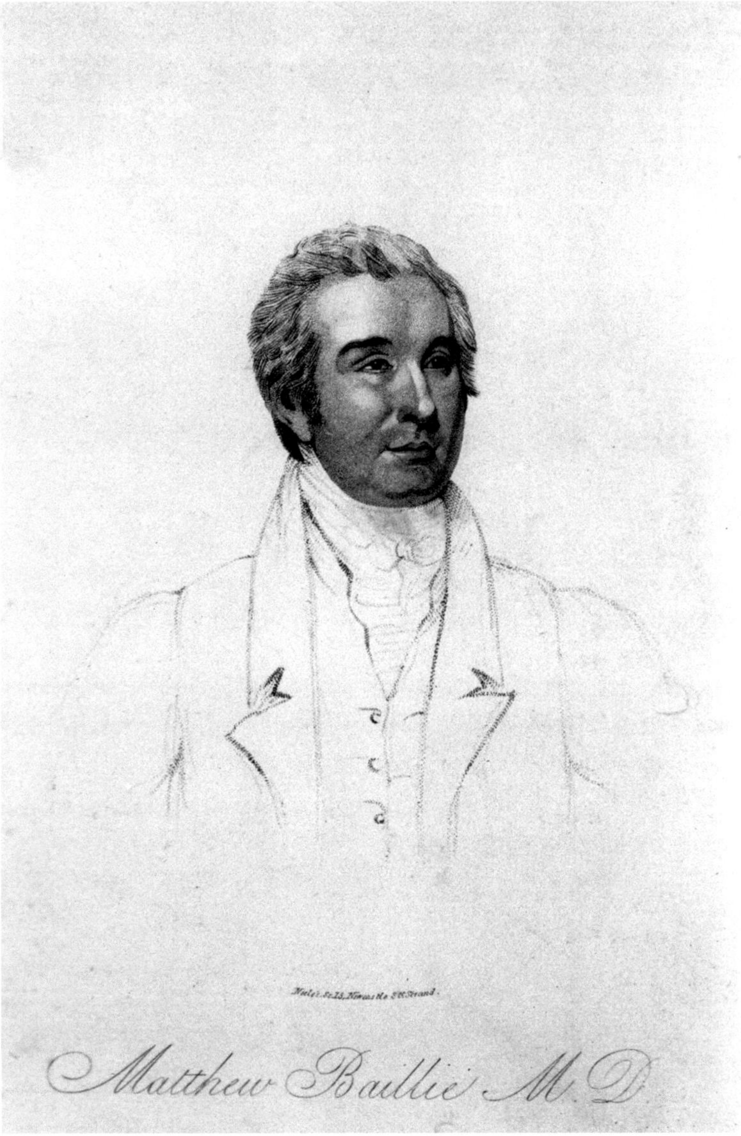

Figure 10.7 Matthew Baillie (1761 – 1823). Courtesy of the National Library of Medicine.

CHAPTER 11

Stillborn twenty-week-old twin males with discordant body weights. (vindiCate, congenital)

"Thus we can see that these authors had worked out their conclusions far better than their arguments." The Universal History of Numbers. Georges Ifrah (1947 –) [1]

11.1 The Autopsy

11.1.1 Case history

A 25-year-old G1P0 (i.e. it was her first pregnancy and she had never given birth) woman presented with vaginal spotting at about 20 weeks gestation. Fetal ultrasound two weeks earlier had shown a monochorionic diamniotic twin pregnancy. Ultrasound detected a 15% discordance between the twins' weights, abnormalities in the flow of blood in their umbilical arteries, and polyhydramnios (increased amniotic fluid) on one side and oligohydramnios (decreased amniotic fluid) on the other side. A diagnosis of twin-twin transfusion syndrome had been made. Ultrasound at the time of presentation showed intrauterine fetal death and the stillborn twin fetuses were delivered.

11.1.2 Postmortem findings

Twin #1 was a 236-gram male fetus. Twin #2 was a 310-gram male fetus. Weights and measures in table 11.1 show that Twin #1 was slightly shorter than his brother, but his organ weights were significantly smaller. Notice that while the brain weights were roughly similar, Twin #2's liver was twice as large as that of Twin #1. This is also reflected in the ratio of the brain to liver weight.

Examination of the placenta is one of the most important parts of a fetal autopsy since the placenta is the organ that supplies the fetus with its nutrition. Only placental fragments were received in this case, but one of the umbilical cords was narrower than the other. Further examination of the two fetuses showed that Twin #2, the larger fetus, had plethoric features including hemorrhagic ascites, leptomeningeal congestion, subarachnoid hemorrhage, and plethoric viscera. Histologic examination of the lungs of Twin #1, the smaller fetus, contained intra-alveolar squamous cells.

11.1.3 Case summary

A fetus this age will normally have a brain to liver weight ratio near 3, but the smaller twin had a ratio of 5. When a fetus is deprived of normal nutrition, physiological mechanisms will try to preserve the brain. Consequently, the liver suffers relative to the brain, and the brain to liver weight ratio is a measure of intrauterine growth restriction. A fetus in utero is floating in and "breathing" amniotic fluid, but its oxygen and nutrition come through its umbilical cord. If there is a so-called "asphyxial event", e.g. the umbilical cord is wrapped around the fetal neck, or the placenta is partially infarcted, then the fetus has a choking response, even though it is not really breathing yet. This reaction causes some fetal skin cells that are floating in the amniotic fluid to become lodged in the lung's air sacs (alveoli) where they are visible under the microscope at autopsy.

There was extensive evidence for the twin-twin transfusion syndrome in this case, and I considered that to be the cause of death. Evidence included that the stillborns were monochorionic twins and so could have vascular anastomoses between their circulations, the history of oligohydramnios in one fetus and polyhydramnios in his twin, the discordant weights and measures between the two twins (especially the discordant brain to liver weight ratios), the observation that one umbilical cord was narrower than the other, the relative plethora or congestion of the larger twin, and the histologic evidence of asphyxia in the smaller twin.

11.2 Discussion

11.2.1 Twin-Twin Transfusion Syndrome

Twins may be monozygotic, forming from a single ovum, or dizygotic forming from two separate ova. Monozygotic twins are so-called identical twins and dizygotic twins are termed fraternal twins. Monozygotic twins may have a monochorionic placenta or a dichorionic placenta. Monochorionic twins have a placenta that formed when fetal tissue split between 4 and 13 days after fertilization. Dichorionic twins have a placenta that formed when fetal tissue split before 4 days after fertilization. Both types of twins may be together in a single amniotic sac, monoamniotic, or each in their own separate amniotic sac, diamniotic twins. About 75% of identical twins are monochorionic and all monochorionic placentas occur in monozygotic twins. Monochorionic twins have connections between some of their placental blood vessels, and in about 15% of cases, there is unbalanced blood flow through these anastomoses leading to the twin-twin transfusion syndrome (TTTS, figures 11.1, 11.2). The underlying etiology is unknown. The syndrome is characterized by oligohydramnios on the side of the twin who is the relative transfusion donor and polyhydramnios on the side of the twin who is the relative transfusion recipient. As the disorder progresses the donor fetus becomes relatively smaller, the recipient fetus becomes plethoric and may develop heart failure with secondary total body edema (hydrops fetalis). These abnormalities have been put into a staging system with stage I being oligohydramnios and stage V being the death of one of the twins [2]. The mortality of TTTS is between 60 and 100%. Treatment has included serial reduction amniocentesis, amniotic septostomy, and laser or radiofrequency ablation of vascular anastomoses. The risk of TTTS is increased in twins with a velamentous cord insertion (the umbilical cord enters the surface of the placenta through the fetal membranes) and in twins that only have a single umbilical cord artery [2,3].

11.3 Medical history

11.3.1 Twin-twin transfusion syndrome

Vascular anastomoses were identified in placentas as early as the 17th century by several different anatomists and there is evidence that discordant twins, possibly representing twin-twin transfusion syndrome, were known in antiquity. Christian Friedrich Schatz (1841 – 1920, figure 11.3), a German gynecologist, described a case of typical twin-twin transfusion syndrome in 1886 and determined that it was due to placental vascular anastomoses between the two twin circulations by injecting a colored solution into the vessels. He called the portion of the circulation that was shared by the two fetuses the "third circulation". This finding agreed with the work of other placentologists of the 19th century including the Austrian anatomist Josef Hyrtl (1810 – 1894) who had published a study of placental vascular anatomy 16 years earlier. The twins that Schatz described had marked edema and a distended bladder in one twin and the other showed marked atrophy. He deduced that the larger twin had polyhydramnios from excessive urination [4].

11.4 Laboratory medicine

11.4.1 Laboratory evaluation of the fetus

Historically, almost completely protected from laboratory testing, the fetus in utero can now have specimens evaluated in the laboratory using several different techniques. Umbilical cordocentesis or ultrasound guided percutaneous blood sampling are used to sample fetal blood. Even tiny fetal blood specimens may represent a relatively significant blood loss and complications of the procedure range from bradycardia in 3 – 11% and fetal death in 1 – 6% of cases. There has also been some difficulty in establishing normal ranges for analytes measured because of the dearth of normal specimens available. Another problem in the analysis of these specimens is ensuring that they come from the fetus and not the mother. Techniques for distinguishing between fetal and maternal blood include the Kleihauer-Betke test in which weak acid elutes fetal hemoglobin (HbF) but not maternal hemoglobin (HbA), the fact that the mean corpuscular volume (MCV) is higher in fetal red blood cells, and the use of flow cytometry using an antibody to HbF. Most recently tests have been developed to identify cell-free fetal DNA in the maternal circulation. This fetal DNA can be used to identify fetal sex and chromosomal abnormalities. Some ethical considerations have been raised because a simple maternal phlebotomy specimen could theoretically be used for non-clinical applications such as determining fetal sex and fetal paternity [5].

11.5 Study questions

1. What is the most common cause of fetal intrauterine growth restriction (formerly called fetal growth retardation)?

2. What are the causes of fetal intrauterine growth restriction occurring in only one twin? In other words, what is the differential diagnosis for findings suggesting twin-twin transfusion syndrome?

3. Why is the brain to liver weight ratio elevated in a fetus with placental insufficiency?

4. Some maternal phlebotomy specimens to detect fetal DNA have unexpectedly contained aneuploid cells of maternal origin. Where might these cells be coming from?

5. Why is there concern about fetuses that are small for gestational age?

11.6 References

1. Ifrah G. The universal history of numbers. From prehistory to the invention of the computer. New York: John Wiley & Sons, Inc; 2000

2. Bianchi DW, Crombleholme TM, D'Alton ME, Malone FD. Twin to twin transfusion syndrome. Fetology. Diagnosis and management of the fetal patient. New York: McGraw - Hill Medical; 2010. p. 818 - 834.

3. Dähnert W. Radiology review manual. Philadelphia: Williams and Wilkins; 1996:763.

4. Benirschke K. History of the twin to twin transfusion syndrome. 2004 http://www.tttsfoundation.org/medical_professionals/history_of_TTTS.php. Accessed 2015.

5. Geaghan SM. Fetal laboratory medicine: On the frontier of maternal-fetal medicine. Clin Chem. 2012;58:337 - 352.

6. Umur A, van Gemert MJC, Nikkels PGJ. Monoamniotic-versus diamniotic-monochorionic twin placentas: anastomoses and twin-twin transfusion syndrome. Am J Obstet Gynecol. 2003;189:1325-1329.

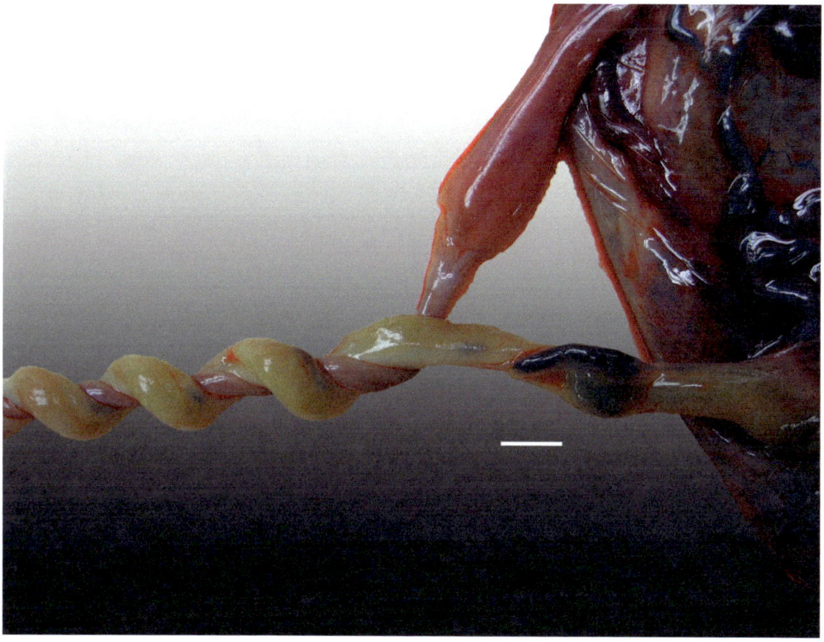

Figure 11.1 Unusual intertwined umbilical cords in a different case of twin-twin transfusion syndrome. Because of the pattern of vascular anastomoses, twin-twin transfusion syndrome is less common in monochorionic-monoamniotic pregnancies. [6] The white bar is 1 cm long.

	Twin 1	Twin 2	$\|\Delta\|$
Body weight (grams)	**236**	**310**	**74**
Crown-Heel length (cm)	**24.8**	**25.9**	**1.1**
Lungs	**6.7**	**9.6**	**2.9**
Kidneys	**1.7**	**3.4**	**1.8**
Liver	**8.6**	**17.3**	**8.8**
Brain	**43**	**45**	**2**
Brain/Liver weight	**5**	**2.6**	**2.4**

Table 11.1. Discordant body weights and measures of the two stillborn twins in Chapter 11.

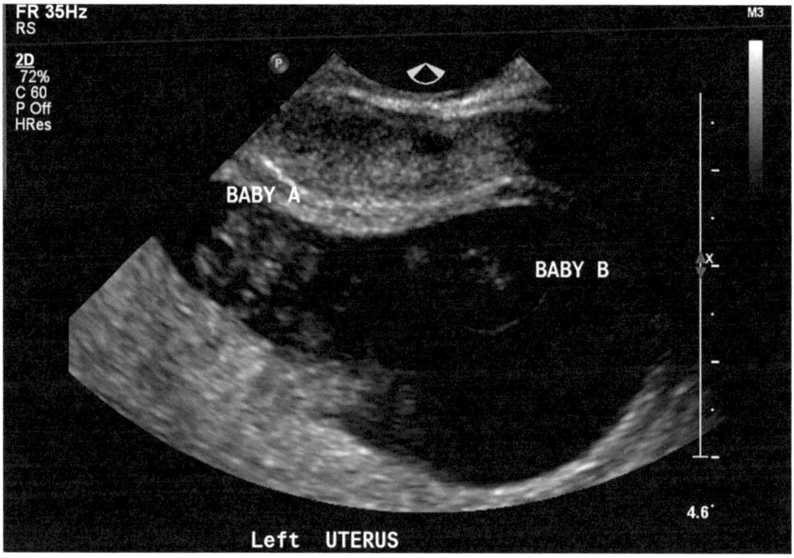

Figure 11.2 An ultrasound image of the uterus from a different case shows a gestational sac containing a twin pregnancy (monoamniotic monochorionic) with decreased size of Baby B relative to Baby A. The finding is concerning for twin-twin transfusion syndrome where Baby A (recipient) pulls blood and nutrients from Baby B (donor) as a result of abnormal arteriovenous communication in the placenta causing restricted growth of the donor baby.

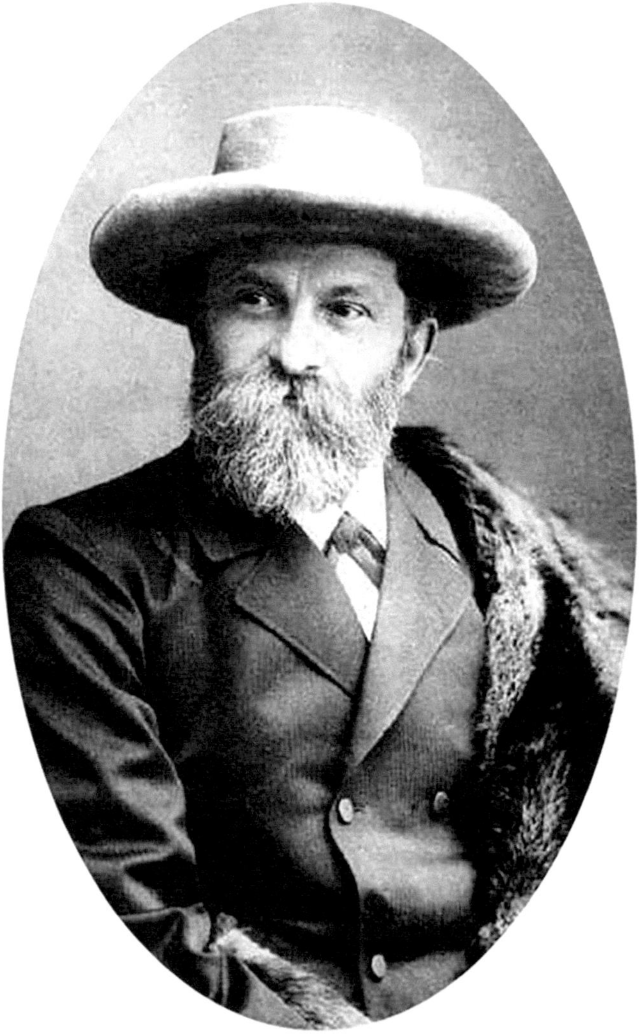

Figure 11.3 Christian Friedrich Schatz (1841 – 1920).

CHAPTER 12

Pulmonary thromboemboli in an elderly man with post-poliomyelitis syndrome. (VINdicate, vascular, infectious, neurological)

"There are no routine autopsies, just routine pathologists." Hans Popper (1903 – 1988)

12.1 The Autopsy

12.1.1 Case History

The patient was a 75-year-old man with post-poliomyelitis syndrome who was confined to a wheelchair. He had a history of systemic hypertension and hyperlipidemia. The patient had had a coronary artery angioplasty many years earlier. His medications included enoxaparin (low molecular weight heparin), oxycodone (narcotic), hydrochlorothiazide (diuretic), esomeprazole (proton pump inhibitor), atorvastatin (statin - HMG-CoA reductase inhibitor), ramipril (anti-hypertensive), and zolpidem (short acting hypnotic). The patient called 911 complaining of difficulty breathing. When the Emergency medical technicians arrived, the patient was having agonal respirations with a respiratory rate of 4 and a heart rate of 30. His EKG showed pulseless electrical activity (An electrical pattern which should be producing a pulse, but is not; also called electromechanical dissociation.). The patient was intubated and cardiopulmonary resuscitation was started. He was brought to the Emergency department. Resuscitatory efforts were unsuccessful.

12.1.2 Postmortem findings

At autopsy, the patient had prominent thoracic scoliosis and some bilateral deformity of the feet. Examination of the heart showed moderate atherosclerosis of the right coronary artery. There was cardiac right ventricular hypertrophy. The liver was congested. Both lungs were slightly heavy. No large thromboemboli were seen at the pulmonary hila, but on cut section, there were multiple thromboemboli in large pulmonary arteries just distal to the hila that were most prominent in the upper lobes bilaterally (figures 12.1, 12.2, 12.3). No pulmonary infarcts were seen. Histologic sections showed pulmonary thromboemboli in all the lung lobes. Some of the emboli had features of early organization indicating that they were about 10 days old. There were some months to years old thromboemboli with recanalization and some atherosclerosis in the pulmonary arteries.

12.1.3 Case summary

The patient had the post-poliomyelitis syndrome and was confined to a wheelchair making him more susceptible to lower leg deep vein thrombi and pulmonary thromboemboli. He was taking enoxaparin and had thromboemboli that were acute, subacute, and chronic. He had right ventricular hypertrophy and hepatic congestion; all indicating long-standing and on-going thromboembolic disease. I attributed his death to pulmonary thromboemboli.

12.2 Discussion

12.2.1 Pulmonary thromboemboli

Deep venous thrombi (DVT) and pulmonary thromboemboli (PE) are two of the most important clinical events that occur in patients with venous thrombosis. About 0.1% of the population will have a DVT, but the incidence is two to four times higher in hospitalized patients. PE is the third leading cause of cardiovascular death. Both DVT and PE may be difficult to diagnose.

DVTs are most common in the lower extremities and the pelvis. About 95% of pulmonary thromboemboli come from lower extremity venous thrombi. The triad of vessel wall injury, stasis and hypercoagulability often referred to as Virchow's triad (see below) lead to platelet aggregation and trigger the formation of a thrombus. Risk factors for a DVT are those that affect the elements of Virchow's triad and include recent surgery, trauma, local infection, paralysis, immobility, pregnancy (with both venous stasis and hypercoagulability), indwelling intravenous lines, high-estrogen oral contraceptives, and malignancy.

Typical presenting features of a DVT of the leg include swelling and tenderness. About 40% of patients with an isolated DVT have asymptomatic pulmonary thromboemboli, so patients with DVT or PE are clinically considered to have both unless proven otherwise. Patients with a PE may have the sudden onset of dyspnea and tachycardia. Other signs and symptoms include chest pain, hemoptysis, hypoxemia, and syncope. Other disorders may mimic PE including pneumonia and myocardial infarct.

Most PEs are clinically silent. If more than 60% of the pulmonary circulation is obstructed, then sudden death, right heart failure, or cardiovascular collapse occur. If small end-arteriolar pulmonary branches are obstructed, then hemorrhage or infarction may occur. Chronic PEs may lead to pulmonary hypertension and right heart failure. Only about 10% of PEs cause a pulmonary infarct; most of these are in the lower lung lobes. Typically, a pulmonary infarct is wedge-shaped with the occluded vessel at the apex of the infarct (figure 12.4). An acute infarct is hemorrhagic. A fibrinous exudate develops on the overlying pleural surface. Over time the infarct scars and becomes a depressed or contracted wedge-shaped area in the lung.

Since DVT and PE are often difficult to diagnose, various algorithms have been published that assign a score for each finding, e.g. a point for heart rate greater than 100, a point for a prior history of DVT etc., and permit the determination of a pre-test probability for the likelihood that the patient has a PE or a DVT [1].

Based on the pretest probability, tests for the presence of a DVT including ultrasound and venography or a PE including ventilation-perfusion scan and pulmonary angiography may be done.

Patients with DVT or PE are treated with anticoagulants. Thrombolytic therapy may be used for patients with PE who are hemodynamically unstable and surgical embolectomy in patients who fail thrombolysis.

Some patients at high risk for PE may have a metal filter resembling an umbrella with no fabric on it inserted in their inferior vena cava just below the renal veins. The filter is intended to catch thromboemboli before they reach the lungs. It was originally developed by Lazar Greenfield. Since the original device, other retrievable versions have been developed, because the frequency of complications increases over time if the filter is left in place. Current guidelines for the use of vena cava filters include patients who cannot be anticoagulated or have had PEs while on anticoagulation. (figure 12.5)

The pathologist needs to distinguish between true pulmonary thromboemboli that formed antemortem and postmortem clots that form after death and are, of course, of no clinical importance. The blood stops circulating in the body after death and the blood settles and clots. Postmortem clot has a lower glistening red part, historically noted to resemble currant jelly, and a tan-yellow upper part historically noted to resemble chicken fat. True antemortem thrombi are a more uniform color or, if mixed, their components do not resemble postmortem settling. Thromboemboli also tend to stick in the vessel when examined and they look as if they formed in another vessel (they did!), not the pulmonary artery in which they are currently lying [2 – 4].

12.2.2 Post-poliomyelitis syndrome

Myelitis of the anterior horn (poliomyelitis, acute infantile paralysis) is described in William Osler's 1892 textbook [5] as "an affection occurring most commonly within the first three years of life, characterized by fever, loss of power in certain muscles, and rapid atrophy." Osler comments that the cause of the disease is unknown, but that it had been attributed to cold, the irritation from dentition, overexertion, and to the nurse letting a child fall. He further stated that the child was usually attacked while in full health and that it was more common in boys than girls and in the warmer months. He also mentioned that several instances of occurrences in epidemic form had been reported. Osler stated that the outlook for complete recovery was bad, and that "there is no other disease in which the physician is so often subject to unjust criticism". Probably the most famous of those afflicted was President Franklin Roosevelt.

Poliomyelitis is now known to be an infectious disease caused by the poliovirus, which was first isolated by Karl Landsteiner (1868-1943, Austrian physician and Nobel prize laureate who discovered the ABO blood groups) in 1908. It is a human enterovirus. About 90% of infections cause no symptoms, a small percentage of infected patients have an acute illness with fever, gastrointestinal symptoms, neck stiffness, and arm and leg pain that usually lasts for 7 - 14 days. In less than 1% of infected patients, there is inflammation of the anterior horn of a portion of the spinal cord with the destruction of motor neurons, leading to an area of paralysis. Some of these patients recover, but some have persistent muscle atrophy and weakness, and a few percent of affected children and up to 30% of affected adults die. A protective killed-virus vaccine was developed in the US by Jonas Salk (1914 – 1995) in the 1950s. In the US in 1952 there were 58,000 cases of whom 3,145 died and 21,269 had some degree of persistent paralysis. The vaccine was introduced in 1955 and in 1964 there were 121 cases. During this time, Albert Sabin's (1906 – 1993) live attenuated virus oral vaccine was also introduced in the US and elsewhere. The oral vaccine has had continued widespread use to attempt to eliminate the disease worldwide. In 2013, there were only 416 reported cases in the world.

Post-poliomyelitis syndrome (PPS) is a condition characterized by slowly progressive weakness and atrophy in muscles that were affected by poliomyelitis years after recovery from the original infection. The cause of PPS is unknown and there is no accepted drug therapy for it. It is theorized that nerve terminals in the motor neuron unit that had compensatory proliferation after the original polio infection slowly degenerate over time. The incidence of PPS is unknown. In the mid-1990s there were about 1 million polio survivors in the US, of whom 443,000 had paralytic polio. It is estimated that 25 - 40% of polio survivors might develop PPS. Some authors state that PPS is not usually life threatening unless affected muscles lead to difficulty with respiration or swallowing, but others maintain that those cases that do not have a progressive downhill course do not represent true examples of PPS [6-8].

12.3 Medical history

12.3.1 Rudolph Virchow and Virchow's Triad

Rudolph Virchow (1821 – 1902), often called the father of modern pathology, was born in Schivelbein in Pomerania, Prussia. He graduated from a school for military physicians in Berlin in 1843 and became an assistant to Robert Froriep (1804 – 1861) at the Charité hospital. He co-founded the *Archiv für pathologische Anatomie und Physiologie und für klinische Medicin* at age 26. This journal was published as Virchow's Archiv for many years. Virchow's great work of pathology was *Cellular Pathology*, first published in 1858. Among his many accomplishments, Virchow is principally remembered for promulgating the concept that all cells in the body come from other cells and that pathological changes occur at the cellular level. Previously, some workers thought that living tissue could develop from various formative structures or fluids (e.g. termed elementary granules, blastema, cytoblastema etc.). Virchow also discussed pulmonary thromboembolism in detail, "...by the detachment of larger or smaller fragments from the end of the softening thrombus which are carried along by the current of blood and driven into remote vessels. This gives rise to the very frequent process upon which I have bestowed the name of *Embolia*." [9]

That venous thrombosis is attributable to alterations of one or more of three elements, blood flow, the vascular endothelium, and the constitution of the blood itself, is often called Virchow's triad. In an extensive review of the English and French literature on this topic, Dickson showed that the name Virchow's triad was not used until the middle of the 20th century [10]. Furthermore, the elements of the triad were not original to Virchow and he did not express them in a way like their current use. This is probably not surprising since similar findings are commonly discovered on careful examination of any eponym, but the discovery hardly diminishes the importance of Virchow's accomplishments [11 – 13].

12.3.2 Poliomyelitis

There is evidence of acute poliomyelitis in antiquity, including an ancient Egyptian hieroglyphic image showing isolated atrophy and paralysis of a leg. In 1893, Drs. John J. Putnam and E. W. Taylor published a paper entitled "Is acute poliomyelitis unusually prevalent this season?" where they reported 26 cases in the Boston area, but they had only counted 6 in 1892. The first definite US epidemic was in Vermont in the summer of 1894 when there were 132 reported cases of the disease. The idea that most polio infections were inapparent and harmless was recognized by the Swedish epidemiologist, Ivar Wickman (1872 – 1914). Karl Landsteiner and E. Popper attempted to culture from the spinal cord of a 9-year-old child who had died of the disease but grew nothing. They injected material from the cord into rabbits and guinea pigs, also without success. But when they fortuitously chose a pair of old world monkeys (new world monkeys are relatively resistant to polio), one died 8 days after intraperitoneal injection and the other developed flaccid paralysis of the lower extremities. Histologic examination of the spinal cord from the monkey that died resembled poliomyelitis as seen in humans and the authors suggested that polio was caused by a virus [8].

12.4 Laboratory Medicine

12.4.1 Pulse oximetry

The laboratory does not play an elaborate role in the diagnosis of deep vein thrombosis or pulmonary thromboemboli. D-dimers, a fibrin degradation product from mature thrombi, are elevated in patients with deep venous thrombi, but they are non-specific. Their best use is in patients who are thought to not have a DVT. If the D-dimer is negative, then the physician may be able to more completely exclude the possibility of DVT. Pulmonary thromboemboli may be detected in the hospital setting when peripheral oxygen saturation decreases. Oxygen saturation in the hospital is often measured in real time using pulse oximetry, one of the great medical technological success stories. The idea of measuring oxygen saturation with different wavelengths of light was developed in the early 20th century, but a commercial device wasn't available until the 1980s when Takuo Aoyagi, a Japanese bioengineer, developed a method using pulsatile variation in optical density at two different wavelengths of red light. The pulse oximeter is usually clipped to a fingertip or an earlobe. The device has light emitting diodes that operate at wavelengths of 660 and 940 nm. Oxygenated hemoglobin absorbs more light than deoxygenated hemoglobin at 940 nm (infrared), and the situation is reversed at 660 nm. A microprocessor calculates the oxygen saturation from these data. Pulse oximeters were historically sensitive to patient movement and to poor vascular circulation with stasis, but new calculation algorithms have made current generation devices more resistant to these problems. Pulse oximetry also becomes inaccurate when hemoglobin is binding to something other than oxygen, e.g. carbon monoxide [3, 14].

12.5 Study questions

1. Rudolph Virchow was also known for his achievements in politics and public health. What were these?

2. How does one distinguish between a thrombus formed after death and one formed during life?

3. A competitor of Dr. Salk was Albert Sabin (1906 – 1993), whose laboratory created an oral polio vaccine using an attenuated live virus. What are the advantages and disadvantages of this vaccine?

4. What is an iron lung, and what was it used for?

5. The patient, in this case, was at increased risk for a pulmonary thromboembolus because he was confined to a wheelchair. What other conditions might put one at increased risk for a PE?

12.6 References

1. Wells PS, Anderson DR, Bormanis J, Guy F, Mitchell M, Gray L, Clement C, Robinson KS, Lewandowski B. Value of assessment of pretest probability of deep-vein thrombosis in clinical management. Lancet 1997;350:1795 – 1798

2. Kumar V, Abbas AK, Aster JC. Robbins and Cotran Pathologic basis of disease. Philadelphia: Elsevier Saunders; 2015

3. Bates SM, Jaeschke R, Stevens SM, Goodacre S, Wells PS, Stevenson MD, Kearon C, Schunemann HJ, Crowther M, Pauker SG, Makdissi R, Guyatt GH. Diagnosis of DVT: Antithrombotic therapy and prevention of thrombosis, 9th ed: American College of Chest Physicians evidence-based clinical practice guidelines. Chest 2102;141:e351A-e418S

4. DeWalt DA, Runge MS. Deep venous thrombosis and pulmonary embolism. In: Runge MS, Greganti MA, editors. Netter's internal medicine Philadelphia:Saunders Elsevier;2009.p. 480-488
5. Osler W. The principles and practice of medicine. New York: D. Appleton and Company. 1892:p. 831
6. Halstead LS. Diagnosing polio syndrome: Inclusion and exclusion criteria. In: Silver JK, Gowne AC, editors. Postpolio syndrome. Philadelphia:Hanley and Belfus; 2004.
7. National Institute of Neurological Disorders and Stroke. Post-polio syndrome fact sheet. 2012. http://www.ninds.nih.gov/disorders/post_polio/detail_post_polio.htm
8. Paul JR. A history of poliomyelitis. New Haven, Connecticut: Yale University Press;1971
9. Virchow R. Cellular pathology. Chance F, translator. London: John Churchill; 1860
10. Dickson BC. Venous thrombosis: On the history of Virchow's triad. Univ Toronto Med J. 2004;81:166-171
11. Bagot CN, Arya R. Virchow and his triad: a question of attribution. Br J Hematol 2008;143:180-190
12. Pruell C. Virchow, Rudolf Karl. In: Bynum WFB, Bynum H, editors. Dictionary of medical biography. Westport, Connecticut: Greenwood Press; 2007.p. 1272-1277
13. Talbott JH. A Biographical history of medicine: excerpts and essays on the men and their work. New York: Grune & Stratton; 1970:1211
14. Severinghaus JW, Honda Y. History of blood analysis. VII. Pulse oximetry. J Clin Monitor. 1987;3:135 - 138

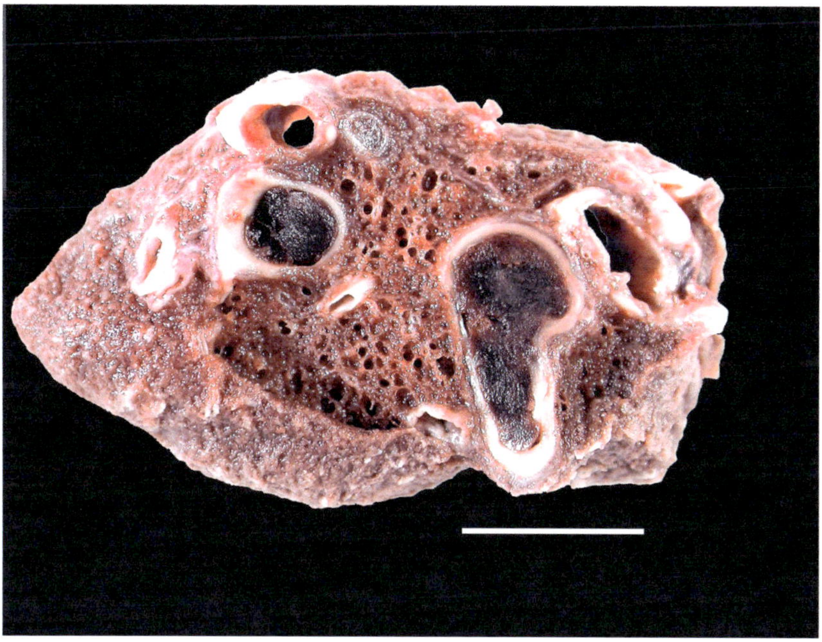

Figure 12.1 A section taken just lateral to the pulmonary hilum showing obstruction of the pulmonary artery branches by a large red thromboembolus. The white bar is 1 cm long.

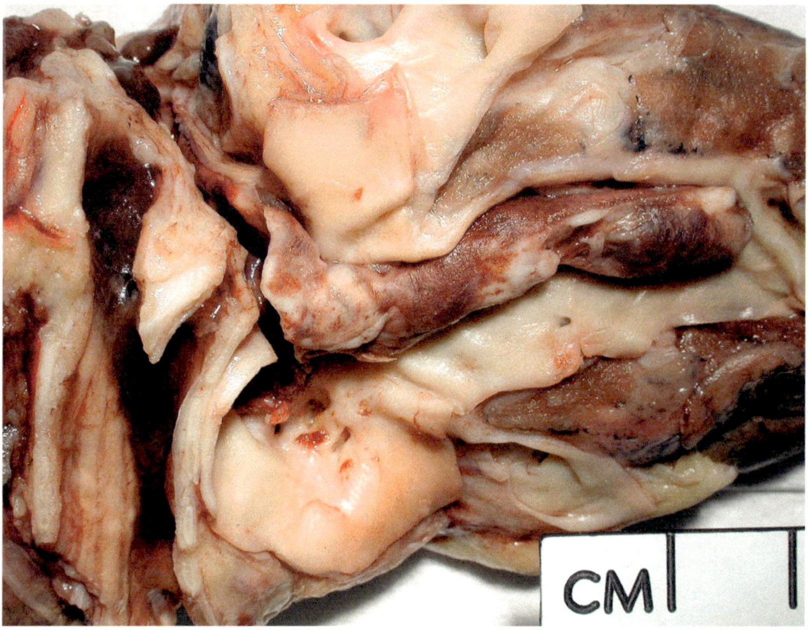

Figure 12.2 A large pulmonary thromboembolus in situ from a different case. The thromboembolus has a dry appearance and its red and white components are mixed unlike a postmortem clot, which would have a superior white part and an inferior glistening red part.

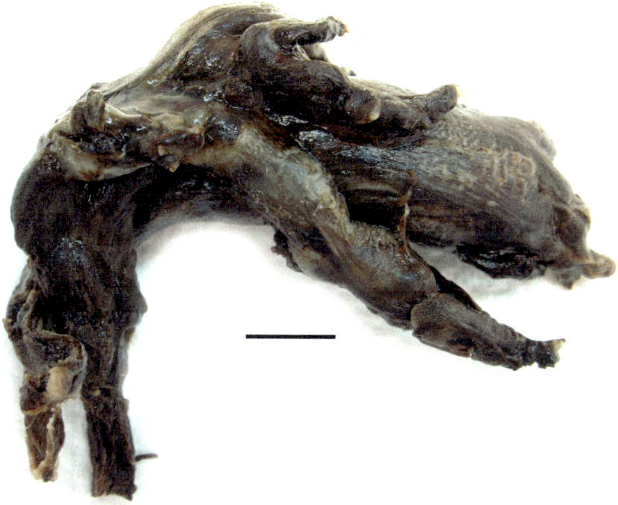

Figure 12.3 A pulmonary thromboembolus from a different case that has been removed for photography. The embolus has a complex shape that is a cast of the veins that they originated from, not the pulmonary artery in which they were found. The black bar is 1 cm long.

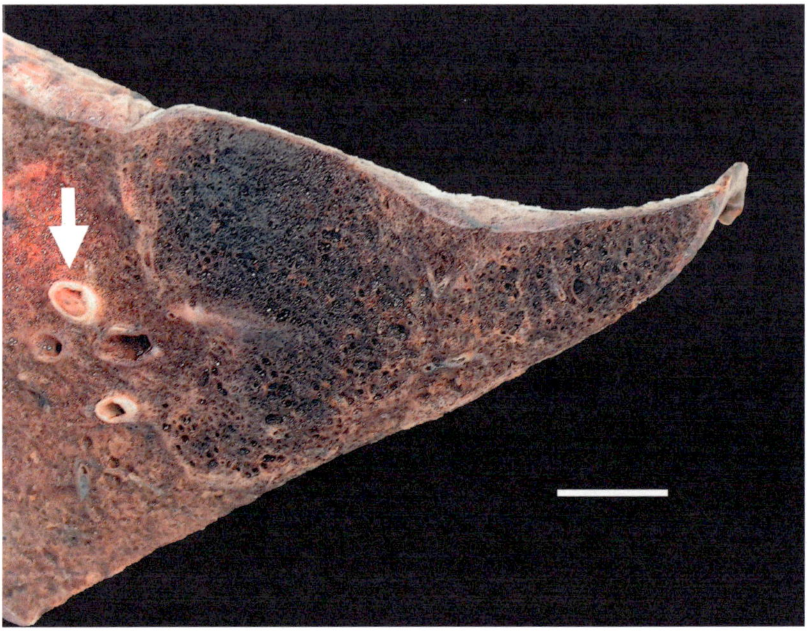

Figure 12.4 A section through a pulmonary infarct from a different case. The white arrow points to the occluded pulmonary artery. The infarct is wedge-shaped and hemorrhagic. The central lighter colored part of the infarct is beginning to organize. The white bar is 1 cm long.

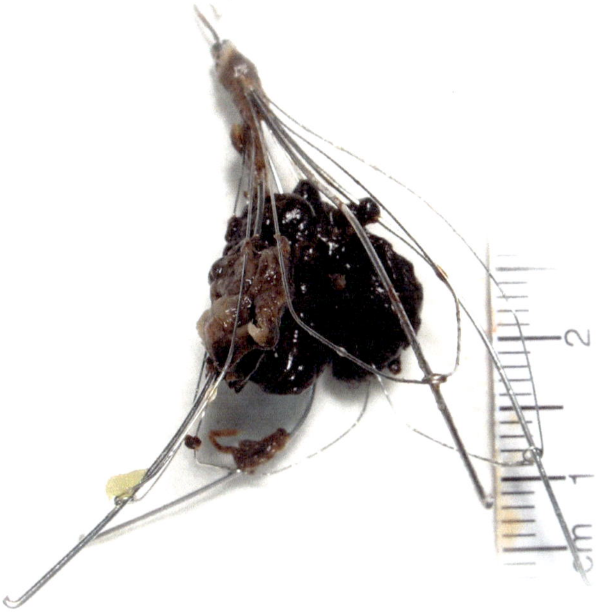

Figure 12.5 An inferior vena cava filter that has been removed from its location just inferior to the renal veins. The filter has both antemortem and postmortem clot in and on it.

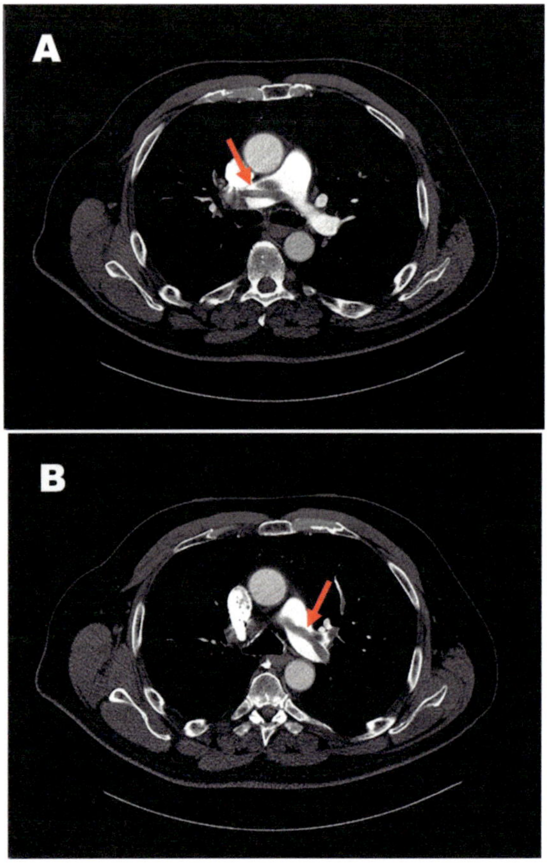

Figure 12.6.A and B Axial contrast enhanced CT pulmonary angiography at the level of the hilum from a different case shows tubular filling defects in the right main pulmonary artery (arrow on left in figure A) and the left main pulmonary artery (arrow on right in figure B) diagnostic of a saddle pulmonary thromboembolus. The embolus typically originates from the deep venous system of a lower extremity and you can see the resemblance to the tubular vein of origin by the shape of the thrombus.

CHAPTER 13

A 70-year-old woman with rheumatic cardiac valve disease and infective endocarditis. (VIndicate, vascular, infectious)

"Supposing is good, but finding out is better." Mark Twain (1835 – 1910)

13.1 The Autopsy

13.1.1 Case history

The patient was a 70-year-old woman with a history of coronary artery disease, diabetes mellitus, severe mitral stenosis, atrial fibrillation, transient ischemic attacks, pulmonary hypertension, and congestive heart failure. She had a history of alcohol abuse and a 40 pack-year smoking history. The patient came to the Emergency department with somnolence and was found to have hyperkalemia, to be hypotensive and acidotic, and to be in acute renal failure with a BUN of 50 (normal = 8 – 25 mg/dL) and a creatinine of 3.8 (normal = 0.6 – 1.5 mg/dL). The patient's medications included fluticasone/salmeterol (for obstructive lung disease), tiotropium (for bronchospasm), omeprazole (to reduce gastric acidity), prednisone 20 mg bid (an anti-inflammatory), moxifloxacin (an antibiotic), digoxin (a cardiac glycoside), fexofenadine (antihistamine), and olmesartan (antihypertensive). The patient became unresponsive and required mechanical ventilation. A chest radiograph showed an infiltrate in her right lung. The patient's peripheral white blood cell count was 18,200 (normal = 4500 – 11,000). She was admitted and she was started on piperacillin/tazobactam for presumed aspiration pneumonia. Dialysis was started. A CT scan of the abdomen showed mild ascites and no evidence of ischemic bowel. A CT scan of the head showed an old lacunar infarct in the cerebellum. A blood culture grew Gram-positive cocci in pairs. She was given norepinephrine to support her blood pressure and vancomycin was added to her antibiotics. An echocardiogram showed a thickened mitral valve compatible with rheumatic heart disease. No deep venous thrombi were detected by ultrasound. The patient died on the second hospital day.

13.1.2 Postmortem findings

At autopsy, the right lung was heavy (1500 grams, normal = 350 – 450 grams) and there was marked confluent bronchopneumonia in the right lower lobe. Coccoid bacteria were visible on the microscopic slides. Some aspirated material was present in the left upper lung lobe. The heart had biventricular hypertrophy. No acute ischemic lesions were seen. The mitral valve was thickened with fusion of the mitral valve chordae and there was mild thickening of the aortic valve leaflets. A partially calcified vegetation was present on the atrial side of the mitral valve leaflet (figures 13.1 - 13.3). There was left atrial dilatation. Sections showed hepatic congestion and changes of pulmonary hypertension. Cultures from the lower lung lobes and from the mitral valve grew abundant Staphylococcus aureus.

13.1.3 Case summary

The gross findings in the heart were those of rheumatic valve disease with superimposed Staphylococcal infective endocarditis. The patient had a large Staphylococcal aureus pneumonia and had sepsis demonstrated in an antemortem blood culture. These findings were the cause of death. Associated findings included pulmonary hypertension with right ventricular hypertrophy and hepatic congestion.

13.2 Discussion

13.2.1 Rheumatic heart disease

There is a tendency to minimize the clinical significance of Group A Streptococcal infections in the modern age of antibiotics. But a cursory review of the diseases associated with Streptococcal infections both before and sometimes after the mid 20th century is sobering. The list includes scarlet fever, acute rheumatic fever, chronic rheumatic cardiac valve disease, peritonsillar abscess, otitis media, mastoiditis, meningitis, impetigo, glomerulonephritis, erysipelas, postpartum endometritis, toxic shock syndrome, and necrotizing fasciitis.

About 3% of patients with acute streptococcal pharyngitis will, without treatment, develop acute rheumatic fever in 2 -3 weeks. Acute rheumatic fever (ARF) is characterized by fever, fatigue, and migratory arthralgias. Criteria for the diagnosis of ARF are called the Jones criteria and include major and minor signs and symptoms and laboratory evidence of Streptococcal infection. Acute rheumatic fever is caused by some strains of group A Streptococci and only follows pharyngitis, although some patients do not have a sore throat. Only about 10% of patients are susceptible to getting ARF after Strep throat. The exact pathogenesis has been mysterious for many years. It is currently thought to be an autoimmune disease, but it is unclear if autoantibodies evoked by the infection, cross-reactive T lymphocytes, or activated T lymphocytes are responsible. Most patients recover from the acute carditis of ARF, but some may die of heart failure and some progress to rheumatic cardiac valve disease. Streptococcal pharyngitis is commonly treated with penicillin to prevent ARF and acute glomerulonephritis (which can also follow impetigo). It is important that patients take the full course of antibiotic to prevent ARF, and not stop the drug when their sore throat goes away.

Rheumatic carditis can affect all three layers of the heart. Histologic examination of the heart in a patient with acute rheumatic carditis may show the Aschoff body, an area of fibrinoid necrosis and associated chronic inflammatory cells. Symptoms of valve dysfunction usually only become manifest 10 to 30 years after the acute disease. The mitral and aortic valves are most often affected. The patients have a characteristic thickening of the valve cusps and fusion of the attached chordae tendineae (figure 13.1) [1,2].

13.2.2 Infective endocarditis

Infective endocarditis (IE) occurs in about one in every 1000 hospital admissions. Before the antibiotic era, it was typically seen in a 35-year-old, but the median age of affected patients is now 55 years. This change is probably attributable to the decreased incidence of rheumatic heart disease and the increased number of intravascular procedures and devices in older patients. The risk of infective endocarditis is increased in patients with abnormal or prosthetic heart valves. Intravenous drug abusers account for 25% of infective endocarditis patients; they are more likely to get disease on their tricuspid valve, but disease in the right heart has a much better prognosis than disease on the left side. The most common microorganism causing infective endocarditis is Streptococcus viridans, a member of the normal oral flora, which is seen in 35% of cases. Staphylococcus is present in 25% and Enterococcus in 10%. Other bacteria and fungi are rare causes. Staphylococcal infective endocarditis often has an acute clinical course. About a third of patients with Staphylococcal endocarditis have a normal cardiac valve. Complications of endocarditis such as perivalvular or myocardial abscess, cardiac conduction defects, and septic emboli are more common in patients with Staphylococcal disease. Untreated infective endocarditis is a fatal illness, so the diagnosis and therapy of the disease are critically important. Patients with endocarditis may have a subacute or a more fulminant acute course. Initial symptoms may be vague and include fever and malaise. A heart murmur may be detectable and peripheral septic emboli may produce peripheral lesions (figure 13.4) including hemorrhagic lesions in the retina (Roth's spots), painful subcutaneous nodules on the end of the digits (Osler's nodes), or non-tender hemorrhagic spots on the palms and soles (Janeway lesions). About a third of patients have central nervous system changes including stroke and more rarely meningitis. Blood culture and echocardiography are the most important specific diagnostic techniques. Transthoracic echocardiography is only 60% sensitive for the detection of vegetations, but transesophageal ultrasound is between 75 and 100% sensitive [3-5].

13.3 Medical history

13.3.1 Cardiac valve disease

Giovanni Morgagni made some comments about cardiac valve disease in his collection of autopsies. He described mitral stenosis, aortic stenosis, and aortic regurgitation. Morgagni also described vegetative endocardial lesions. Some 17th century reports of cardiac pathology are confused by the description of intracardiac postmortem clot as polyps. Matthew Baillie mentioned a connection between rheumatic fever (acute articular rheumatism) and heart disease in 1797. He got the idea from a patient of his, Dr. David Pitcairn, who mentioned it in a 1788 lecture. J. B. Bouillaud (1796 – 1881) described rheumatic cardiac valve disease in detail in 1836, although he seems to have grouped rheumatic and infective heart disease together. He coined the term endocarditis. Trousseau recommended that endocarditis be called "Maladie de Bouillaud", but that name was used instead for rheumatic fever. An article describing how microorganisms in the blood could attack heart valves, by E. Winge from Oslo, was published in 1867. A few years later Samuel Wilks (1824 – 1911) described abscesses in non-cardiac organs that he called "arterial pyaemia as a result of embolization". William Osler gave a lecture on so-called malignant endocarditis in 1885 in which he described both an acute and chronic course for infective endocarditis. The subacute course was described several years later and was known to be associated with Streptococcus viridans. The full history of rheumatic heart disease has yet to be written because its precise cause is still unknown. A microbial connection to rheumatic heart disease was investigated as early as 1887 by A. Mantle in the British Medical Journal [6,7].

13.4 Laboratory Medicine

13.4.1 Evaluation of the patient with suspected endocarditis

In patients with infective endocarditis, a microorganism is detectable in one of the first two sets of blood cultures in 90% of patients. Negative cultures may occur in patients who have been previously treated with antibiotics and those with a slow-growing fastidious or unusual organism. At least three sets of blood cultures should be done in the first 24 hours. Sterile technique is always important in the collection of blood cultures, but a contaminant with Staphylococcus might be especially disturbing in a patient suspected of having infective endocarditis. Patients with infective endocarditis may have other associated laboratory findings, but they are non-specific and aren't useful for making the diagnosis. These findings include elevation of the erythrocyte sedimentation rate, anemia of chronic disease (in 80%), rheumatoid factor (50%), proteinuria (50%), and hematuria (40%); the last two from immune complexes or renal infarction.

Laboratory tests are necessary to confirm prior Streptococcal infection in patients with suspected rheumatic carditis. Antistreptolysin O, anti-DNAase B, and a latex agglutination test (Streptozyme) which is made of a mixture of Streptococcal antigens are used.

Streptozyme is a screening test for antibodies to several different streptococcal antigens, including NADase, DNase, streptokinase, streptolysin O and hyaluronidase.

Patients make an antibody to streptolysin O in about 1 week after their infection. The antibody peaks in 2 – 4 weeks and it may persist for up to a year. The ASO test can be done by nephelometry, hemolysis inhibition, and latex agglutination. Elevated titers are seen in about 85% of patients with acute rheumatic fever and 95% of patients with glomerulonephritis. Sequential ASO assays are usually done to identify a rising antibody titer, but a single positive anti-DNase B test is evidence of a Streptococcal infection. Anti-DNAase B has the same sensitivity as the ASO test; if used together with ASO it is 95% sensitive [2,8].

13.5 Study questions

1. Why do IV drug abusers have an increased risk of infective endocarditis? Is there a way to decrease their risk?

2. Patients with a prosthetic heart valve have a 2% risk of getting infective endocarditis. These can be divided into those occurring within the first two months of surgery and those that occur later. Staphylococcal infections are more common early and Streptococcal infections are more common late. Why might this be so?

3. What is the difference between Janeway's spots and Osler's nodes?

4. Why are patients with prosthetic heart valves sometimes asked to take antibiotics before they have dental procedures?

5. What would you expect to hear on auscultation with a stethoscope in a patient with a vegetation on their aortic valve?

13.6 References

1. Edwards MM, O'Gara PT, Lilly LS. Valvular heart disease. In: Lilly LS, editor. Pathophysiology of heart disease. Philadelphia: Lippincott Williams & Wilkins; 2007. p. 197 - 198.

2. Whitnack E. Streptococci. In: Schaechter ME, NC Eisenstein, BI Medoff, G, editor. Mechanisms of microbial disease. Philadelphia: Lippincott Williams & Wilkins; 1999. p. 143 - 152.

3. Cobbs GC, Saccente M. Endocarditis, intravascular infections, pericarditis and myocarditis. In: Humes HD, editor. Kelley's textbook of internal medicine. Philadelphia: Lippincott William and Wilkins; 2000. p. 1931-1938.

4. Patterson KB, Patterson C. Infective endocarditis. In: Runge MS, Greganti MA, editor. Netter's internal medicine. Philadelphia: Saunders Elsevier; 2009. p. 663 - 670.

5. Pelletier LL. Endocarditis. In: Porter RS, Kaplan JL, editors. The Merck manual of diagnosis and therapy. Whitehouse Station, NJ: Merck Sharpe & Dohme Corp; 2011. p. 2193 - 2199.

6. Acierno LJ. The history of Cardiology. New York: Parthenon; 1994. p. 65.

7. Krumbhaar EB. History of the pathology of the heart. In: Gould SE, editor. Pathology of the heart. Springfield, Illinois: Charles C. Thomas; 1960. p. 3.

8. Jacobs DS, Oxley DK, DeMott WR. Laboratory Test Handbook. Hudson (Cleveland), Ohio: Lexi-Comp, Inc; 2001

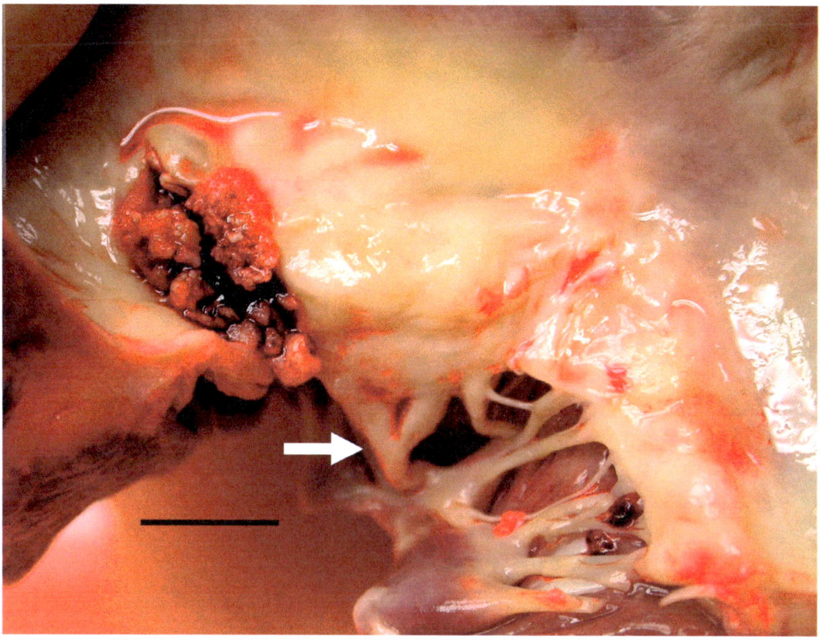

Figure 13.1 The patient's mitral valve with a vegetation of infective endocarditis in its usual location on the atrial side of the valve leaflet slightly back from the edge of the leaflet. The string-like structures that attach to the bottom of the valve leaflets are called the chordae tendineae. There is prominent thickening of the chorda tendineae at the arrow; a characteristic feature of old rheumatic heart disease. Compare to figure 13.2. The black bar is 1 cm long.

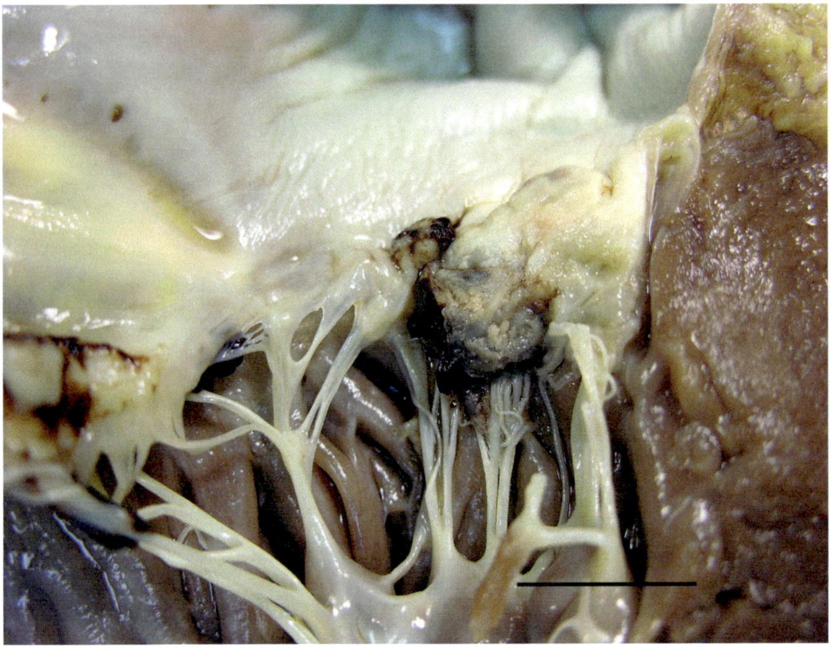

Figure 13.2 A valve vegetation in a different patient with infective endocarditis. This patient did not have rheumatic heart disease. The black bar is 1 cm long.

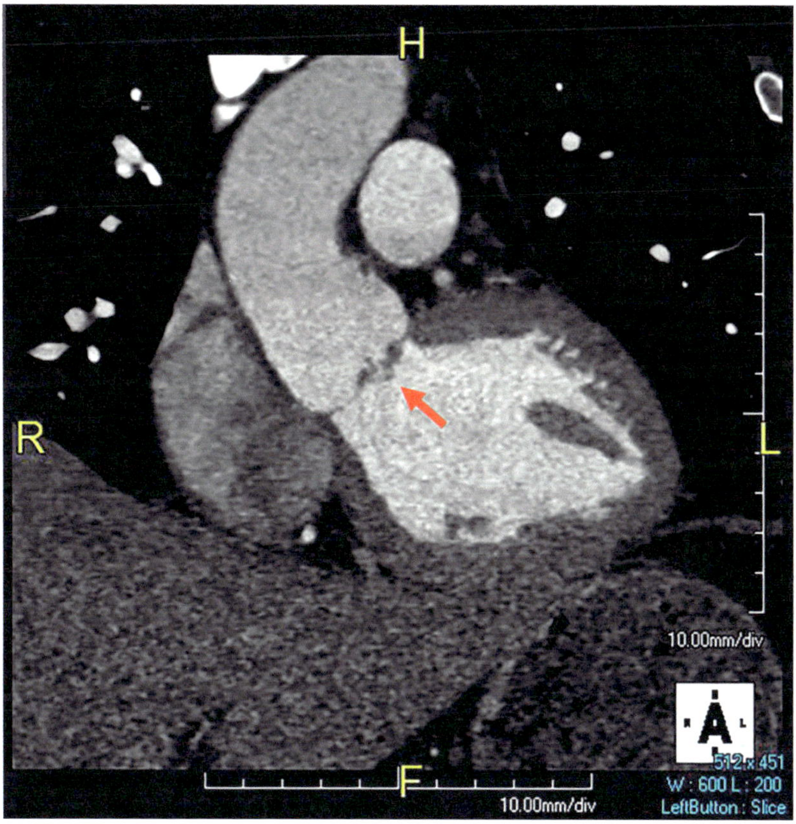

Figure 13.3 A multiplanar reformatted sagittal image contrast enhanced CT through the aortic valve from a different febrile patient shows nodular thickening of the aortic valve leaflets (arrow) highly suggestive of the valve vegetations of endocarditis.

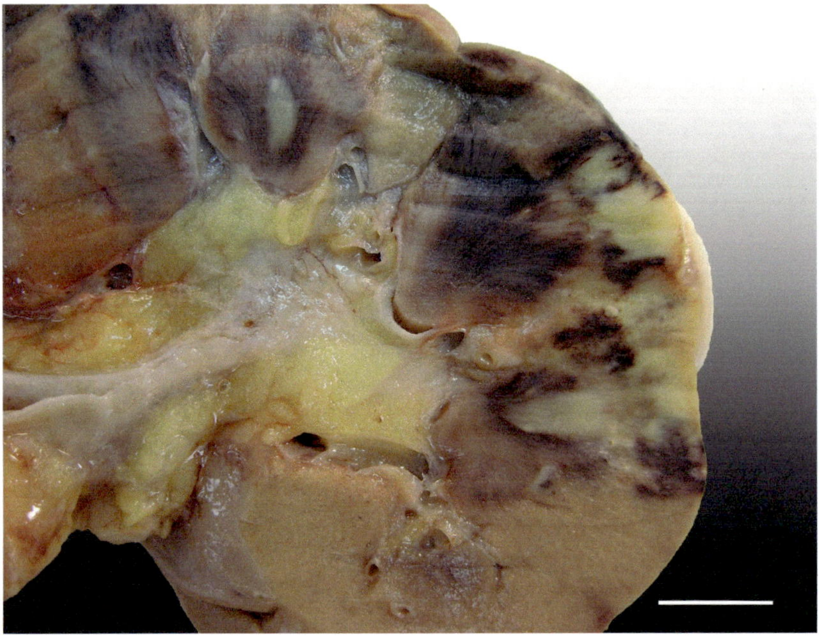

Figure 13.4 A section of the kidney in a different case of infective endocarditis. The kidney has been partially infarcted from embolic material from the cardiac valve vegetations, and it shows red and yellow discoloration. The white bar is 1 cm long.

CHAPTER 14

A 50-year-old man with pancreatitis. (vindIcate, idiopathic)

"Medicine being a compendium of the successive and contradictory mistakes of medical practitioners, when we summon the wisest of them to our aid, the chances are that we may be relying on a scientific truth the error of which will be recognized in a few years' time." Marcel Proust (1871 – 1922), The Guermantes Way.

14.1 The Autopsy

14.1.1 Case history

The patient was a 50-year-old man who had been short of breath for a few days when he became lethargic and then unresponsive. He was brought to the hospital where he had a systolic blood pressure of 70 (normal = 120 mm Hg) and coffee-ground emesis. The patient was given norepinephrine and required intubation and mechanical ventilation. The initial diagnostic impression was septic shock and the patient was placed on antibiotics empirically. A CT scan showed radiographic features of pancreatitis. The patient's serum lipase was as high as 1726 (normal = 20 – 250 U/L) in the first month of his hospitalization. He remained hospitalized until his death three months later. His lipase one month after admission was 239. The etiology of the patient's pancreatitis was unknown. He had not used alcohol for several years. He had no history of abdominal trauma. An abdominal ultrasound showed sludge in his gallbladder, but not stones and no dilatation of the common bile duct. The patient's diagnosis, after his initial tests were done, was systemic inflammatory response syndrome secondary to acute pancreatitis. He was noted to have a splenic vein thrombus and dissection of the superior mesenteric artery. The patient's course was complicated by persistent hypotension, renal and liver failure and atrial fibrillation. He had stabilized to some degree, but several days before his death he developed abdominal pain, abdominal distension, and fever. His white blood cell count went from 10,500 to 24,100 (normal = 4500 – 11,000 cells/cubic mm) and his differential white blood cell count was 28% band forms (normal = 0 – 5%). CT scan had earlier shown a pseudocyst (figures 14.1, 14.2) and now showed a peripancreatic phlegmon (an inflammatory mass). Paracentesis was done and the fluid was exudative, but no microorganisms were identified. The patient died after about 15 weeks in the hospital.

14.1.2 Postmortem findings

Postmortem examination confirmed the presence of acute pancreatitis with a pancreatic pseudocyst. There was extensive fat necrosis in and adjacent to the pancreas (figure 14.3) with some hemorrhagic discoloration. There was extensive tan, green, and yellow exudate on the peritoneal surface and there was perforation of the jejunum with a 2.5 cm mural defect (figures 14.4, 14.5).

No gallstones were present. The liver weighed 3150 grams (normal = 1500 g) and there was marked steatosis. Sections of lung showed diffuse alveolar damage with focal organization. There was bilateral renal cortical scarring; histologic sections of kidney showed acute tubular necrosis. Examination of the heart showed an organizing obstructive thrombus in the right coronary artery overlying a ruptured atherosclerotic plaque and there were areas of myofiber eosinophilia in the right ventricle only, compatible with acute myocardial infarct. The features of the organizing thrombus were compatible with an age of about 7 days, but the abnormal area in the myocardium was more compatible with an age of 24 hours and may have been an agonal event.

14.1.3 Case summary

The patient had acute pancreatitis of unknown cause. His prominent hepatic steatosis suggested the possibility of alcoholism, but steatosis might also have been due to poor nutrition from his long illness. The digestive power of the damaged pancreas and its associated inflammatory reaction caused surrounding vascular changes with venous thrombosis and dissection of the superior mesenteric artery and ultimately perforation of the jejunum and peritonitis. I attributed the patient's death to acute peritonitis from bowel perforation secondary to acute pancreatitis.

14.2 Discussion

14.2.1 Pancreatitis

The pancreas is examined late during a typical autopsy. It is a 12 – 15 cm long deep central retroperitoneal organ that seems to be hidden away. The pancreas is surrounded by the duodenum at its head and is often very close to the splenic hilum at its tail. The stomach is above and anterior and the pancreatic head is crossed anteriorly by the root of the transverse mesocolon. It lays over the abdominal aorta and inferior vena cava (the largest artery and vein in the body), and the portal vein, splenic artery and vein, and the superior mesenteric artery and vein are intimately associated with it. The exocrine pancreas secretes the enzymes that digest food. These pass through the pancreatic duct and the ampulla of Vater into the duodenum. The endocrine pancreas (the islets of Langerhans) secretes various hormones including insulin.

Normally the body is protected from the action of pancreatic enzymes. They are secreted as proenzymes that aren't active until they reach the duodenum where they are activated by trypsin. Trypsin itself is activated in the duodenum by locally secreted enteropeptidase, and the exocrine pancreas makes trypsin inhibitors. Pancreatitis occurs when this protective system is disrupted or overwhelmed.

Pancreatitis occurs in acute and chronic forms. The annual incidence in the US is 10 – 20 cases per 100,000 people. It has a wide range of severity and presenting signs and symptoms, and it may be notoriously difficult to diagnose. Mild cases of pancreatitis often resolve with supportive care, but patients with necrotizing pancreatitis have a mortality of 10%, and, if there is both necrosis and infection, the mortality rate is over 25%. There are many causes of pancreatitis, but in the US 80% of cases are due to either alcohol or gallstones. About 10% of cases are from a more unusual cause, e.g. trauma, mumps, autoimmunity, hypertriglyceridemia, or drug reaction, and the remaining 10% are idiopathic. The male to female ratio is 1:3 in those with gallstone pancreatitis and 6:1 in those with alcoholism. Chronic pancreatitis may develop after acute pancreatitis, but it more often develops insidiously.

Patients with acute pancreatitis often present with the sudden onset of epigastric pain associated with nausea and vomiting. The pain may radiate to the patient's back. The differential diagnosis is lengthy and includes many of the causes of an acute abdomen such as a perforated gastric ulcer, ischemic bowel, bowel obstruction, acute biliary colic, myocardial infarct, and ectopic pregnancy. Diagnostic features include elevation of serum amylase and serum lipase to more than 3 times the upper limit of normal and CT scan showing characteristic radiographic changes in the pancreas. Gallstones may be identified by abdominal ultrasound or with endoscopic retrograde cholangiopancreatography (ERCP). There is no specific medical treatment for acute pancreatitis that has been shown to be useful. Patients are treated with supportive care. Bile duct stones may be removed with ERCP and surgery may be useful, usually after the patient has recovered from the acute illness, to remove the gallbladder. Surgical debridement may be necessary for patients with necrosis and infection since the prognosis is otherwise very poor (see the medical history discussion below).

The prognosis of patients with pancreatitis may be difficult to judge and this is reflected by the existence of published prognostic scoring techniques including that of Ranson and BISAP (the bedside index for severity in acute pancreatitis); the APACHE II system for prognosis in ICU patients is also used.

The leaking enzymes in acute pancreatitis cause edema, inflammation, hemorrhage, and thrombosis in and adjacent to the pancreas. The death of pancreatic and peripancreatic fat cells along with the action of the enzyme lipase leads to the formation of fatty acids that combine with calcium. This process is the same chemical process that occurs in the manufacture of soap and is called fat saponification. Grossly visible chalky yellow-white areas correspond to these areas of fat necrosis (figure 14.3).

Complications of pancreatitis include infection of necrotic pancreatic tissue, a systemic inflammatory response that may lead to multi-organ failure, and the formation of a pancreatic pseudocyst which may itself be complicated by rupture, hemorrhage, or infection [1 – 3].

14.3 Medical history

14.3.1 Pancreatitis

A case of acute pancreatitis was described in 1652 by the Dutch anatomist Nicolaes Tulp (1593 – 1674). Tulp was also the mayor of Amsterdam and the subject of a famous painting by Rembrandt, "The anatomy lesson of Dr. Nicolaes Tulp". Acute pancreatitis was not the subject of much written comment until 1842, when Heinrich Claessen, a physician in Cologne proposed it as a distinct entity. Additional small numbers of cases were reported in the next 50 years and Edwin Klebs , a student of Virchow and professor in Bern, first postulated that pancreatitis was due to the "corroding qualities" of pancreatic secretions. In 1882 Nicolaus Friedreich, also a student of Virchow, suggested a classification of pancreatitis based on autopsy findings. He separated cases into those characterized by hemorrhage, gangrene, or abscess formation. But the first detailed study and classification of the disease was by Reginald Fitz (1843 – 1913, figure 14.6) in a lecture and subsequent paper presented in 1889.

Fitz was born in Chelsea, Massachusetts. He left Harvard in his junior year to work in a Michigan copper mine, but he returned to graduate at age 21. He wrote to his family, "I find that it will be much pleasanter to become a professional man and live moderately and free from care than to become rich and have my mind continually harassed with care and anxiety". Fitz graduated from medical school and went to Europe where he studied with Rokitansky, Joseph Skoda (1805 – 1881), and Virchow.

He returned to Boston in 1870 and was made an instructor in pathology at Harvard. Eight years later, at age 35, he was appointed to the Shattuck professorship in pathological anatomy. Fitz was noted to be a demanding lecturer. The surgeon John Blake remembered that "he had a habit of tilting his head backward, closing his eyes, talking with extreme rapidity and fluency, never missing a word, for 61 minutes in the hours…it was as if he read a carefully prepared lecture from the inside of his eyelids."

Fitz is best remembered for his 1886 study in which he suggested the use of the term appendicitis, but in the paper from his 1889 lecture (also published as a book and available at books.google.com) he reviewed the literature and presented 53 patients with pathologically documented acute pancreatitis. He separated his cases into those with hemorrhage, those with hemorrhage and suppuration, and those with disseminated fat necrosis. He mentioned gallstones, alcohol, perforating gastric ulcer, and trauma as causes and he described abscess and pseudocyst as complications. Fitz observed that "It is evident that all treatment, at the outset, can be nothing but palliative. With the formation of pus in the omental cavity comes the opportunity for the surgeon." Fitz did mistakenly believe that he had a patient who had discharged his entire gangrenous pancreas from his bowels and had recovered and was well 17 years later.

Surgery of the pancreas was restricted to treatment of trauma and drainage of abscesses until the beginning of the 20th century when Berkeley Moynihan (1865 – 1936) and others began using laparotomy and gauze drainage to treat patients with acute necrotizing pancreatitis. This became the therapy of choice for 30 years despite a surgical mortality rate between 60 and 80%. When the serum test for amylase was described in 1929 and showed that there were less severe cases of pancreatitis that responded to non-invasive therapy, surgical intervention for acute necrotizing pancreatitis became uncommon. Surgery was popular again in the 1960s and 70s, but the mortality rate remained high. In recent times surgery has become uncommon again but guided by CT scan and better intensive care unit therapy surgical mortality rates are between 10 and 20% [4 – 7].

14.4 Laboratory medicine

14.4.1 Evaluation of the patient with suspected pancreatitis

In 1929, R. Elman, a surgical resident working under Evarts Graham at the Barnes hospital in St. Louis, proposed that a serum test for amylase could be used for the diagnosis of acute pancreatitis, a difficult diagnosis then and now. Amylase is a group of hydrolases made in the exocrine pancreas and salivary glands that is elevated in the serum of about 80% of patients with acute pancreatitis within 12 hours of the onset of symptoms. More than 200 methods exist for its measurement. It is usually ordered in combination with serum lipase, which is somewhat more sensitive and specific than amylase for the diagnosis of pancreatitis. Amylase may also be elevated in patients with inflammation of a salivary gland, e.g. mumps, perforated gastric ulcer, bowel obstruction, cholecystitis, cirrhosis, aortic dissection, appendicitis, cerebral trauma, burns, diabetic ketoacidosis, and certain non-pancreatic carcinomas (especially of the esophagus, lung and ovary). Patients with severe acute pancreatitis often have amylase and lipase levels that are 3 – 5 times the upper limit of normal, but amylase may be elevated as high as 25 times normal in patients with a metastatic carcinoma producing it. Other causes of elevation of amylase include pregnancy, tubo-ovarian abscess, ectopic pregnancy, in patients with macroamylasemia, renal failure, alcoholics, and secondary to many different drugs. Narcotics may cause spasm of the sphincter of Oddi and increase amylase levels, and more than 20 drugs have been associated with cases of pancreatitis. Patients with hypertriglyceridemia have false depression of their amylase level.

Tests for urine amylase are not used much, but they may be useful in certain clinical situations. Patients with macroamylasemia have complexes of amylase and immunoglobulins in their blood that are not present in the urine. Patients with renal failure have elevation of their serum amylase, but their urine amylase is normal. Urine amylase remains elevated after serum amylase has returned to normal in patients with acute pancreatitis and it may be useful to assist in the diagnosis of pancreatic pseudocyst [8,9].

A urine dipstick for trypsinogen-2 is available, and it is moderately sensitive and specific for the diagnosis of acute pancreatitis.

Elevation of alanine aminotransferase (ALT) to more than 3 times the upper limit of normal is indicative of gallstone etiology in a non-alcoholic patient from a typical patient population [10].

14.5 Study questions

1. What are the two most common causes of pancreatitis in the US?

2. Why would surgery have occasionally become popular for the treatment of severe acute pancreatitis, if the surgical mortality was so high?

3. Is elevated serum amylase specific for pancreatitis?

4. Reginald Fitz took some time off school to work in a copper mine in Michigan. Where was copper mined in Michigan in the 19th century?

5. In which clinical situations might a test for urine amylase be useful?

14.6 References

1. Hruban RH, Iacobuzio-Donahue CA. The Pancreas. In: Kumar V, Abbas AK, Aster JC, editors. Robbins and Cotran pathologic basis of disease. Philadelphia: Elsevier Saunders; 2015. p. 883 - 896.

2. Grimm IS. Pancreatitis. In: Runge MS, Greganti MA, editor. Netter's internal medicine. Philadelphia: Saunders Elsevier; 2009. p. 394 - 398.
3. Freedman SD. Pancreatitis. In: Porter RS, Kaplan JL, editors. The Merck manual of diagnosis and therapy. Whitehouse Station, NJ: Merck Sharp & Dohme, Corp.; 2011. p. 140 - 145.
4. Talbott JH. A biographical history of medicine: excerpts and essays on the men and their work. New York: Grune & Stratton; 1970:1211.
5. Leach SD, Gorelick FS, Modlin IM. Acute pancreatitis at its centenary. The contribution of Reginald Fitz. Ann Surg. 1990;212:100 - 113.
6. Bradley EL, III, Dexter ND. Management of severe acute pancreatitis: A surgical odyssey. Ann Surg. 2010;251:6 - 17.
7. Pannala R, Kidd M, Modlin IM. Acute pancreatitis: a historical perspective. Pancreas. 2009;38:355 - 366.
8. Jacobs DS, Oxley DK, DeMott WR. Laboratory Test Handbook. Hudson (Cleveland), Ohio: Lexi-Comp, Inc; 2001
9. Bailey DN, Herold D. Laboratory diagnosis of pancreatic disease. UCSD Lab Medicine. 2010
10. Tenner S, Dubner H, Steinberg W. Predicting gallstone pancreatitis with laboratory parameters: A meta-analysis. Am J Gastroenterol. 1994;89:1863 - 1866.

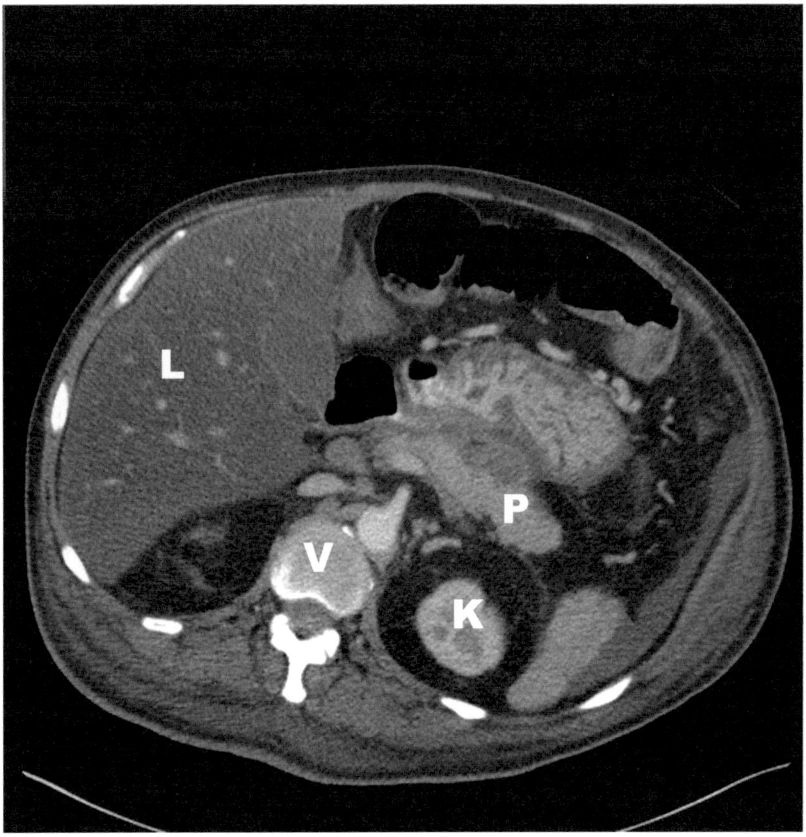

Figure 14.1 One level of a CT scan through the patient's pancreas with contrast. There is evidence of peripancreatic inflammation and an area of decreased density that was interpreted by some as a pseudocyst. The scan highlights the retroperitoneal deep central location of the pancreas. L = liver, P = pancreas, V = vertebral body, K = superior end of the left kidney.

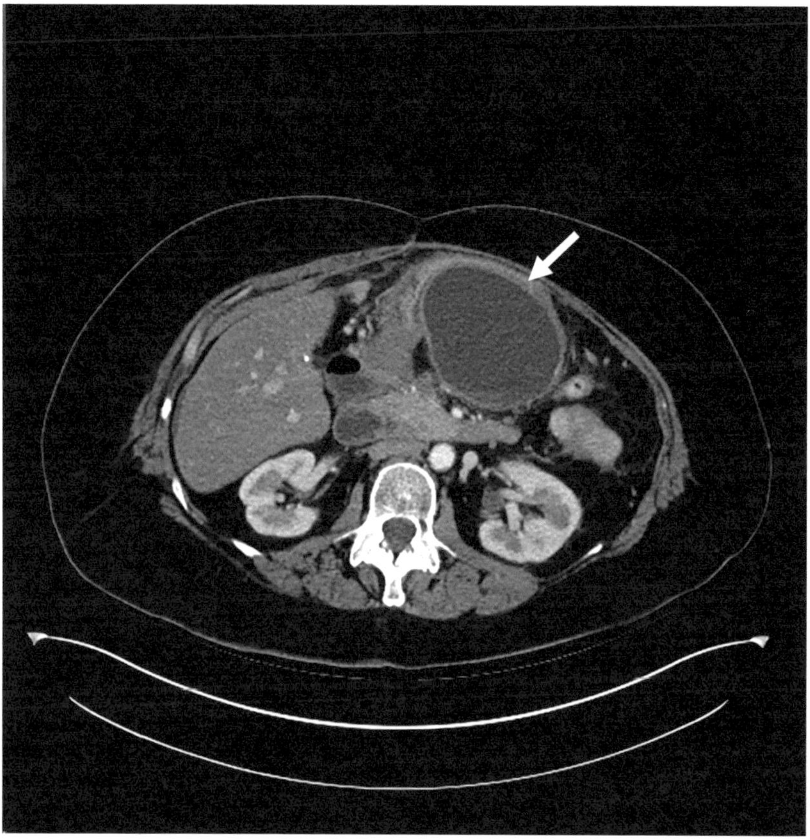

Figure 14.2 An axial contrast enhanced CT at the level of the kidneys in a different case of pancreatitis shows a round fluid collection with thick enhancing walls inferior and anterior to the pancreas compatible with a pseudocyst pushing and compressing the stomach anteriorly (arrow).

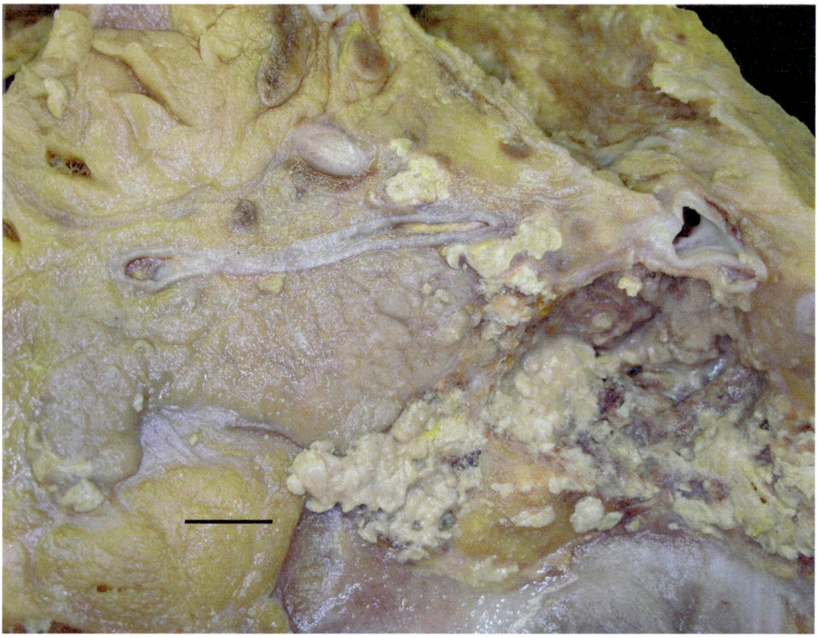

Figure 14.3 An en face section through the pancreas with abundant chalky yellow material indicating fat necrosis from leaking pancreatic enzymes. The black bar is 1 cm long.

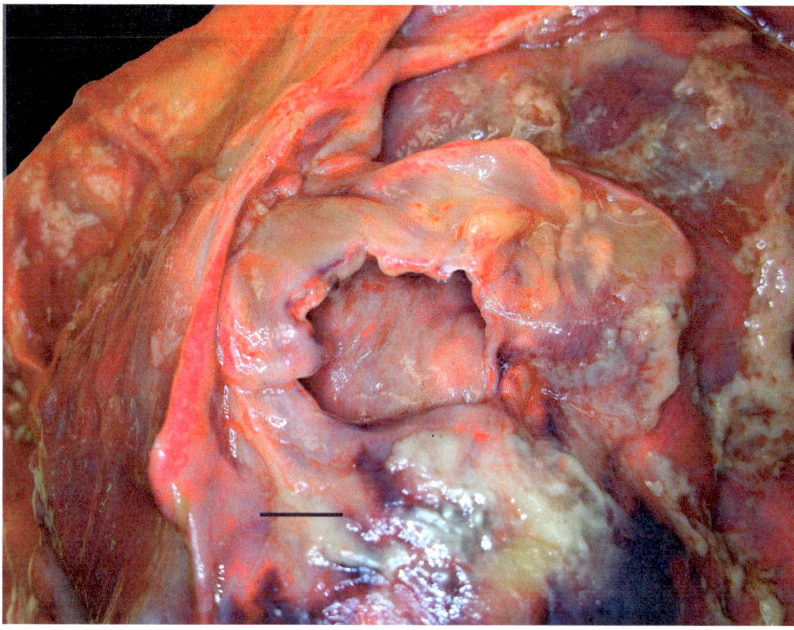

Figure 14.4 A large defect in the wall of the jejunum with adjacent exudate. The black bar is 1 cm long.

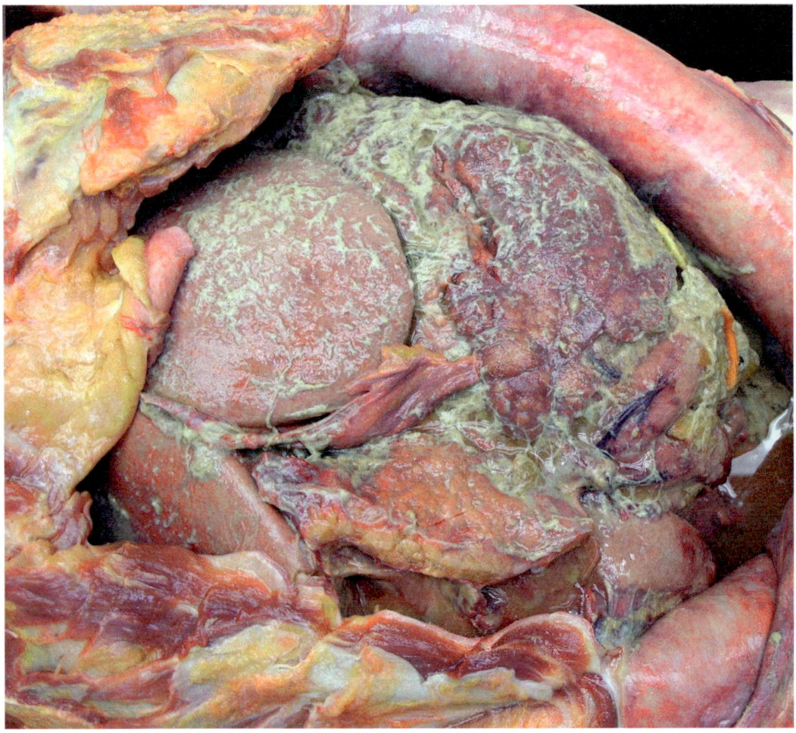

Figure 14.5 The patient's abdomen with the viscera in situ. There is green exudate and some food on the peritoneal surface.

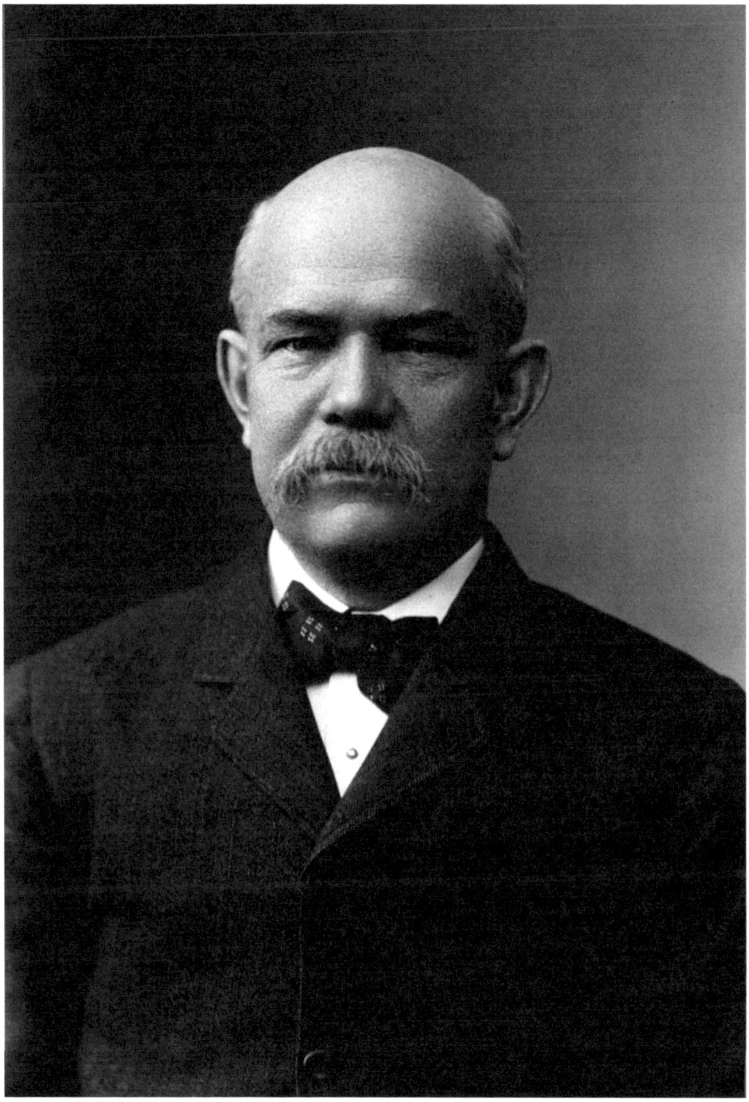

Figure 14.6 Reginald Fitz (1843 – 1913). Courtesy of the National Library of Medicine.

CHAPTER 15

A 50-year-old woman with broncho-pulmonary Aspergillosis. (vIndicate, infectious)

Quando il Fatto parla Ragione tace, perche la Ragione e figlia del Fatto, non il Fatto figlio della Ragione. (When Fact speaks, Reason is silent, because Reason is the child of Fact, not Fact the child of Reason). The motto of Agostino Bassi (1773 – 1856).

15.1 The Autopsy

15.1.1 Case history

The patient was a 50-year-old woman with a history of chronic obstructive lung disease, hypertension, and tobacco use. She had a one-week history of fever and a dry cough. She had been given a diagnosis of acute bronchitis and treated with the antibiotic levofloxacin, but did not improve. A chest radiograph was said to show no active disease, but her peripheral arterial oxygen saturation dropped to 80% and she was sent to the Emergency Department to rule out a pulmonary thromboembolus. Tests to rule out an embolus were negative. The patient was treated with antibiotics, oxygen, and a nebulizer and was admitted to the hospital. Three days later she had another episode of oxygen desaturation and was given 6 liters of oxygen per minute by nasal cannulae and then continuous positive airway pressure ventilation. She had a decrease in her mental status and was intubated and transferred to the intensive care unit. The patient had severe bronchospasm causing difficulty in mechanical ventilation, and a tracheal aspirate on hospital day #7 grew Aspergillus fumigatus. The patient's medications included vancomycin, ceftriaxone, voriconazole (an antifungal agent), acyclovir (an antiviral agent), and a steroid. Pulmonary infiltrates were worsening on chest radiograph. She developed renal failure and a Gram-negative rod was isolated from a bronchial specimen and the patient was thought to have a bacterial super-infection. The patient died on the 10th hospital day.

15.1.2 Postmortem findings

The patient's autopsy was limited to the examination of the chest contents. Her left lung weighed 1350 grams and her right lung weighed 1000 grams (normal ≈ 350 – 500 grams each). On cut section, the bronchi showed mural thickening with a luminal greenish exudate (figure 15.1). There were small military foci of tan-white discoloration and firmness in all lung lobes. In addition, some areas had a more lobar pattern of consolidation (figure 15.2). A frozen section from the right main bronchus done during the autopsy showed fungal hyphae. The patient's heart was unremarkable. Histologic sections confirmed the presence of a necrotizing pseudomembranous Aspergillus tracheobronchitis with tissue invasion (figure 15.3). Aspergillus pneumonia was also present. No eosinophils or Charcot-Leyden crystals were seen. There was no evidence of hypersensitivity pneumonitis, cavity formation or Aspergilloma.

15.1.3 Case summary

The patient had a history of fever and dry cough one week prior to receiving any steroid therapy suggesting that she had pseudomembranous necrotizing Aspergillus tracheobronchitis at the time that she presented to the hospital. This type of tracheobronchitis has a very poor prognosis and some authors claim that it is uniformly fatal [1]. The patient was thought to have severe bronchospasm limiting her ventilation, but it is possible that she had some degree of bronchial obstruction by her pseudomembranous exudate [2]. Most cases of Aspergillus pneumonia occur in immunocompromised patients, but rare cases in immunocompetent patients have been well described [3,4]. I attributed the patient's death to pseudomembranous necrotizing Aspergillus tracheobronchitis and pneumonia.

15.2 Discussion

15.2.1 Aspergillosis

Aspergillus species are a ubiquitous filamentous mold that may cause an opportunistic infection when its spores are inhaled. Patients at increased risk of infection often have neutropenia, are receiving steroid therapy, are taking immunosuppressive drugs for organ transplantation, have a hereditary disorder of neutrophil function, or have AIDS. Aspergillus prefers to grow in cavities like the nasal sinuses or a lung cavity from old tuberculosis or bronchiectasis. Infection of these cavities tends to be a local problem, but if invasion of surrounding tissue occurs, often in immunosuppressed patients, then treatment is difficult and the prognosis is grim. The locally growing "fungus-ball" or Aspergilloma may need to be resected, usually because of hemorrhage, since antifungal agents will not reach the organism. The most common organism causing invasive pulmonary disease is Aspergillus fumigatus, but A. flavus, niger, and terreus may also cause infection. Systemic infection may involve almost any organ; disease of the heart valve and brain are common sites. The antemortem diagnosis of Aspergillosis may be difficult [5,6].

15.3 Medical history

15.3.1 Fungal disease

Infection of an animal by fungus had been illustrated or described in the mid-seventeenth to early eighteenth centuries, but the first great investigator was Agostino Bassi (1773 – 1856, figure 15.4), an Italian lawyer who retired to his father's farm when poor eyesight forced him to give up his administrative position. Bassi had many interests and his teachers included Lazzaro Spallanzani who had published important papers disproving spontaneous generation of fungi. In 1807 Bassi began to investigate muscardine disease that had damaged the silkworm industry in Italy and France. He subjected silkworms to many environmental changes but failed to reproduce the disease. In 1816, stimulated by the observation of some natural epidemics, Bassi began to investigate the possibility that muscardine disease was caused by an "extraneous germ". He examined the white efflorescence that developed on the dead silkworms under his microscope and found it to be a "plant of the cryptogamic kind, a parasitic fungus". There are now known to be many types of muscardine disease affecting different insects, often named for their color and caused by different fungi. The white muscardine that Bassi studied is caused by Beauveria bassiana. Other important early workers in the field of mycology were Robert Remak (1815 – 1865), a German physician who discovered that the skin disease favus was caused by a fungus after he successfully inoculated himself with it, and David Gruby (1810 – 1898), a Hungarian physician, who discovered the fungal etiology of several different human skin diseases and of *mouget* (oral thrush in infants). Gruby later left research for his medical practice; his patients included Franz List, Frederic Chopin and George Sand. Rudolph Virchow described human pulmonary Aspergillosis in 1856 [7].

15.4 Laboratory medicine

15.4.1 Aspergillus

Aspergillus is a septate hyaline mold, a large group of saprophytic fungi that contains many different possible pathogens. Aspergillus species can be found in soil, composted leaves, and stored grain. The hyphae of Aspergillus species are septate and divide at a 45-degree angle. They are best seen in tissue sections using a PAS or silver stain. It is important to remember that not all fungi with septate hyphae that divide at 45 degrees are Aspergillus. Some patients may mount a granulomatous reaction to Aspergillus. These granulomas may contain small fragments of Aspergillus hyphae. The fruiting head of Aspergillus may be seen in fungus balls where the oxygen tension is relatively high, and the histologic features of these conidiophores may be helpful in making a specific diagnosis. Aspergillus mold grows quickly on culture medium, unlike the dimorphic fungal pathogens. The color and morphology of the colonies and the morphologic details of the conidiophores under a dissecting microscope should permit speciation [8]. Other diagnostic tests include serum galactomannan, a component of Aspergillus conidial cell walls. This test is specific for Aspergillus, but it is relatively insensitive, and it is not used much for the detection of early disease [5].

15.5 Study questions

1. Where might one come into contact with Aspergillus?

2. Name a component of the immune system that is important for the control of an Aspergillus infection.

3. For many years, mushrooms were thought to be associated with or caused by thunder. Why might people have thought this was so?

4. Both Drs. Remak and Gruby had difficulty getting academic appointments because of their religion. Why would anyone think that one's religion would affect his or her performance as a professor?

5. Serum galactomannan might not be ordered for the diagnosis of Aspergillosis since it might be too insensitive to detect an infection quickly. Why would the patient's clinicians be in a hurry to make a diagnosis?

15.6 References

1. Tasci S, Glasmacher A, Lentini S *et al.* Pseudomembranous and obstructive Aspergillus tracheobronchitis - optimal diagnostic strategy and outcome. Mycoses. 2006;49:37-42.
2. Routsi C, Kaltsas P, Bessis E, Rontogianni D, Kollias S, Roussos C. Airway obstruction and acute respiratory failure due to Aspergillus tracheobronchitis. Crit Care Med. 2004;32:580-582.
3. Clancy CJ, Nguyen MH. Acute community-acquired pneumonia due to Aspergillus in presumably immunocompetent hosts: clues for recognition of a rare but fatal disease. Chest. 1998;114:629-634.
4. Maurer C, Collon T, Bodiguel V, Cymbalista M, Adotti F, Piquet J. [Aspergillus bronchitis in an immunocompetent patient]. Rev Pneumol Clin. 2001;57:221-224.
5. Sugar AM. Fungi. In: Porter RS, Kaplan JL, editors. The Merck manual of diagnosis and therapy. Whitehouse Station, NJ: Merck Sharpe & Dohme Corp.; 2011. p. 1329.
6. Peppercorn A, Serody JS. Fungal infections. In: Runge MS, Greganti MA, editor. Netter's Internal Medicine. Philadelphia: Saunders Elsevier; 2009. p. 735 - 744.
7. Ainsworth GC. Introduction to the history of Mycology. New York: Cambridge University Press; 1976:163.

8. Iwen PC. Mycotic Diseases. In: MacPherson RA, Pincus MR, editors. Henry's Clinical Diagnosis and Management by Laboratory Methods. Philadelphia: Elsevier Saunders; 2011. p. 1182 - 1185.

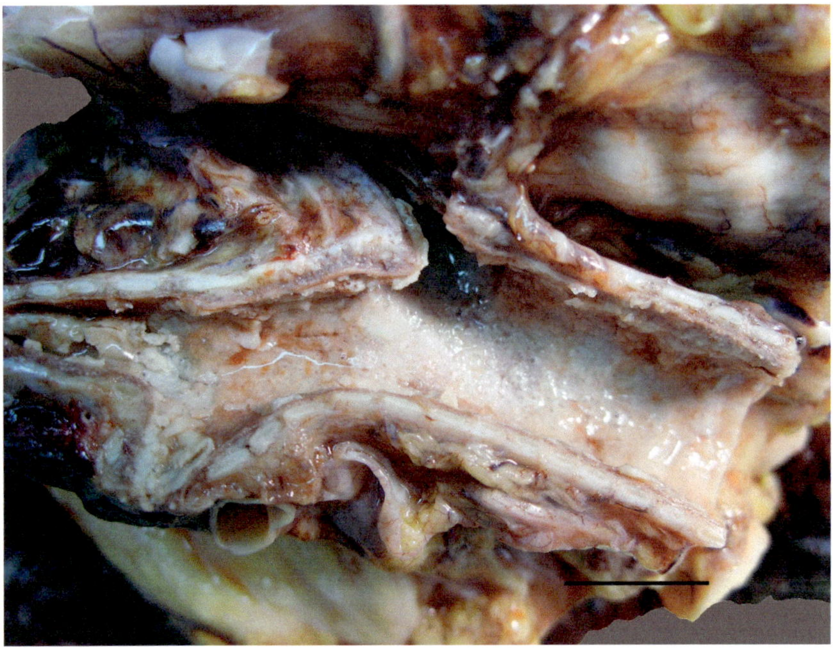

Figure 15.1 A main bronchus with exudate on the mucosal surface. The exudate was slightly green on original gross examination. The black bar is 1 cm long.

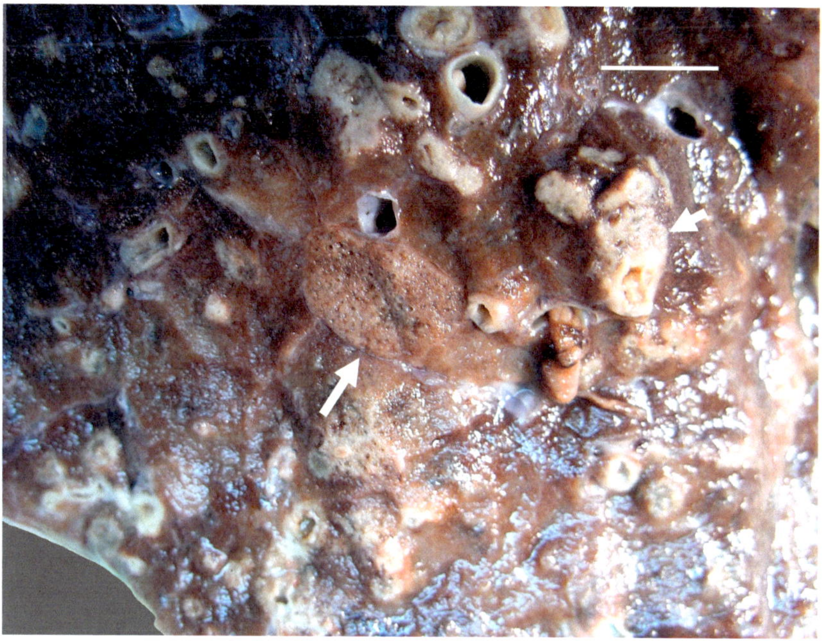

Figure 15.2 A section of one of the patient's lungs. The bronchial walls are thickened and there are peribronchial white areas (short white arrow on right). There is a central brown area with thickened alveolar walls that was firm to palpation (long white arrow). These represent the invasion of the lung by Aspergillus and pneumonia respectively. The white bar is 1 cm long.

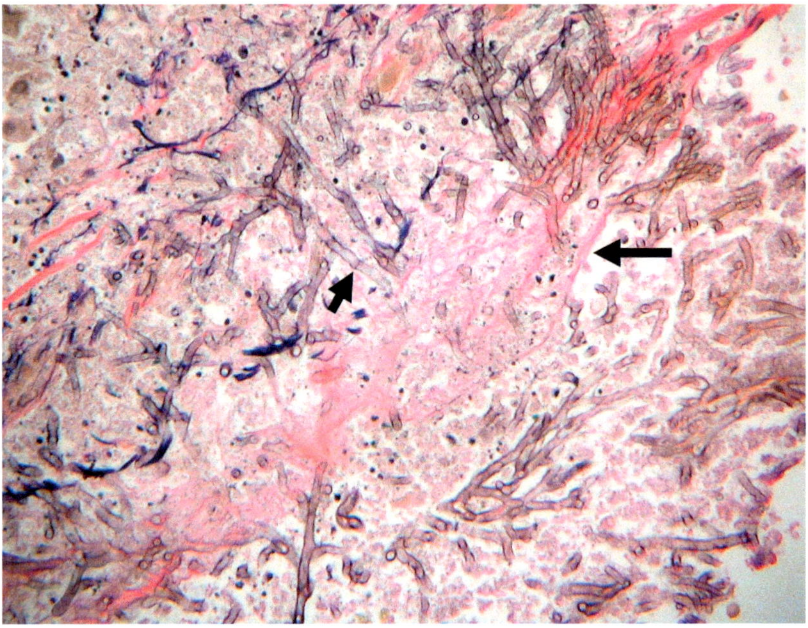

Figure 15.3 A histologic section of the bronchial wall. The long arrow points to what is left of the bronchial epithelial basement membrane; the fungal hyphae invade into underlying necrotic tissue. The short arrow points to a septum in a fungal hypha. This is a silver stain to highlight the fungi. The original magnification is 200x.

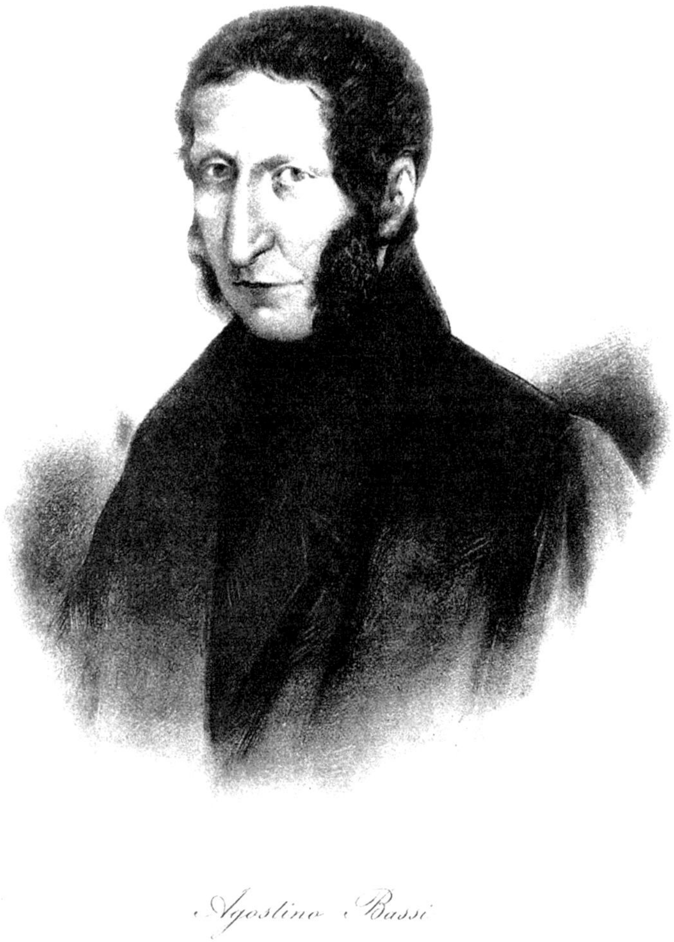

Figure 15.4 Agostino Bassi (1773 – 1856). Courtesy of the Wellcome Library Collection.

CHAPTER 16

A 60-year-old woman with aortic dissection. (Vindicate, vascular)

"The fool questions what he sees, but not what he knows. The wise man questions what he knows, not what he sees." Huang Po (c. 840)

16.1 The Autopsy

16.1.1 Case history

The patient was a 60-year-old woman who was found apneic and unresponsive while seated at home. She had a history of hypertension, chronic obstructive lung disease, and she had had two brain aneurysms that were treated with clips. She smoked cigarettes and her medications included atorvastatin/amlodipine (for high cholesterol and high blood pressure), benazepril (ACE inhibitor, anti-hypertensive), Adderall (psychostimulant), clonidine (anti-hypertensive), paroxetine (antidepressant), Combivent inhaler (albuterol/ipratropium for COPD), lorazepam (anti-anxiety), temazepam (hypnotic for insomnia), and oxcarbazepine (anti-epileptic). The patient had been awake and, apparently, without complaint about 30 minutes prior to being discovered unresponsive. When the emergency medical technicians arrived, her EKG showed pulseless electrical activity. She was brought to the hospital Emergency department, but could not be resuscitated.

16.1.2 Postmortem findings

At autopsy, the pericardial space contained a moderate amount of clotted blood. The heart weighed 510 grams (normal = 350 grams) with biventricular hypertrophy. The patient had moderate calcific coronary artery atherosclerosis, but the coronaries were widely patent and there was no gross evidence of a myocardial infarct. The ascending aorta also showed moderate atherosclerosis and there was a 1 cm long transverse tear in the aortic intima, 1.8 cm above the aortic valve (figures 16.1, 16.2). There was an area of hemorrhagic discoloration on the epicardial surface of the heart near the aortic root. The aorta had a mural dissection extending from the root of the aorta to just distal to the origin of the left subclavian artery. Other findings included a 1.5 cm deep well-demarcated scar in the left renal cortex, atherosclerosis of the basilar artery, and a metal clip on the anterior circle of Willis. Histologic examination of the heart confirmed the presence of myocardial hypertrophy with mild replacement type fibrosis and without evidence of acute myocardial ischemia. Sections of the aorta showed no vasculitis, no changes diagnostic of so-called cystic medial necrosis, and no detectable changes with an elastic stain. Sections of lung showed abundant hemosiderin in intra-alveolar histiocytes.

16.1.3 Case summary

The postmortem findings were diagnostic of aortic dissection associated with a tear in the proximal aorta and extending to just beyond the origin of the left subclavian artery. This type of dissection can be classified as DeBakey type I and Stanford type A. It is the most common type of dissection and the type that, in the acute stage, may be associated with perforation into the pericardial space; a fatal event. The patient had biventricular cardiac hypertrophy indicating hypertensive heart disease, the most common risk factor for aortic dissection. Some patients with certain connective tissue disorders (e.g. Marfan's syndrome and Ehler-Danlos syndrome) are at increased risk for aortic dissection, and since the patient had a history of cerebral artery aneurysms, this possibility was considered. But no other signs of these disorders were found. The presence of hemosiderin in the patient's pulmonary intraalveolar histiocytes suggested the possibility of some degree of heart failure, but another explanation was that she smoked cigarettes.

16.2 Discussion

16.2.1 Aortic dissection

The aorta is the largest artery in the body and it has elastic properties. The wall of the aorta comprises three layers, the endothelial lining, the muscular media, and the outer fibrous adventitia. Aortic dissection is the idiopathic formation of a tear in the lining of the artery with penetration of blood into the wall and separation of the laminar layers. About 50% of the tears occur in the ascending aorta, but they may occur anywhere along its course. The age distribution of aortic dissection is bimodal. Most patients are in their sixth and seventh decade and have hypertension. Males outnumber females four to one. Some patients with a connective tissue disorder (e.g. Marfan's syndrome or Ehler-Danlos syndrome) are also at increased risk for aortic dissection but tend to present in their third to fifth decades. Aortic dissection may rarely occur in pregnancy. Bicuspid aortic valve and coarctation of the aorta are also risk factors. Patients often present with the sudden onset of tearing chest or back pain. The dissection may cause aortic regurgitation and cut off circulation in branch arteries leading to associated signs and symptoms such as loss of a peripheral pulse, discordant blood pressure readings in the right and left arms, ischemic bowel, or spinal ischemia leading to paraparesis. The dissection may perforate into the pericardial space (as described in the case above) causing cardiac tamponade, or into the pleural space or the abdominal cavity. Aortic dissection is a grave illness, 20% of patients die before they reach the hospital and as many as 35% die of operative or perioperative complications. The disease has been classified based on the location and extent of the dissection (The DeBakey and Stanford classification systems); in general, the cases are divided into those that occur in the ascending aorta and those that occur more distally. The prognosis is better for cases with distal dissection. The diagnosis is usually made radiographically or by transesophageal ultrasound (figure 16.3). Chest radiograph often shows widening of the mediastinum. Multiplanar transesophageal ultrasonography is highly sensitive and specific for the diagnosis. Computed tomography angiography and magnetic resonance angiography are also excellent tests for aortic dissection. The treatment usually involves aggressive control of the patient's blood pressure and serial imaging to monitor the progression of the dissection. Surgical repair of the aorta and placement of a synthetic graft are frequently necessary, especially in dissection of the ascending aorta. Some patients with distal dissections are treated with endovascular stents.

It has been presumed for many years that patients with aortic dissection have an abnormal arterial wall that leads to a weakened area susceptible to penetration by blood at high pressure, but the exact nature of the abnormality is not known [1,2].

16.3 Medical history

16.3.1 Aortic aneurysm and dissection

The distinction between aortic aneurysm and aortic dissection was only made in the 20th century; the term dissecting aortic aneurysm is still commonly used. Peripheral aneurysms were known in antiquity. Antonio Scarpa's (Italian anatomist, 1752 – 1832, figure 16.4) treatise on aneurysms in 1808 attributed the original description to Jean François Fernel (French physician, 1497 – 1558) in 1542. In 1628 Daniel Sennert (German physician and chemist, 1572 – 1637) described a case of aortic dissection that he thought was the mechanism of the formation of all aortic aneurysms.

G. B. Morgagni also described a case of aortic dissection that penetrated the pericardial sac [3]. He described the process of dissection as

"...the blood had, by degrees, made itself a way through one of the intervals of this kind, and had come out under the external coat of the artery; and first by drawing it from the internal coats, and then by raising it, as a large kind of ecchymosis...and finally, by distending it more and more, had burst through this external coat in one place, and had poured itself out within the pericardium."

Perhaps the most famous decedent with a diagnosis of aortic dissection, who died with findings quite like those seen in the case presented above, was King George II of Great Britain. The 76-year-old King had his usual morning hot chocolate on October 25th, 1760 then went to use the toilet. His valet de chamber heard a groan and found the King lying unresponsive on the floor with a facial laceration. An autopsy was performed the next day and the pericardium contained a pint of coagulated blood. A 1.5-inch long transverse fissure was found in the ascending aorta through which blood had passed to the external surface of the aorta [4].

J. P. Maunoir (French physician, 1768 – 1861) gave the first detailed and accurate description of aortic dissection in 1802, but many physicians adhered to the concept of Sennert that dissection preceded all aneurysms. Laénnec believed this as well and coined the term 'dissecting aneurysm' (anévrisme disséquant) in the second edition of his great work on auscultation in 1826. That the dissection passed between layers of the aortic media was shown by C. W. Pennock (1799 – 1867) in 1839. [5]

16.4 Laboratory medicine

16.4.1 Aortic dissection

The diagnosis of aortic dissection is made by clinical signs and symptoms and using various imaging techniques as described above. Patients with aortic dissection may have slight anemia from blood loss. Lactate dehydrogenase may be elevated, especially in those with mesenteric ischemia. Troponin might be helpful in distinguishing a myocardial infarct from aortic dissection, but would be confounded by a patient with both dissection and myocardial ischemia. There has been interest in the development of blood tests for the detection of aortic dissection, and various assays have been tested. D-dimer, a fibrin degradation product, has been shown to be sensitive for the detection of aortic dissection, but it has poor specificity and may be elevated in pulmonary thromboembolism, trauma, recent surgery, and similar conditions. Smooth muscle myosin heavy chain is a sensitive and specific test for the detection of aortic dissection, but it is only useful in the first three hours after the onset of symptoms and it is more sensitive for proximal lesions. Studies using the calcium binding protein calponin have shown that both the acidic and basic isoforms are elevated in patients with aortic dissection. An assay for soluble elastin has shown elevation in patients with re-entry type dissection, but not in patients with a "closed" type aortic dissection. There is also some evidence that Transforming growth factor beta is elevated in patients with aortic dissection. At present, blood tests do not play a large role in the diagnosis of aortic dissection [6].

16.5 Study questions

1. Why might a patient's hemoglobin be decreased in the presence of aortic dissection?

2. How is the antemortem diagnosis of aortic dissection made?

3. What famous French physician coined the term, "dissecting aneurysm"?

4. King George II of Britain died of a ruptured aortic dissection. What systemic illness is King George III thought to have suffered from?

5. What is the difference between a Stanford type A and a Stanford type B dissection?

16.6 References

1. Hallett JW, Jr. Aortic dissection. The Merck Manual of diagnosis and therapy. Whitehouse Station, NJ: Merck Sharp & Dohme Corp.; 2011. p. 2212 - 2214.

2. Mitchell RN. Blood vessels. In: Kumar V, Abbas AK, Aster JC, editors. Robbins and Cotran Pathologic basis of disease. Philadelphia: Elsevier Saunders; 2015. p. 491 - 500.

3. Morgagni G. The Seats and Causes of Diseases. Alexander B, translator. London: A. Millar and T. Cadell; 1769. Volume 1, pp. 803-804, letter XXVI, Article 17

4. Leonard JC. Thomas Bevill Peacock and the history of dissecting aneurysm. Br Med J. 1979;2:260 - 262.

5. Acierno LJ. The history of Cardiology. New York: Parthenon; 1994:65.

6. Listijono DR, Pepper JR. Current imaging techniques and potential biomarkers in the diagnosis of acute aortic dissection. J R Soc Med Sh Rep. 2012;3

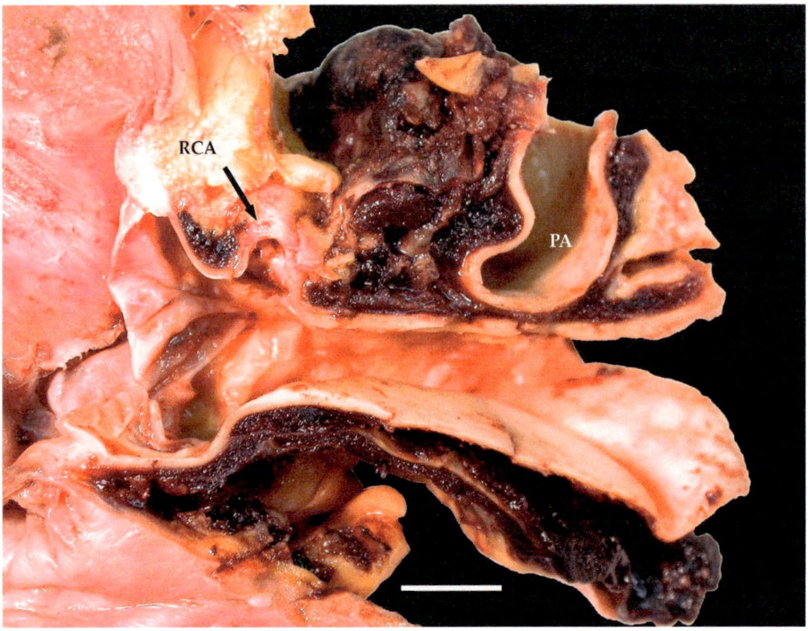

Figure 16.1 A section through the aortic root. The band of hemorrhage in the wall of the aorta, which is best seen in the lower half of the image, is the dissection. RCA = origin of the right coronary artery. PA = pulmonary artery. The white bar is 1 cm long.

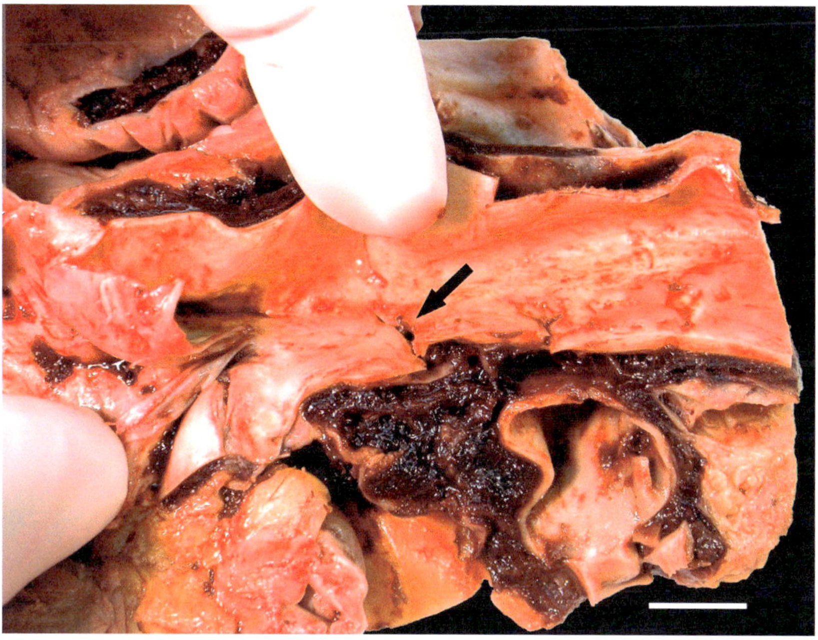

Figure 16.2 A section through the aortic root with the lumen exposed. The black arrow points to the intimal tear and entry point of the dissection. The white bar is 1 cm long.

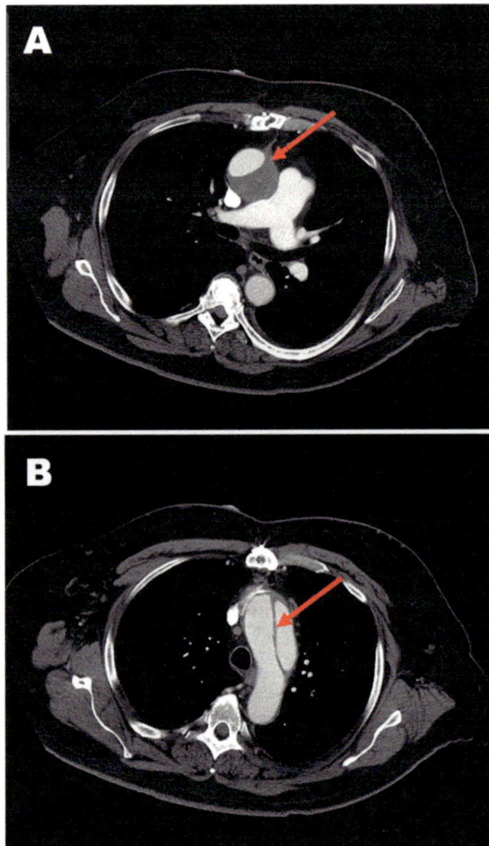

Figure 16.3.A An axial contrast enhanced CT at the level of the pulmonary arteries from a different case shows a crescentic-shaped low-density lesion (red arrow) within the anterior/ascending aortic arch consistent with an intramural hematoma vs a dissection flap with clot and compatible with a Type A aortic dissection.

Figure 16.3.B An axial contrast enhanced CT at the level of the aortic arch shows a dissection flap (red arrow) within the lumen diagnostic for aortic dissection. Two lumens form as a result of the flap, a true lumen and a false lumen (under the arrow's head). The false lumen can be occluded by thrombus as seen in figure 16.3.A.

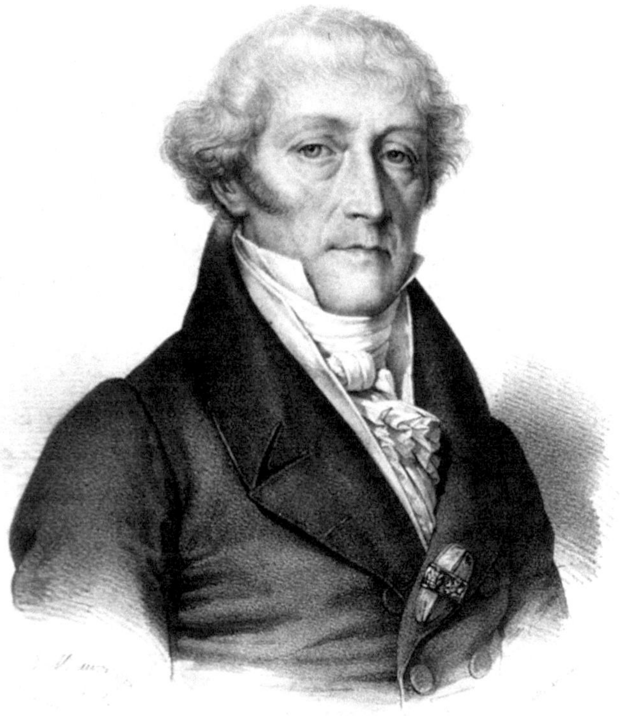

Figure 16.4 Antonio Scarpa (1752 – 1832). Courtesy of the National Library of Medicine.

Chapter 17

A 60-year-old man with amyloidosis. (viNdiCAte, Type AL amyloid can be considered of neoplastic origin, type ATTR can be classified as congenital, type AA is often seen in rheumatoid arthritis, an autoimmune disease.)

"The road to medical knowledge is through the pathological museum and not through an apothecary's shop." William Withey Gull (1816 – 1890, a great physician by many standards, but accused of being the serial killer Jack the Ripper in some works of literature, long after his death).

17.1 The Autopsy

17.1.1 Case history

A 60-year-old man with end-stage renal disease and a history of amyloidosis was admitted to the hospital with splenomegaly and abdominal tenderness. A previous workup had shown that the patient had a primary AL type amyloid. The patient had had a stem cell transplant several months prior. His left ventricular ejection fraction was 25% (normal > 55%) and he was said to have hyperlipidemia. A diagnosis of peritonitis and sepsis with a Gram-negative bacillus was made and the patient was treated with antibiotics. A peritoneal fluid culture grew an Alcaligenes species. He had thrombocytopenia that was thought to be due to sepsis. The patient was treated with antibiotics and was doing better, but had some runs of ventricular tachycardia. He elected to discontinue his dialysis on the twelfth hospital day and died a few days later.

17.1.2 Postmortem findings

At autopsy, the patient had 4 liters of cloudy yellow ascitic fluid. The spleen weighed 450 grams (normal = 150 grams) and had a waxy consistency on cut section (figure 17.1). The left lung weighed 375 grams, but the right lung weighed 675 grams (normal = 350 grams). No definite gross pulmonary consolidation was seen. The heart weighed 650 grams (normal = 350 grams) with left and right ventricular hypertrophy. No coronary artery disease was present.

Histologic examination showed interstitial and vascular wall amyloid deposition in all the examined organs except the brain (figures 17.2, 17.3). The patient had acute bronchitis and acute bronchopneumonia in the left lower, right upper, and right middle lung lobes.

Immunohistochemical stains on a portion of the patient's spleen were said to be equivocal for amyloid type. An antemortem evaluation of biopsy tissue had shown AL type amyloid.

17.1.3 Case summary

The patient had a history of end-stage renal disease and a more recent diagnosis of amyloidosis. Some patients with a long history of renal dialysis accumulate the protein beta-2 microglobulin in their body and develop a secondary amyloidosis from it, but this patient had had an antemortem workup from a previous tissue biopsy that showed AL type amyloidosis. Beta-2 microglobulin type amyloid has become uncommon with the use of modern dialysis filters, and patients with primary AL amyloidosis often progress to renal failure. There was no evidence of multiple myeloma or obvious plasmacytosis at autopsy, but those findings are often absent in patients with AL amyloidosis. The bacteria Alcaligenes faecalis can be a dialyzer contaminant, but in this case, it was the probable cause of the patient's sepsis.

17.2 Discussion

17.2.1 Amyloidosis

Amyloidosis is a group of diseases all characterized by extracellular deposition of one of various insoluble proteins. The deposited materials have certain constituents in common, and about 95% of the material in all of them consists of a non-branching 7.5 to 10 nm diameter fibril that stains homogeneously pink on hematoxylin and eosin stain and metachromatically red with the Congo red stain. In the 19th century, the gross staining properties of the material in the organs of patients with the disease were thought to be similar or even identical to those of starch (amylose) and the disease has been called amyloidosis since then. The protein in amyloidosis may be any one of over 20 different proteins. The proteins are not toxic, but as they accumulate over time, they cause damage to the surrounding cells of the involved organs.

The different diseases that make up amyloidosis can be classified in various ways. A common system is to divide it into primary amyloidosis, the most common form, due to the deposition of immunoglobulin light chains (AL amyloid); secondary amyloidosis due to the deposition of AA amyloid, a degradation product of the acute phase reactant serum amyloid A; familial amyloidosis due to the deposition of an abnormal plasma protein, usually abnormal transthyretin (ATTR amyloid); and several other even rarer forms. Amyloid may accumulate locally in the islets of Langerhans in patients with type 2 diabetes mellitus, in the thyroid gland in patients with medullary carcinoma, and in the brain in patients with Alzheimer's disease. Patients on chronic dialysis for renal failure may develop amyloidosis that contains beta-2 microglobulin, a component of the major histocompatibility complex.

There are about 2500 new cases of AL type amyloidosis in the US each year. These patients make an abnormal monoclonal immunoglobulin light chain that accumulates in the body. Common sites of deposition include the skin, nerves, gastrointestinal tract, the tongue, kidneys, liver, spleen, and blood vessels, but amyloid may accumulate in any organ. These patients have a clone of plasma cells that produce the abnormal light chains, but most of them do not have a demonstrable tumor. Only a minority of the patients has the diagnostic features of multiple myeloma, a malignant tumor of plasma cells.

Secondary amyloidosis is due to the accumulation of AA protein, which is a degradation product of a circulating acute phase reactant. These patients either have a chronic inflammatory disease or a malignancy. The inflammatory disease has historically included tuberculosis, bronchiectasis, osteomyelitis, and leprosy, but in modern times most of these patients have inflammatory bowel disease or rheumatoid arthritis. About 3% of patients with rheumatoid arthritis have amyloidosis, but in only about half of those patients is the protein deposition of any clinical significance. The most common malignancies associated with AA amyloidosis are renal cell carcinoma and Hodgkin's lymphoma.

Familial amyloidosis has many forms, but the most common is due to hepatic production of an abnormal form of transthyretin (prealbumin), a circulating protein that binds to retinol and the thyroid hormone thyroxin. These patients often present with a neuropathy and may also get carpal tunnel syndrome from amyloid deposition. Patients with the autosomal recessively inherited Familial Mediterranean Fever may also get amyloidosis.

The diagnosis of amyloidosis is made by tissue biopsy and light microscopic examination using special stains, most often Congo red. Patients with suspected AL amyloid usually have serum and urine protein electrophoresis and they may have a bone marrow biopsy to identify a monoclonal plasma cell population. Scintigraphy with radiolabeled serum amyloid P may be useful for diagnosis and to follow patients with amyloidosis.

The prognosis of primary AL amyloidosis is poor with a median survival time of two years. Patients with myeloma and AL amyloidosis have an even shorter median survival time. These patients may be treated with chemotherapy and some patients may receive an autologous stem cell transplant. Patients with secondary AA amyloidosis have a better prognosis, especially if the underlying inflammatory or malignant disorder can be treated. Patients with familial ATTR amyloidosis often survive untreated for 10 - 15 years. They have hepatic production of the abnormal protein and may be treated with liver transplantation [1,2].

17.3 Medical history

17.3.1 Amyloidosis

Several case reports from the 17th through the 19th century might have been amyloidosis. Thomas Bartholin (1616 – 1680), the Danish physician who was the first to describe the human lymphatic system, reported the case of a woman whose spleen was so hard that it could only be cut with difficulty. Other case reports in the 18th and 19th centuries described skin masses and enlargement of the liver, spleen, or kidneys, all with a gray waxy albuminous quality. In 1842 Carl von Rokitansky commented that some patients with tuberculosis, syphilis, or mercury poisoning had enlargement of the liver due to the infiltration by a gray albuminous, gelatinous, lardaceous substance.

The term amyloid was coined by Matthias Schleiden (1804 – 1881), a German botanist, in 1838 to describe a normal starch-like constituent of plants. Rudolph Virchow (figure 17.4) discussed amyloidosis in his lecture of April 17, 1858. Virchow used the term amyloid and commented that he was referring to the same material that was called lardaceous (or literally bacon-like) in Vienna and waxy in Edinburgh. He discussed the use of the iodine test for starch on amyloid and some similar substances at autopsy or on histologic sections. A solution of iodine/potassium iodide will form a blue or dark purple color with amyloid, giving an appearance similar to the reaction seen with starch, and causing some confusion at the time.

It was discovered in the late 19th century that some of the newly discovered aniline dyes would stain amyloid a color that was slightly different from the color of the dye in the bottle. This phenomenon was called metachromasia and examined in detail, most importantly for leukocytes, by Paul Ehrlich (1864 – 1915). Methyl violet stains amyloid metachromatically and was used by André-Victor Cornil in 1875 to show that amyloid was an extracellular material. Congo red was one of many aniline dyes developed for the textile industry at Bayer in Germany at the time of the 1884 – 1885 Berlin West Africa Conference when many dyes received names referencing Africa (e.g. Sudan black). Bayer initially had no interest in the dye and it was later produced by AGFA. In 1922, Bennhold described the use of Congo red as a metachromatic stain for amyloid and it is still used for this purpose today. Bennhold also described a proposed test in which patients were injected with intravenous Congo red and had its disappearance from the plasma and accumulation in amyloid deposits quantified.

The English physician Henry Bence Jones (1813 – 1873, figure 17.5) described a protein in urine in patients with multiple myeloma in 1847. This protein is now known to be immunoglobulin light chain, the same material that forms AL amyloid. A. Magnus-Levy (1931) raised the question of Bence Jones protein as the 'mother substance' of amyloidosis. In a later publication, he noted that amyloidosis could occur in patients with both large and small amounts of Bence Jones protein and suggested that there was decreased metabolism of the protein in patients with amyloidosis. It is now thought that the particular amino acid sequence in some patient's monoclonal light chains makes them susceptible to abnormal folding and predisposed to form the beta-pleated sheet conformation of amyloid [3-5].

17.4 Laboratory medicine

17.4.1 Alcaligenes

Alcaligenes is a genus of Gram-negative bacilli that was originally isolated from feces and the most commonly isolated species of the genus is Alcaligenes faecalis. The organism is, however, widely present in water and soil and can be found in moist environments in the hospital including dialyzer equipment. Alcaligenes is motile, strictly aerobic and both oxidase and catalase positive. It has been found in some urinary tract and respiratory tract infections and in some cases of bacterial sepsis [6,7].

17.4.2 Speciation of amyloidosis

For many years pathologists were happy with a simple diagnosis of amyloidosis, but since the disease is now understood in more detail, and amyloid can be any one of more than 20 different proteins, a more specific diagnosis is necessary. Patients with disease from amyloid due to immunoglobulin light chains may be treated with chemotherapy or bone marrow transplantation, but patients with increased hepatic production of an abnormal transthyretin may be treated with liver transplantation; clearly the distinction is critical.

Immunohistochemical stains for AA protein, immunoglobulin light chains lambda and kappa, amyloid P component, and beta-2 microglobulin are available. Amyloid P is present in all types of amyloid, but it is also found in normal connective tissue. Antibodies available for immunoglobulin light chain tend to stain the non-variable end of the protein, and some patient's AL protein will not stain. Beta-2 microglobulin antibodies may be adequate, but they are difficult to validate and use in the laboratory without control materials for this rare condition. Because of these problems, and the increasing number of types of rare amyloid proteins, some large medical centers may perform more elaborate tests including chemical analysis to show protein size and amino acid sequencing [8 – 10].

17.5 Study questions

1. How did amyloidosis get its name?

2. What does metachromatic mean?

3. Which organs are usually affected in patients with primary (AL) type amyloidosis?

4. How may patients with primary (AL) type amyloidosis be treated?

5. Does Alcaligenes faecalis occur anywhere besides feces?

17.6 References

1. Kumar V, Abbas AK, Aster JC. Robbins and Cotran Pathologic basis of disease. Philadelphia: Elsevier Saunders; 2015
2. Cohen AS. Amyloidosis. In: Porter RS, Kaplan JL, editors. The Merck Manual of Diagnosis and Therapy. Whitehouse Station, NJ: Merck Sharp & Dohme Corp.; 2011. p. 905 - 907.
3. Kyle RA. Amyloidosis: A convoluted story. Br J Haematology. 2001;114:529 - 538.
4. Steensma DP. "Congo" red: Out of Africa? Arch Pathol Lab Med. 2001;125:250 - 252.
5. Virchow R. Cellular Pathology. Birmingham, Alabama: Gryphon editions, Ltd.; 1860:204.
6. Jorgensen JH, Pfaller MA. A clinician's dictionary of pathogenic microorganisms. Washington, D.C: ASM Press; 2004:273.
7. Tille PM. Bailey & Scott's Diagnostic Microbiology. St. Louis: Elsevier Mosby; 2014

8. Miller RT. Immunohistochemistry in Amyloidosis. http://www.pro-path.com/companies/press-clippings/26-newsletters/261-immunohistochemistry-in-amyloidosis-september-2004. 2004
9. Kaplan B, Martin BM, Livneh A, Pras M, Gallo GR. Biochemical subtyping of amyloid in formalin-fixed tissue samples confirms and supplements immunohistologic data. Am J Clin Pathol. 2004;121:794-800.
10. Gertz MA. The classification and typing of amyloid deposits. Am J Clin Pathol. 2004;121:787-789.

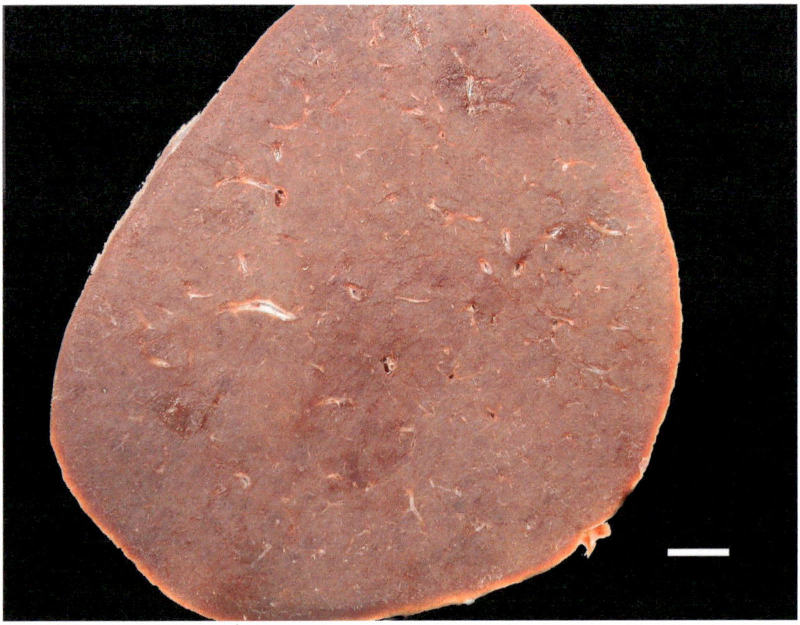

Figure 17.1 The cut surface of the patient's spleen showing enlargement and an unusual uniform waxy quality. Some amyloidosis patients have deposition of amyloid in the Malpighian corpuscles and the resulting white nodularity is called sago spleen (sago is a tapioca-like flavorless starch used in cooking that comes from the sago palm). The spleen, in this case, is like those that have been called waxy or lardaceous spleen. The white bar is 1 cm long.

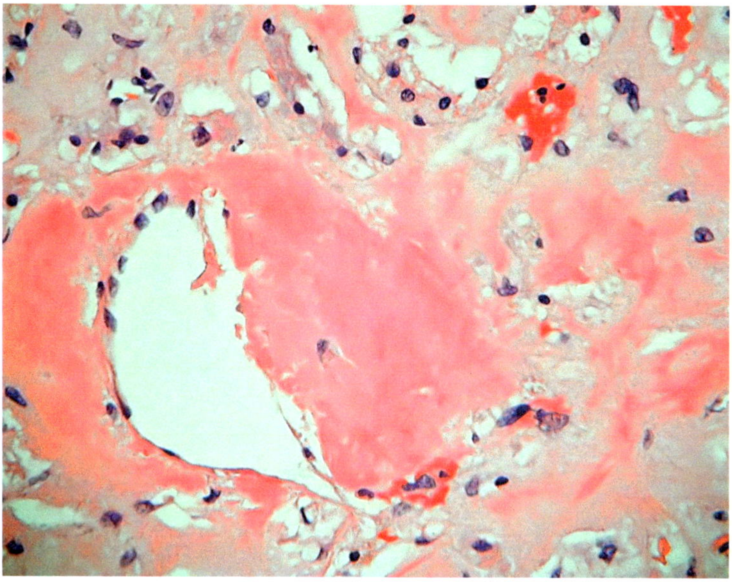

Figure 17.2 A histologic section of the patient's adrenal gland showing deposition of perivascular extracellular material that stains homogeneously pink with a standard hematoxylin and eosin stain. (Original magnification x 200, H&E stain)

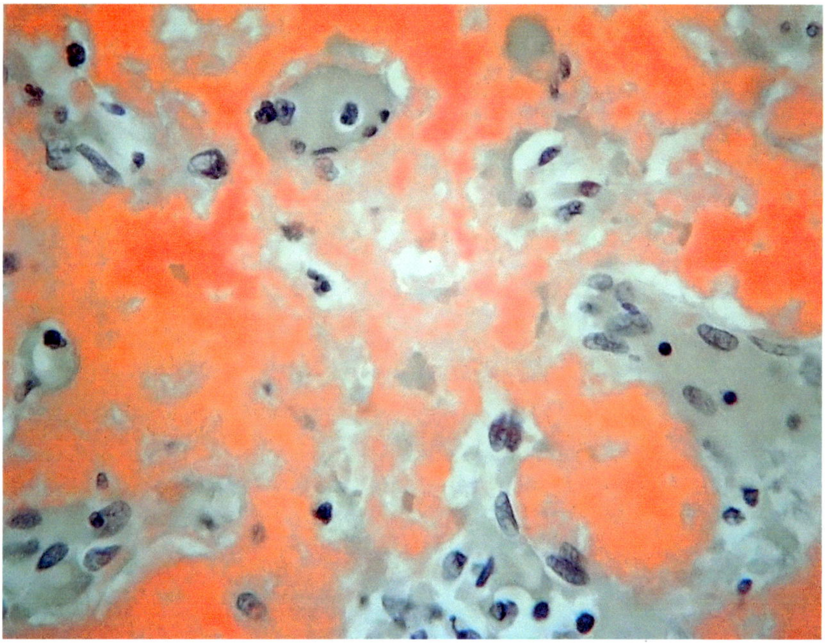

Figure 17.3 A histologic section of the patient's adrenal gland showing red metachromatic staining of amyloid by Congo red. (Original magnification x400, Congo red stain)

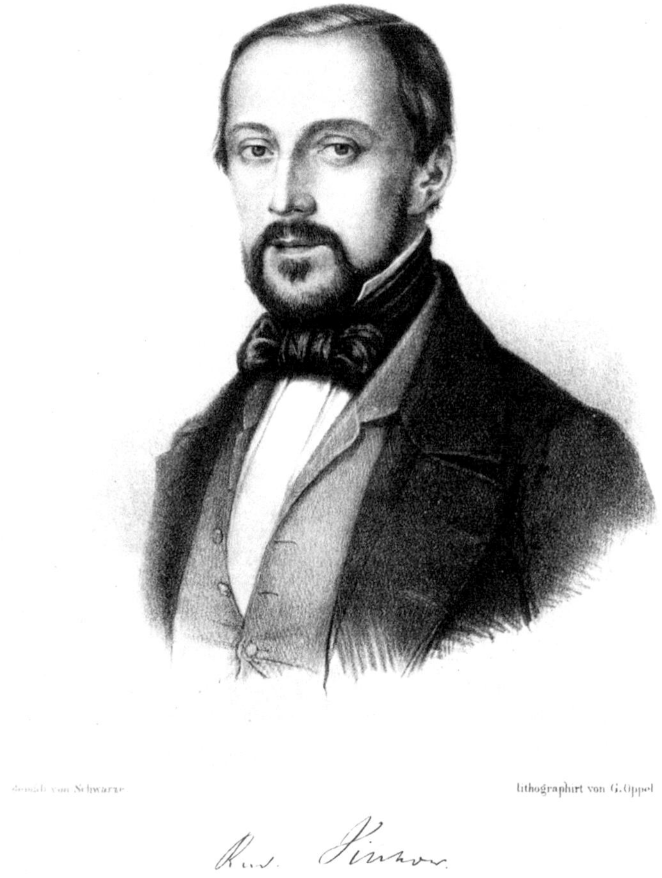

Figure 17.4 Rudolph Virchow (1821 – 1902). Courtesy of the National Library of Medicine.

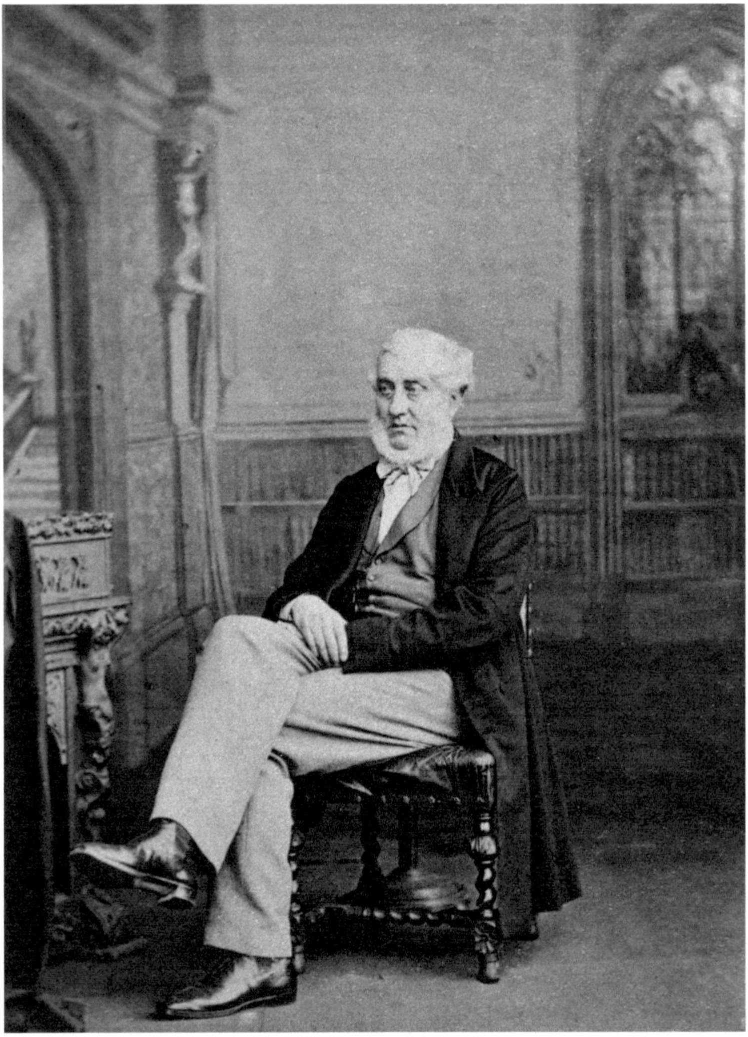

Figure 17.5 Henry Bence Jones (1813 – 1873). Courtesy of the National Library of Medicine.

CHAPTER 18

A 19-week stillborn fetus with placental abruption and maternal cocaine use. (vinDiCate, drug, congenital)

"I was making frequent use of cocaine at that time ... I had been the first to recommend the use of cocaine, in 1885, and this recommendation had brought serious reproaches down on me." Sigmund Freud (1856 – 1939), The Interpretation of Dreams

18.1 The Autopsy

18.1.1 Case history

The patient's mother was a 30-year-old G4P0120 woman (She'd been pregnant four times, she had had one child that was delivered prematurely and two abortions, and recall that the medical term abortion means a preterm loss from any cause.). She was seen for a level 2 ultrasonographic examination at

19 weeks gestation and was noted to have cervical dilatation. A level 2 ultrasound is more detailed than a level one ultrasound; fetal measurements, the placental location and detailed views of the fetal viscera are made. She was sent to the hospital where she had spontaneous onset of labor and had vaginal delivery of a stillborn female fetus. The patient's mother (recall that at the autopsy of a stillborn fetus, the fetus is called the patient) had had the usual prenatal care tests and was rubella immune, RPR negative (a test for exposure to syphilis), HBsAb negative (a test for exposure to hepatitis B), Gonococcus negative, chlamydia negative, and HIV negative. She had a urine toxicology screen that was positive for cocaine. The patient's mother also used ethanol, tobacco, and marijuana. She had mild leukocytosis after delivery. She was afebrile. Permission was granted for an autopsy.

18.1.2 Postmortem findings

The placenta had abundant maternal surface blood clot (figures 18.1, 18.2). Histologic sections of placenta showed mild acute chorioamnionitis (inflammation of the fetal membranes). Examination of the fetus showed no gross abnormality. The fetus weighed 244 grams with a crown-rump length of 16.5 cm. The postmortem measurements were compatible with a 19-week gestation. The internal viscera were all normal weight. The brain to liver weight ratio was 2.6 (normal about 3).

18.1.3 Case summary

The fetus, in this case, was normal, but the placenta had an unusual amount of clotted blood on its maternal surface. The diagnosis of placental abruption is not usually possible by gross examination of the placenta since there is often some clotted blood on the maternal surface in normal placentas. The usual exception is chronic abruption in which the blood accumulates over time and compresses the underlying placental tissue. This case was also an exception since the amount of blood present was much greater than I've seen in a 19-week stillbirth. Cocaine use is a known risk factor for placental abruption, and

I described the cause of death as prematurity due to placental abruption in a background of maternal cocaine use.

18.2 Discussion

18.2.1 Placental abruption

Placental abruption, also called abruptio placentae, is the premature separation of the placenta from the wall of the uterus. The separation occurs either because of traumatic shearing at the interface between the decidua basalis and the placental tissue, e.g. in a motor vehicle accident, or because of ischemic necrosis in this area (figures 18.3, 18.4). Placental abruption occurs in about 0.5% of deliveries and it is characterized pathologically by retroplacental hemorrhage. As many as 15% of all perinatal deaths are caused by abruption. Fetal mortality is associated with the severity of the abruption, the size of the maternal surface that is involved, and the volume of the blood clot. Clinically, these patients have vaginal bleeding in about 80% of cases, and they may have uterine pain, tetanic uterine contractions and/or abnormal fetal heart rate in 20% of cases. Very rarely placental abruption can cause maternal death, either from blood loss or disseminated intravascular coagulation. The risk of preterm labor and stillbirth are increased. Abruption has a bimodal distribution by maternal age with the highest incidence in young and older mothers.

Many different maternal and placental conditions have been associated with an increased risk of placental abruption. Important ones include maternal cigarette smoking, acute chorioamnionitis, trauma, a prior history of abruption, retroplacental leiomyoma of the uterus, maternal hypertension (especially with preeclampsia), and thrombophilia (e.g. patients with the lupus anticoagulant or an abnormal clotting factor). There has been some controversy whether cocaine can cause placental abruption. [1] The usually proposed mechanism has been vasoconstriction and resultant ischemia and necrosis. There are many case reports and small series reporting an association, and a meta-analysis of 33 studies from 2001 [2] showed that both placental abruption and premature rupture of membranes were associated with cocaine use [3 – 6].

18.2.2 Cocaine

Bitter-tasting plant-derived nitrogen-rich chemical compounds have been sometimes called alkaloids since the 19th century. Some of these compounds have drug-like properties, including mind-altering activity, like cocaine. Cocaine comes from the South American plant Erythroxylum coca, an 8 – 10-foot-high bush with thin green leaves and red berries. It is a derivative of the alkaloid ecgonine. Cocaine hydrochloride is water-soluble and can be absorbed through the mucous membranes or used intravenously. Cocaine is a stimulant that causes a strong feeling of euphoria, a feeling of unreality, and agitation. It is highly addictive. Like other mind-altering drugs of abuse, the precise mechanism of action of cocaine is not known, but it increases the release of multiple different neurotransmitters, including norepinephrine, serotonin, and dopamine and it may inhibit their reuptake at the neuronal synapse. It appears to act especially on the limbic system of the brain and on the sympathetic nervous system. Cocaine is a local anesthetic and is still used for that purpose on mucosal surfaces by otorhinolaryngologists. Freebase and crack cocaine are alkalinization products of cocaine. They are not water-soluble and are usually smoked. After intravenous injection or inhalation, there is a sensation of euphoria in 3 to 5 minutes. The drug is most often snorted, a pathway of delivery that has intermediate effects between oral use and IV injection, with peak serum levels in 20 – 60 minutes and effects that may last for hours. Cocaine is rapidly metabolized by liver esterases (leading to the smaller effect of an oral dose), plasma cholinesterase, and by non-enzymatic hydrolysis. It has a half-life of 1-2 hours and cocaine and its metabolites are usually eliminated from the body by 48 hours.

In addition to being powerfully addictive, cocaine has multiple dangerous properties. It can cause cardiac arrhythmia and up to 25% of myocardial infarcts in patients 18 – 45 years of age have been attributed to cocaine. Cocaine is a vasoconstrictor, and chronic use by snorting can lead to erosion and eventual destruction of the nasal septum. Chronic use can also lead to depression and psychosis. It is estimated that about 25 million Americans have used cocaine at least once.

As mentioned above, cocaine has been associated with placental abruption, but it also easily crosses the placenta into the fetal circulation and is present in breast milk. Infants receiving cocaine in this way may develop growth and mental retardation and drug addiction [7,8].

18.3 Medical history

18.3.1 Placental abruption

A classification of the types of maternal hemorrhage occurring at birth that distinguished between those cases that were inevitable and due to the placenta having grown across the internal cervical os (placenta previa) and those that were due to "accidental" early separation of the placenta (abruptio placentae) was first described by the English physician Edward Rigby (1747 – 1821, figure 18.4). Rigby was born in Lancashire, England in 1747. He was apprenticed at age 14 to the surgeon Mr. Martineau in Norwich and continued his medical training in London. He had a surgical practice in Norwich and later studied obstetrics under Franz Karl Naegele (1778 – 1851) in Heidelburg. Rigby was, apparently, a practicing surgeon and did not receive his medical degree until he was 67 years old. Rigby was elected mayor in 1805 and is said to have introduced vaccination for smallpox in Norwich. His famous paper, "An Essay on the uterine hemorrhage, which precedes the delivery of the full grown foetus. London, Joseph Johnson, 1775" was published in six editions and was translated into French and German.

Rigby wrote:

"causes of *accidental hemorrhage* include blows, falls, to some peculiar laxity of the uterine vessels from badness of habit, or fever, or to the influence of the passions of the mind suddenly exited, such as fear, anger, &c."

The placenta may happen to be so situated that when the full term of pregnancy arrives, "a flooding *necessarily* accompanies it and without the intervention of any of the above accidental circumstances".

Rigby's son, also called Edward Rigby, was a prominent obstetrician in the first half of the 19th century and the first president of the Obstetrical Society of London [9,10].

18.3.2 Cocaine

The famous explorer, after whom the New World continents are named, Amerigo Vespucci (1454 – 1512) saw people chewing coca leaves when he arrived in Venezuela in 1499 and was astonished by their condition and single-minded devotion to the process. These people were, of course, developing a serum level of cocaine much lower than that obtained by cocaine addicts today. There is a scene on a 2500-year-old pot from northern Peru that depicts people chewing coca leaf.

Angelo Mariani (1838 – 1914) was a Corsican pharmacist who produced a coca wine in Paris eventually called vin Mariana that had become very popular by 1870. Medications were commonly prescribed as wine tonics at the time. In 1884, one list of materia medica had 154 wine tonics shown. Mariani was a great self-promoter and sold his wine in a characteristically shaped bottle. His cousin, Charles Fauvel (1830 – ?) was an otorhinolaryngologist who used coca tincture to anesthetize the throat of his patients. Cocaine then began to be added to other medications and treatments, e.g. dandruff shampoos and soft drinks. In 1884, Sigmund Freud (1856 – 1939), the future father of psychoanalysis, published a review of the subject in "On Coca". He recommended seven possible uses for cocaine: as a mental stimulant, for digestive disorders, as an appetite stimulant in wasting diseases, for morphine and alcohol addiction, for asthma, as an aphrodisiac and as a local anesthetic. Freud's article was a review of the literature; he had little experience himself with the drug, yet. He may have been unaware that all the articles he cited concerning the use of cocaine for the control of morphine or alcohol addiction were published in the Therapeutic Gazette whose editor, George Davis, was one of the directors of the Parke, Davis pharmaceutical company. Parke, Davis & Co. of Detroit marketed a liquid coca extract and some of the articles published in the Therapeutic Gazette were payed for by the drug company. Freud recommended the use of cocaine for his friend Ernst von Fleischl-Marxow who had become a morphine addict after using the drug while recovering from a thumb amputation. It was widely thought at the time that stimulants could work to counter the effects of narcotics, but cocaine did not, and does not, work as a treatment for morphine addiction and von Fleischl-Marxow eventually died of complications of his addictions. There were soon some published criticisms of the use of cocaine for morphine addiction and Freud responded that it was important to use cocaine orally, not by intravenous injection. It is true that oral administration of cocaine leads to a much lower blood level of the drug than injection. Cocaine was apparently not used intranasally until around 1905. The first case report of erosion of the nasal septum from snorting cocaine was in 1910. Freud's friend Karl Koller published an article the same year that "On coca" appeared, describing the use of cocaine as a topical ocular anesthetic. Another great physician whose life was affected by cocaine was the surgeon William Halstead. Halstead noticed Koller's work while he was working at Roosevelt hospital in New York and within a year, he and his group had performed 1000 nerve blocks with injected cocaine for anesthesia during surgery. A student of Halstead, Leonard Corning, invented spinal anesthesia with cocaine. Halstead eventually became addicted to cocaine. William Welch, the famous pathologist and one of the founders of the Johns Hopkins medical school, chartered a boat and took Halstead on a Caribbean cruise to try to cure him of his addiction. This was unsuccessful and Halstead entered Butler hospital in Providence for treatment. He, unfortunately, became addicted to morphine during that treatment and, according to William Osler, Harvey Cushing (1869 – 1939, the father of modern neurosurgery), and others, Halstead remained addicted to cocaine and morphine until his death in 1922 [11,12].

18.4 Laboratory medicine

18.4.1 Placental abruption

There are no good blood tests for the detection of placental abruption. Maternal serum alpha-fetoprotein, beta HCG, and inhibin-A have been tried, and there is an increased risk of placental abruption when these analytes are elevated, but they are non-specific and ultimately not useful except, perhaps, in very specific clinical circumstances. The acid elution test for the detection of fetal hemoglobin in erythrocytes in the maternal circulation has also been tried to detect placental abruption, but the test is not useful. This is probably because the retroplacental blood clot in abruption does not increase the likelihood of fetal erythrocytes entering the maternal bloodstream [3,13,14].

18.4.2 Cocaine

Patients who are poisoned with cocaine often have leukocytosis, hypokalemia, and hyperglycemia. Since some of the effects of cocaine toxicity are countered by benzodiazepines, it is common to also find these drugs in patient's urine specimens due to self-medication. Gas chromatography – mass spectroscopy can detect cocaine metabolites for up to 48 hours after the drug was used. The more commonly used immunoassays can usually only detect them for 24 – 36 hours. Patients using crack cocaine usually have very high serum levels of the drug, and the parent compound, cocaine itself, can sometimes be detected for several hours by thin layer chromatography [7,8].

18.5 Study questions

1. Why did Sigmund Freud think that cocaine might work as a therapy for morphine addiction?

2. Why did Edward Rigby call placental abruption, accidental bleeding?

3. How many risk factors for placental abruption can you name?

4. If some Obstetrics texts say that placental abruption may be difficult to identify with certainty clinically, and one must sometimes defer to the pathologist's examination of the placenta, and if some Pathology texts say that

the gross diagnosis of placental abruption may be difficult or impossible, what does this indicate about the diagnosis of placental abruption?

5. Why may tests for the detection of fetal blood in the maternal circulation not be helpful for the diagnosis of placental abruption?

18.6 References

1. Fox H. Pathology of the Placenta. Philadelphia: W.B.Saunders; 1997:125.
2. Addis A, Moretti ME, Ahmed SF, Einarson TR, Koren G. Fetal effects of cocaine: an updated meta-analysis. Reprod Toxicol. 2001;15:341-369.
3. Kay HH. Placenta previa and abruption. In: Gibbs RS, Karlan BY, Haney AF, Nygaard I, editors. Danforth's obstetrics and gynecology. Philadelphia: Wolters Kluwer/Lippincott Williams & Williams; 2008. p. 385 - 399.
4. Hulse GK, Milne E, English DR, Holman CD. Assessing the relationship between maternal cocaine use and abruptio placentae. Addiction. 1997;92:1547 - 1551.
5. Naeye RL. Disorders of the placenta, fetus and neonate. Philadelphia: Mosby Year Book; 1992:213.
6. Lewis SH, Benirschke K. Overview of placental pathology. In: Lewis SH, Perrin E, editors. Pathology of the placenta. New York: Churchill Livingstone; 1999. p. 15 - 16.
7. Liang IE. Cocaine poisoning. In: Linden CH, Rippe JM, Irwin RS, editors. Manual of overdoses and poisonings. Philadelphia: Lippincott Williams & Wilkins; 2006. p. 84 - 87.
8. Pincus MR, Abraham NZ. Toxicology and therapeutic drug monitoring. In: McPherson RA, Pincus MR, editors. Henry's clinical diagnosis and management by laboratory methods. Philadelphia: Elsevier Saunders; 2011. p. 331 - 364.
9. Lee S, editor. Dictionary of national biography. London: Smith, Elder and Company; 1896:301.
10. Speert H. Obstetric and gynecologic milestones. New York: The Parthenon publishing group; 1996:311.

11. Karch SB. A brief history of cocaine. New York: Taylor and Francis; 2006
12. Markel H. An Anatomy of Addiction. Sigmund Freud, William Halstead, and the Miracle Drug Cocaine. New York: Pantheon Books; 2011
13. Atkinson AL, Santolaya-Forgas J, Matta P, Canterino J, Ovelese Y. The sensitivity of the Kleihauer-Betke test for placental abruption. J Obstet Gynaecol. 2015;35:139 - 141.
14. Tikkanen MI, Hämäläinen E, Nuutila M, Paavonen J, Ylikorkala O, Hiilesmaa V. Elevated maternal second-trimester serum alpha-fetoprotein as a risk factor for placental abruption. Prenat Diagn. 2007;27:240 - 243.

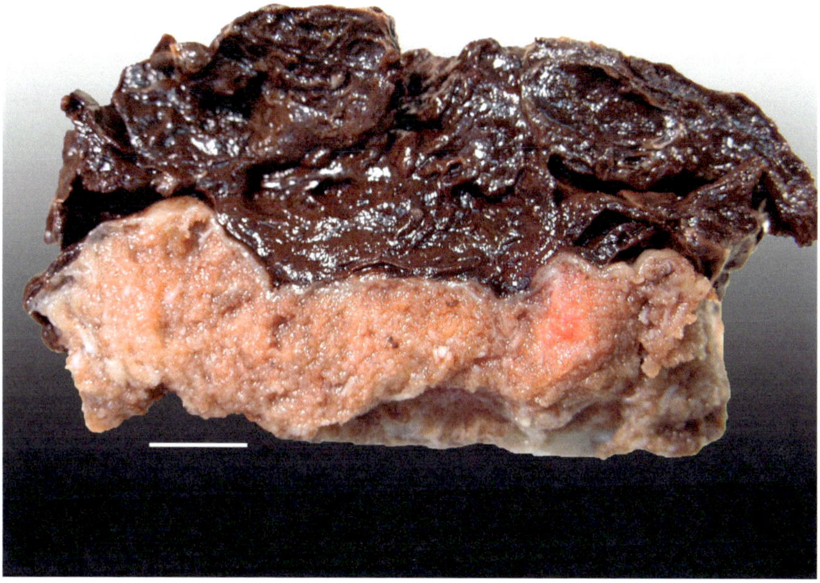

Figure 18.1 The placenta in the case presented in this chapter had abundant fresh appearing blood clot on its maternal surface. The photograph of that placenta was less enlightening than the one shown here. This is an image of a portion of the placenta from a different case with a more chronic placental abruption. The clot has a laminated appearance and some brownish discoloration and there is compression of the underlying placental tissue. The white bar is 1 cm long.

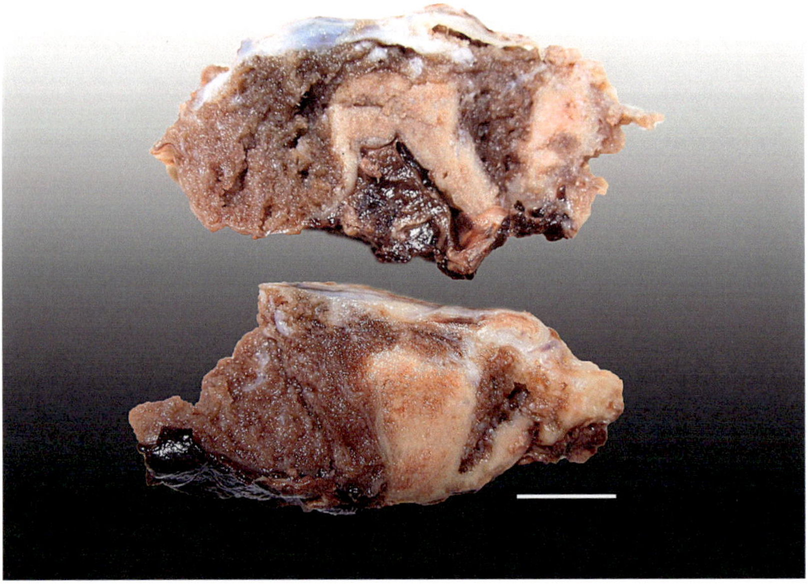

Figure 18.2 This is another image from the case shown in figure 18.1. Some portions of the placenta have central infarcts. These are seen grossly as firm areas with tan to yellowish discoloration. This change is sometimes seen normally at the edge of a placenta, but it is always abnormal in the central placental tissue, where central is defined by the location of the insertion point of the umbilical cord. The top surface in these pictures is the fetal side of the placenta, and the bottom surface is the maternal side. There is a thin layer of adherent blood clot on the maternal surfaces of both pieces. The white bar is 1 cm long.

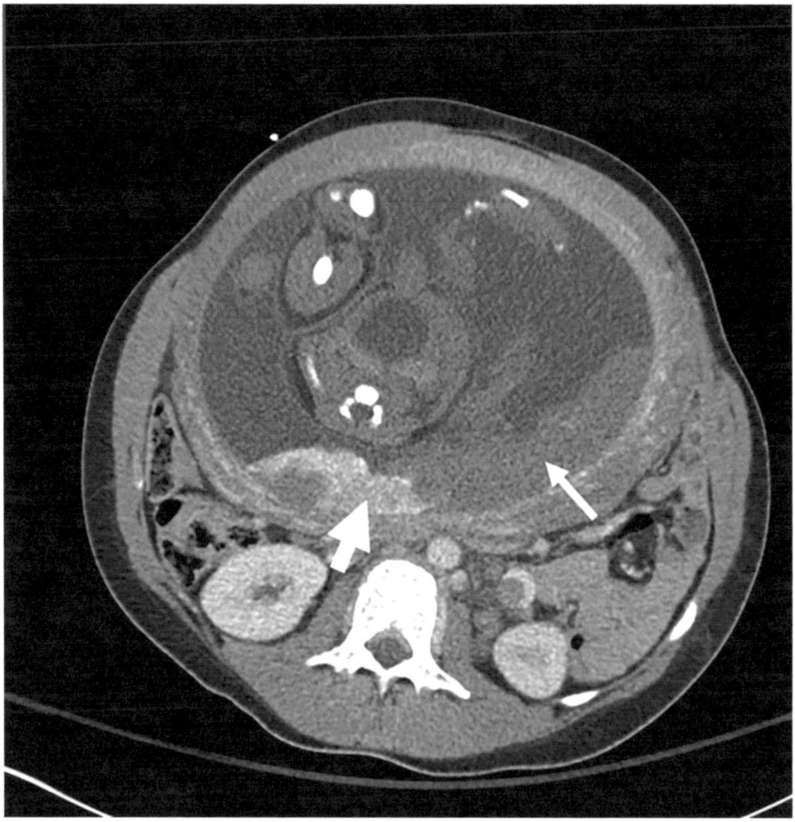

Figure 18.3 An axial contrast enhanced CT through the level of the kidneys from a different case shows a gravid uterus with a posterior placenta with hypo-enhancement (thinner arrow on the right) and a region of normal enhancement (thicker arrow on the left) concerning for placental abruption.

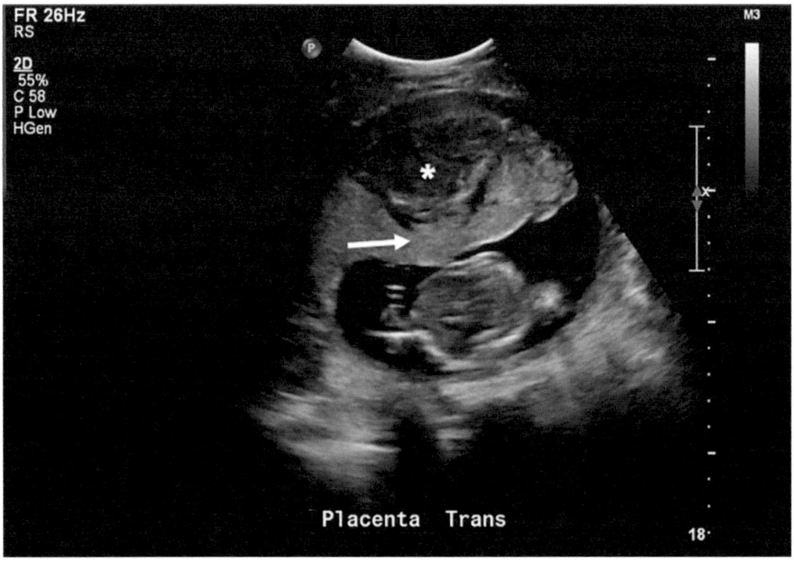

Figure 18.4 Ultrasound of the gravid uterus shows an anterior placenta (arrow) and a hypoechoic mass (asterisk) below the placenta concerning for a subchorionic hemorrhage suggesting placental abruption.

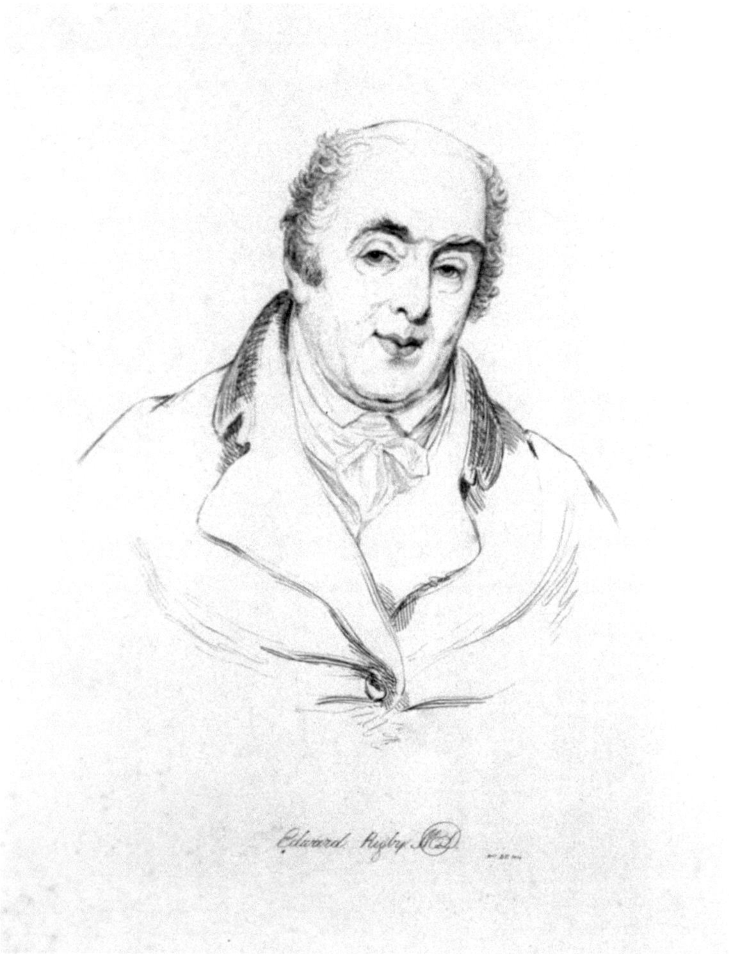

Figure 18.5 Edward Rigby (1747 – 1821). Courtesy of the National Library of Medicine.

CHAPTER 19

A 70-year-old woman with a recent total hip arthroplasty. (VindicaTe, vascular, trauma)

"Most men die of their remedies and not of their illnesses." Moliére (1622 – 1673), The Imaginary Invalid

19.1 The Autopsy

19.1.1 Case history

The patient was a 70-year-old woman who had polio as a child. She had severe osteoarthritis with avascular necrosis and subluxation of her right femoral head. Other problems included gastroesophageal reflux disease, hiatal hernia, systemic hypertension, and emphysema. The patient had a previous history of pneumonia, Clostridium difficile colitis, and seizures. She had smoked less than 1 pack of cigarettes/day for many years previously. The patient was admitted from a nursing home and had a right total hip arthroplasty performed. Low molecular weight heparin was given as prophylaxis against thromboembolic disease. On postoperative day #4 she had the sudden onset of hypotension then loss of consciousness and code blue was called. The patient had a narrow complex cardiac rhythm and no pulse, but resuscitation was successful and she had normal mental status. Cardiac ultrasound showed a dilated right heart and hypokinesis and increased pulmonary arterial pressure to 100 mm Hg (normal = 9 – 18 mm Hg). CT angiogram of the lungs showed no evidence of a thromboembolus, but there was a 2.7 x 2.4 cm area of increased lung density in the right base. The patient had cardiac arrest on the same day and resuscitatory efforts were unsuccessful.

19.1.2 Postmortem findings

At autopsy, the right lung weighed 600 grams and the left lung weighed 550 grams. There was a firm red roughly wedge-shaped mass near the base of the right lower lung lobe measuring 2.5 x 4 x 2 cm. Gross features of emphysema were present and most marked in the apices bilaterally (figure 19.1). The kidneys weighed just 75 grams each and had marked cortical scarring. An Oil Red O stain was performed on a frozen section of lung tissue.

Histologic sections showed prominent intravascular lipid in sections of the lung (figures 19.2, 19.3). The firm area in the right lower lung lobe showed acute intra-alveolar hemorrhage. This area also showed bronchiolitis obliterans and non-necrotizing granulomas containing vegetable material. (figures 19.6, 19.7)

Sections of kidney showed segmental nephron sclerosis with moderate chronic inflammation. There were arteriolar intimal thickening and some elastic lamina reduplication.

19.1.3 Case summary

The patient was an elderly woman with emphysema who had a right total hip arthroplasty. The surgery went well, but the patient had the sudden onset of hypotension with increased pulmonary arterial pressure on the third postoperative day. A pulmonary embolus was excluded by CT angiogram.

Postmortem examination showed prominent intravascular lipid in the lungs. There was no evidence of an acute myocardial infarct. There was only moderate atherosclerosis in the proximal right coronary artery. There was no evidence of a pulmonary thromboembolus.

Other findings included right lower lobe aspiration pneumonia and marked arterionephrosclerosis.

Patients who die after bone surgery often show pulmonary intravascular lipid, so this finding alone does not indicate fat embolism syndrome, but the clinical story, the absence of significant coronary artery disease, and the absence of pulmonary thromboemboli suggested fat embolism syndrome (FES) as the cause of death. This patient had no petechiae, but some have commented that this is only seen in 20 – 50% of patients with fat embolism syndrome. The patient's condition was probably exacerbated by her emphysema. [1]

19.2 Discussion

19.2.1 Fat embolism syndrome

The classic features of fat or lipid embolism syndrome are mental status changes, respiratory distress, and a petechial rash that occur 24 to 48 hours following bone trauma. The incidence is between 0.5 and 3% of patients with fracture of a long bone, and the incidence is much higher in patients with multiple bone fractures. [1] It has been reported in 33% of patients with bilateral femoral fractures. [2] The incidence is much lower in children, presumably because there is less lipid in the bone marrow of children than in adults. Most patients recover with supportive care, but there is a mortality of 5 – 15%. [2]

The diagnosis of fat embolism syndrome is often difficult. Fat embolism has been documented following bone fracture and bone surgery in patients who do not have the syndrome and are asymptomatic, and a significant fraction of patients with the syndrome do not have all the classic findings. The diagnosis is often made using the criteria of Gurd [3] in which the patient must have one major feature (of respiratory insufficiency, cerebral involvement, or petechial rash), four minor features (of pyrexia, tachycardia, retinal changes, jaundice, or renal changes) and fat macroglobulemia (large droplets of fat in the blood)). Unfortunately, as stated above, blood fat droplets are common in patients with trauma who do not have the syndrome. Because of the poor performance of these criteria, others have been described including a semiquantitative scoring system and a system using just measured respiratory features (figures 19.4, 19.5). [2]

The pathogenesis of FES is unknown. The two commonly mentioned theories are the mechanical and the biochemical. Mechanical obstruction of vessels would account for all the symptoms and signs in these patients, but it is not clear why some patients have fat embolism, but no symptoms and why there is a delay in onset of symptoms after bone fracture. In the biochemical theory, the symptoms are due to the toxicity of fatty acids in plasma from the degradation of the embolized fat. There is experimental evidence in animals that neutral fat is not toxic by itself. [2]

In a typical case, patients usually have hypoxia and tachypnea after a symptom-free interval. The chest radiograph may show multiple bilateral areas of increased density in the lung fields called the snowstorm appearance. Lung function usually resolves over a period of a week.

The mental status changes start as restlessness, confusion, or somnolence and may progress to coma. Very rarely mental status changes may occur in patients who have no respiratory findings. The characteristic skin rash may require some searching to detect. The axillae, anterior neck and chest, conjuctivae, oral cavity, and periumbilical skin are common locations. Both the mental status changes and rash usually resolve completely.

The fat embolism syndrome is more common in cases of closed fractures than open ones. It has been known for many years that early splinting is important in the prevention of the syndrome. Some authors think that the incidence of fat embolism syndrome has declined in the last 50 years because of the increased use of open reduction and internal fixation of fractures. The use of intravenous fluids at the time of fracture is also thought to be beneficial. [1] Steroids have been used in some patients with FES, but there has been no change in mortality. [4]

Tissue that is processed for examination under the microscope usually passes through the solvent xylene to remove lipid so that the tissue can be infiltrated by paraffin and cut on a microtome. Consequently, a typical hematoxylin and eosin stained slide used in the pathology laboratory has no lipid in it. The pathologist might notice the empty bubble-like spaces in blood vessel spaces that formerly contained lipid, but if the diagnosis of fat embolism syndrome is suspected, it is best to take fresh tissue and cut a frozen section. The frozen section can then be stained for lipid using Oil Red O or Sudan Black.

19.2.2 Aspiration pneumonia

Patients with difficulty swallowing, loss of a normal gag reflex, after repeated vomiting, during anesthesia, or while unconscious may aspirate oral and gastric contents into their lungs. The result is a mixed bacterial and chemical pneumonia that is often necrotizing. Aspiration pneumonia can be anywhere in the lungs, but because of the course of the bronchi in the reclining patient, the right middle and lower lung lobes are often affected. Massive aspiration is associated with adult respiratory distress syndrome and the histologic pattern called diffuse alveolar damage. A characteristic histologic feature of aspiration pneumonia is the presence of intra-alveolar histiocytes with ingested foreign, often vegetable, material from the gastric contents. Culture of the sputum or a biopsy often grows multiple organisms including both aerobes and anaerobes from the oral cavity. The bronchiolitis associated with aspiration may organize and resemble bronchiolitis obliterans – organizing pneumonia. The necrotizing pneumonia may progress to abscess formation with a significant risk of mortality. Lesser amounts of chronic micro-aspiration usually do not cause significant lung disease. [5]

19.3 Medical history

19.3.1 Fat embolism syndrome

Fat embolism was widely reported in trauma patients in the mid to late 19th century. One of the best early reviews was published in 1913 by a famous pathologist from my alma mater, Aldred Scott Warthin (1866 – 1931). Dr. Warthin attributed the first reported case of fat embolism (but not fat embolism syndrome) to Zenker who in 1862 reported the case of a railway worker who was crushed between two train cars and died immediately from exsanguination. In 1873 Bermann reported the case of a tinsmith who fell from a roof and fractured his femur. The patient had deterioration and death following a symptom-free interval, and the case is often presented as the first report of fat embolism syndrome. In his review of FES, Duis claimed that there were several reports of FES by others prior to 1873.

Aldred Scott Warthin was born in 1866 in Greensburg, Indiana (figure 19.8). In 1877, he received a Teacher's diploma of Music from the Cincinnati Conservatory, but he continued his education and acquired Doctor of Medicine and Doctor of Philosophy degrees from the University of Michigan. While in medical school he supported himself by teaching music and as a church organist. During three consecutive Summers, Dr. Warthin studied with the pathologist Ernst Ziegler at Freiburg (Ziegler's famous pathology text is still available as a reprint; one of the English translations was by Dr. Warthin). While studying in Europe, Warthin studied hypnotism (the craze of the times) and conducted an experiment in which he attempted to make his subjects sensitive to music by hypnotic suggestion. He played Wagner's Flight of the Walküre for them and recorded their physiological responses. Warthin found the responses so dramatic that he recommended that the experiment never be repeated. In 1896 Warthin became a demonstrator in medicine and assistant to Professor George Dock. Warthin performed all the autopsies at the time. He did 12 autopsies and saw 158 diagnostic specimens in 1896. In 1920, there were 131 autopsies and 5,419 diagnostic specimens. Warthin became professor in 1903 and was on the faculty at the University of Michigan for 40 years. He is best known for his work on the common parotid gland tumor that now bears his name, for the description of the Warthin-Finkeldy giant cell in patients with measles, and for the development of a silver impregnation stain for syphilis that is still used and called the Warthin-Starry stain.

Warthin used his silver stain on all his autopsy patients in 1919 and reported a 40% incidence of positive staining for syphilis! The stain is difficult to interpret and one must be careful not to over-interpret various structures as spirochetes when none are present.

Warthin also did work on the effects of mustard gas after the First World War. He maintained correctly that gastric ulcers only rarely progressed to gastric carcinoma, contrary to the opinion at the Mayo Clinic.

Warthin was, regrettably, also a supporter of the notion of the thymicolymphatic constitution, that some children could have sudden death because an enlarged thymus was pressing on their trachea. This mistake, due to ignorance concerning the appearance of the normal thymus in children on chest radiograph, led to many instances of unnecessary irradiation and surgery. [6,7]

19.4 Laboratory medicine

19.4.1 Fat embolism syndrome

About 70% of patients with FES have anemia and as many as 50% of them have thrombocytopenia. The mechanism for these abnormalities is unknown. Some patients have elevation of their serum lipase and hypocalcemia has also been reported. Fat globules have been described in cytologic specimens from urine, sputum, and blood in patients with FES. In 1970, Alan Gurd reported a technique in which the patient's serum was passed through a Millipore microfilter and stained for fat. Various reports have also attempted to find some specificity in MRI examination of the patient's brain and CT examination of the patient's lungs. Unfortunately, there is no good specific test for FES and it can only be suspected based on the patient's findings and clinical circumstances. [2]

19.4.2 Aspiration pneumonia

Some have recommended the use of fat stains on sputum to identify lipid-bearing macrophages in cases of aspiration pneumonia, but just as in the fat embolism syndrome, this finding is non-specific. [5]

19.5 Study questions

1. Why isn't the finding of fat emboli in the lung at autopsy sufficient to make a diagnosis of fat embolism syndrome?

2. Which three organ systems are classically affected in patients with the fat embolism syndrome?

3. Can the fat embolism syndrome occur in patients without bone trauma? How many such reported cases can you find?

4. A. S. Warthin had training in music before becoming a physician. Can you name any famous musicians who had training in medicine?

5. What circumstances might predispose a patient to develop aspiration pneumonia?

19.6 References

1. ten Duis HJ. The fat embolism syndrome. Injury. 1997;28:77 - 83.
2. Gupta A, Reilly CS. Fat embolism. Cont Edu Anaesth Crit Care and Pain. 2007;7:148 - 151.
3. Gurd AR, Wilson RI. The fat embolism syndrome. J bone Joint Surg [Br]. 1974;56B:408-416.
4. Bederman SS, Bhandari M, McKee MD, Schemitsch EH. Do corticosteroids reduce the risk of fat embolism syndrome in patients with long-bone fractures? A meta-analysis. J Can Chir. 2009;52:386-393.
5. Katzenstein AA. Katzenstein and Askin's Surgical Pathology of Non-neoplastic Lung Disease. Philadelphia: Saunders Elsevier; 2006:445.

6. Davenport HW. Not just any medical school. The science, practice and teaching of Medicine at the University of Michigan 1850 - 1941. Ann Arbor: The University of Michigan Press; 1999:117.
7. Long ER. A history of pathology. New York: Dover; 1965:199.

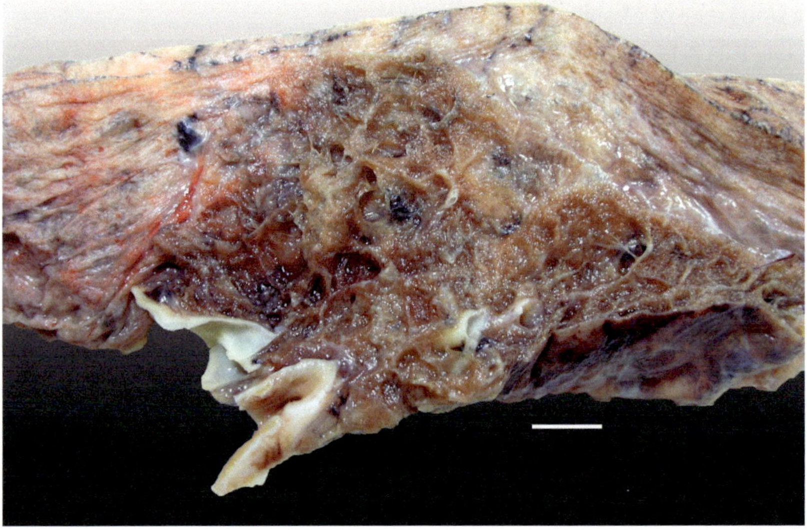

Figure 19.1 An image of one of the patient's lungs shows the characteristic gross features of centrilobular emphysema. The lung looks as if there is decreased tissue centrally with what Ian Donald Stuart (Director of the Autopsy Service at the University of Rochester Medical Center in the 1970's) referred to as the appearance of a collapsed hair net. The white bar is 1 cm long.

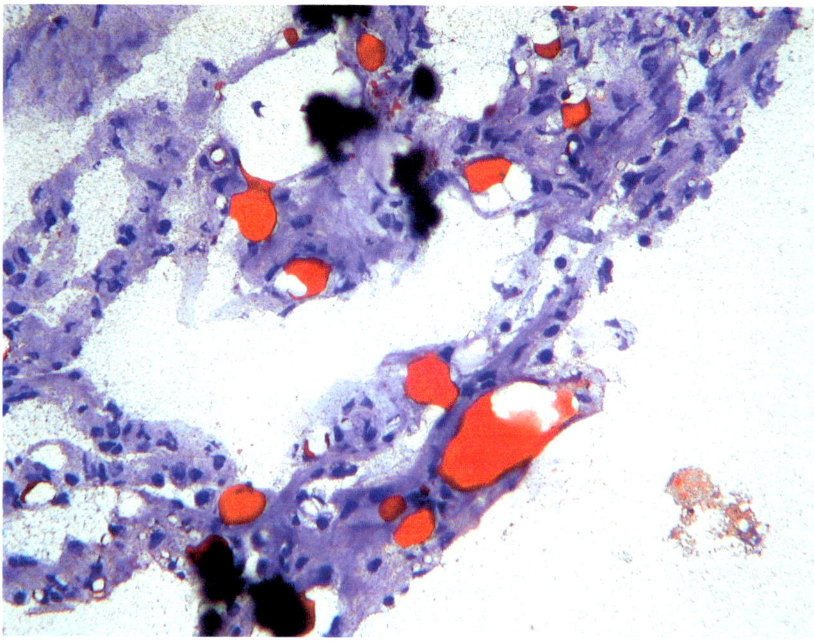

Figure 19.2 A frozen section of the patient's lung stained with Oil Red O. The red material is lipid in the blood vessel lumina. (Original magnification x200)

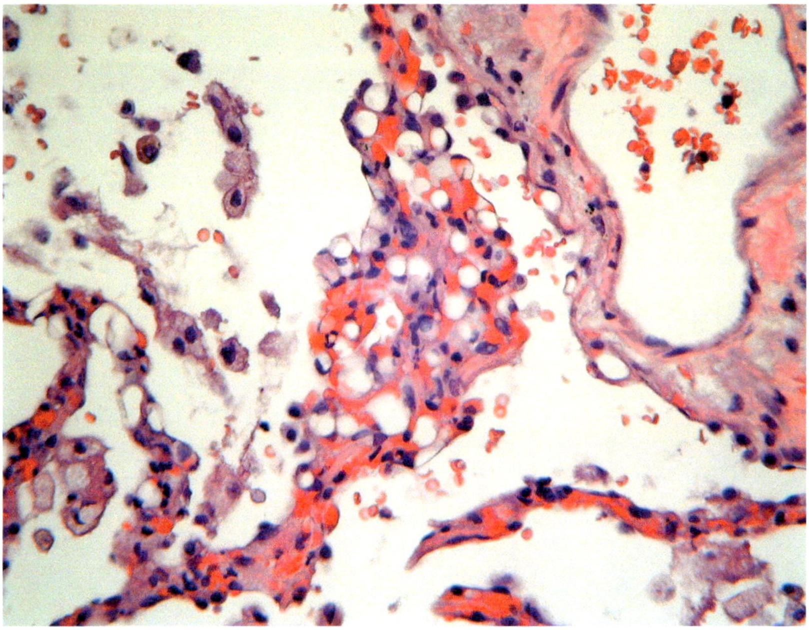

Figure 19.3 An H&E stained section of the patient's lung. The circular spaces in the blood vessels are lipid that was removed when the tissue was processed with xylene. (Original magnification x200)

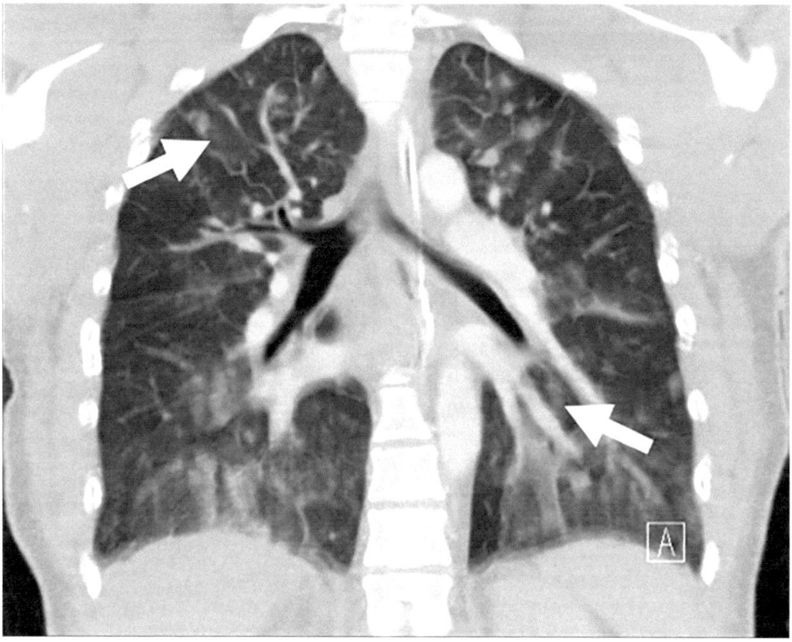

Figure 19.4 A coronal CT in lung window at the level of the carina from a different patient demonstrates patchy bilateral ground glass opacities in the lung parenchyma (arrows), a nonspecific finding that can be seen in pulmonary edema or multifocal pneumonia most commonly, however the clinical history of recent femoral fracture in this patient supported a diagnosis of pulmonary fat embolism.

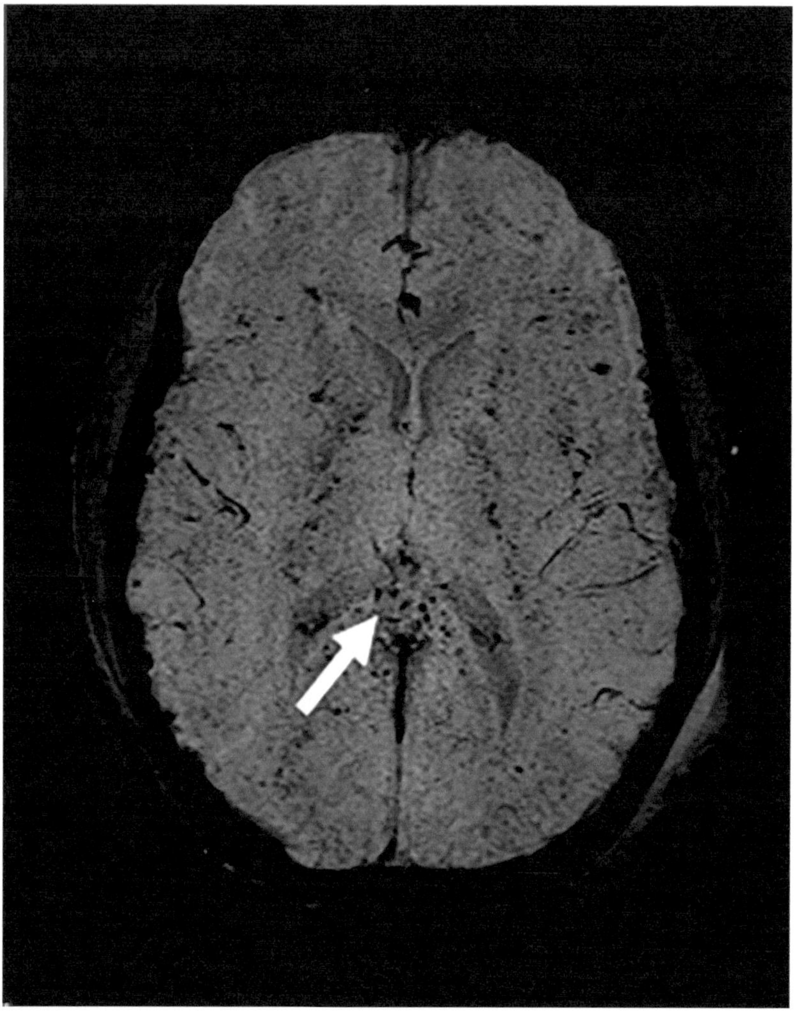

Figure 19.5 A susceptibility weighted sequence axial MRI of the brain from the same patient shown in figure 19.4 at the level of the lateral ventricles shows numerous tiny black dots (arrow) scattered randomly through the brain parenchyma due to tiny micro-hemorrhages from fat emboli.

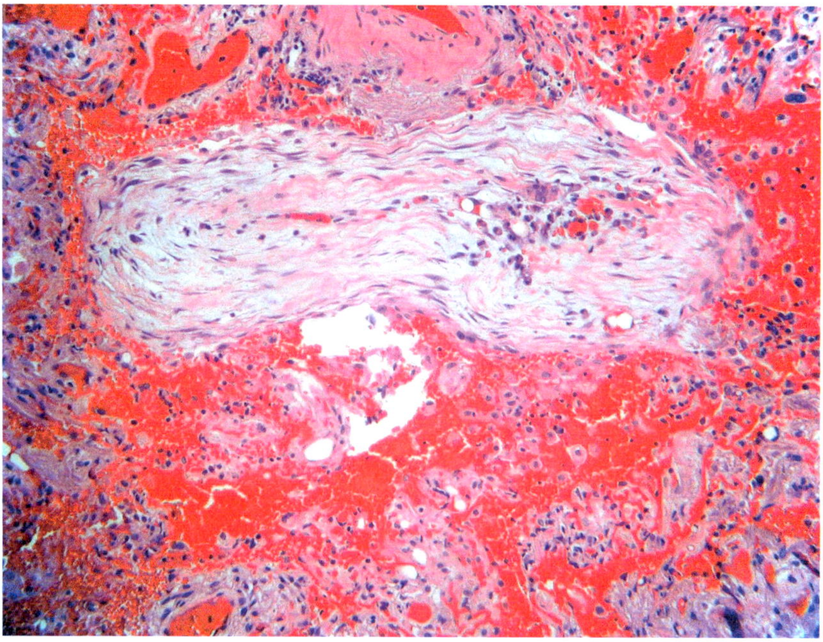

Figure 19.6 A histologic section from the patient's right lower lung lobe. There is acute intraalveolar hemorrhage and there is a large onion-like fibrous structure indicating bronchiolitis obliterans type organization compatible with aspiration pneumonia. (Original magnification x100, H&E stain)

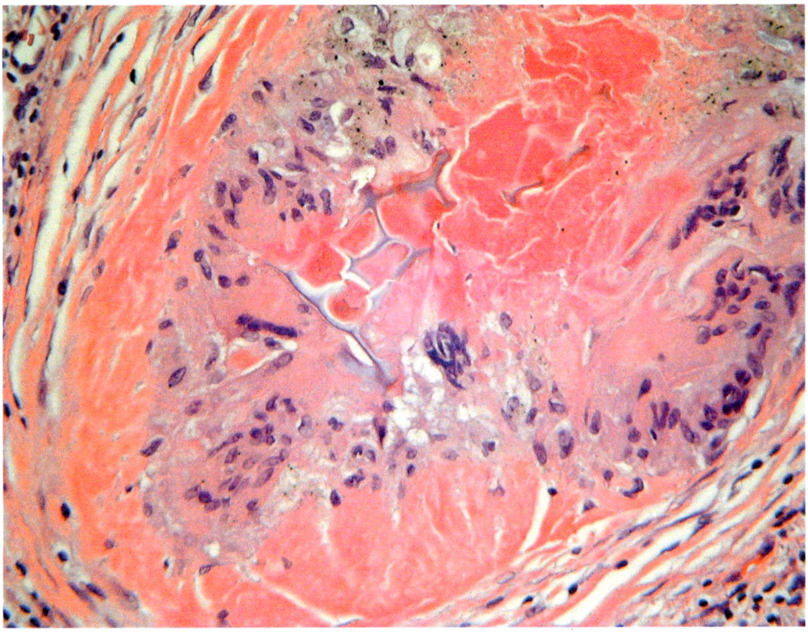

Figure 19.7 A histologic section from the patient's right lower lung lobe showing a granuloma with contained refractile vegetable-like material compatible with aspiration pneumonia. The multinucleated giant cells are reactive cells of histiocytic origin. (Original magnification x200, H&E stain)

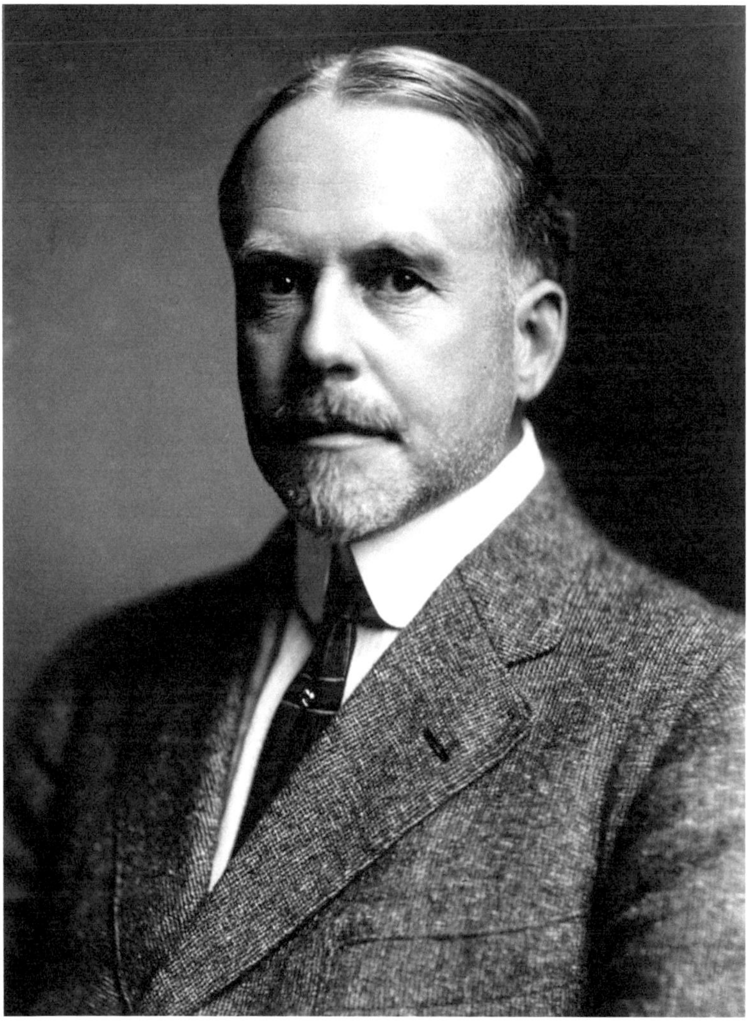

Figure 19.8 Aldred Scott Warthin (1866 – 1931). Courtesy of the National Library of Medicine.

CHAPTER 20

An 80-year-old woman with dementia and bacterial sepsis. (ulndlcate, infectious, idiopathic)

"I've always said that the most useful equipment for a successful surgeon is a pessimistic pathologist." John Rowan Wilson (1919 –)

20.1 The Autopsy

20.1.1 Case history

The patient was an 80-year-old non-ambulatory woman with dementia who was admitted to the hospital from her nursing home for a 24-hour history of fever. She had a medical history of systemic hypertension, hypothyroidism, and osteoarthritis. On her initial examination, she had pyuria (neutrophils in the urine), right lower leg cellulitis, and a peripheral white blood cell count of 29,900 (normal = 3900 – 10,700 cells/microliter). Her peripheral blood white cells were 76% neutrophils and 16% band forms (normal = 50 – 70% neutrophils and 3 – 5% bands). She had a hemoglobin of 8.7 (normal = 12.0 – 15.5 grams/deciliter) and a serum creatinine of 1.3 (normal = 0.5 – 1.1 milligrams/deciliter). Her drugs in the nursing home had included rivastigmine (a reversible anticholinesterase used to treat Alzheimer's disease), hydroxyzine (an antihistamine sometimes used as a sedative), lisinopril (an angiotensin converting enzyme inhibitor used to treat hypertension), and furosemide (diuretic). She was treated with the antibiotics Zosyn (piperacillin and tazobactam), cefepime, and clindamycin.

The patient fractured her right femur during her hospitalization and had open reduction and internal fixation on about the 19th hospital day. She became progressively obtunded and developed oliguria and hypotension over 48 hours following her surgery. She remained afebrile, but her white blood count increased to 97,000 and her creatinine increased to 3.5. The patient died on the 24th hospital day.

20.1.2 Postmortem findings

At autopsy, the patient had bacterial sepsis, pseudomembranous colitis, gross and histologic features of Hashimoto's thyroiditis, and cerebral cortical atrophy with a brain weight of 1000 grams (average normal = 1500 grams). The colonic lumen had confluent tan colored pseudomembranes that were most prominent in the distal colon (figure 20.1). Histologic examination of the colon had a typical appearance for pseudomembranous colitis (figure 20.3). Histologic examination of the brain showed the diagnostic features of Alzheimer's disease, including hippocampal and parahippocampal gyrus senile plaques, neurofibrillary tangles and granulovacuolar degeneration of the pyramidal cells. (figures 20.4 - 20.6)

Postmortem cultures of portions of the patient's spleen and both lower lung lobes grew rare to moderate numbers of Enterococcus faecium.

20.1.3 Case summary

The neuropathologic findings confirmed a diagnosis of Alzheimer's disease. The finding of the same organism in three separate postmortem cultures indicated bacterial sepsis. The patient's pseudomembranous colitis was likely due to colonization by toxin-producing Clostridium difficile following therapy with antibiotics. I attributed the patient's death to bacterial sepsis.

20.2 Discussion

20.2.1 Clostridium difficile pseudomembranous colitis

Clostridium difficile is the most common cause of antibiotic-associated colitis. It accounts for up to 30% of cases of hospital-acquired diarrhea. It is thought to result from loss of the normal bacterial flora of the colon and colonization by a toxin producing strain of Clostridium difficile.

Nursing home residence, debilitating diseases, old age, and a prolonged hospital stay are all risk factors. Diarrhea usually begins 5 to 10 days after antibiotic therapy is started, but it may occur almost immediately or months later. Rare cases may progress to toxic megacolon and require surgery. The diagnosis should be suspected in patients who develop diarrhea after admission to the hospital or who have received antibiotics in the previous few months (figure 20.2).

Surgical and autopsy colon specimens have a characteristic yellowish membranous exudate on the mucosal surface, giving the disorder its name. As the disease progresses the areas of mucosal exudate may coalesce and form a geographic appearing pattern. Histologically the pseudomembrane has a "mushroom cloud" appearance on the luminal surface. Although characteristic for Clostridium difficile colitis, this histologic appearance has been described in many other disorders including ischemic colitis. Many antibiotics have been associated with pseudomembranous colitis, but the highest risk is with penicillins, cephalosporins, clindamycin, and the fluoroquinolones.

Clostridium difficile produces both an enterotoxin and a cytotoxin, called toxins A and B. These high molecular weight proteins bind to specific intestinal mucosal receptors and disrupt normal cell function.

Mild cases may recover after cessation of antibiotic therapy, but cases of moderate severity are usually treated with oral metronidazole or vancomycin. As many as 20% of patients may suffer relapse, and patients who have relapsed once have a 45% risk for another relapse. In fulminant cases, total colectomy may be necessary.

A new investigational therapy with considerable success in some studies, especially for recurrent disease, is fecal microbiota transplantation, in which the patient's colonic flora is replaced using fecal material from a normal donor patient. [1 – 3]

20.2.2 Alzheimer's Disease

Dementia is the acquired loss of some degree of cognitive brain function affecting daily function, lasting for at least months and not associated with loss of consciousness. Dementia has many causes, but Alzheimer's disease (AD) is the most common cause in the elderly. The affected patient typically has the gradual impairment of memory, reasoning, planning, personality, and language ability over the course of 5 to 10 years. The disease is present in only 1% of patients between 60 and 64 years of age, but increases to 40% for those between 85 and 89 years old. Between 5 and 10% of cases are familial. Most familial cases have an early onset, but some do not. The definitive diagnosis of AD requires examination of brain tissue at autopsy, but the diagnosis is usually made clinically and with the help of radiographic examination of the brain. There are some described diagnostic tests based on the detection of certain proteins in the cerebrospinal fluid.

Patients with Alzheimer's disease have the accumulation of Aß protein and tau protein in areas of their brain due to increased production or decreased clearance. The characteristic histopathologic features of AD are due to the accumulation of these proteins and the secondary alteration of surrounding normal structures.

The characteristic histopathologic features of AD are neuritic or senile plaques and neurofibrillary tangles. Plaques are spherical collections of abnormal neuritic processes that surround a core of amyloid protein. The main component of the amyloid core is the protein Aß that forms from amyloid precursor protein (APP). Neurofibrillary tangles are collections of paired helical filaments by ultrastructural examination that are associated with hyperphosphorylated tau protein and are thought to be a component of the cell microtubule system. The tangles often resemble a flame-like cytoplasmic structure in pyramidal neurons when stained with the Bielschowsky silver impregnation stain. The failure to clear the brain of these abnormal proteins and the accumulation of these structures is thought by many to be the etiologic mechanism of the brain abnormality in AD, but although characteristic of AD, these findings are not specific for it. Neurofibrillary tangles, for example, may be quite prominent in the hippocampus of some elderly patients who have no dementia. There is evidence of clinical, pathological, and molecular heterogeneity among the patients with inherited AD. The gene for the production of APP is associated with the Down's syndrome critical region on chromosome 21 and patients with Down's syndrome have a high incidence of AD. Certain alleles of the gene for apolipoprotein E on chromosome 19 are also associated with an increased risk for AD. [4,5]

20.3 Medical history

20.3.1 Alzheimer's disease

Alois Alzheimer (1864 - 1915) was born in Marktbreit am Main in Bavaria (figure 20.7). He trained in Medicine and graduated from Würzberg in 1888 with a dissertation "On the ceruminal glands of the ear". Alzheimer had a special interest in the histopathology of the nervous system. He worked with Franz Nissl (1860 – 1919) at a Frankfurt asylum for the mentally ill and later worked with the great psychiatrist Emil Kraepelin (1856 – 1926) in Heidelberg and then in Munich where he became head of the neuroanatomy laboratory. The original 32-page medical record of Alzheimer's first observed case of the disease that bears his name was found in Frankfurt in 1995. The patient, Auguste D., was a 51-year-old woman with progressive cognitive impairment, hallucinations, delusions and "psychosocial incompetence". Her record includes a complete written account of her medical interviews and photographs of the patient. Mrs. D. died in 1906. At autopsy, Dr. Alzheimer described abundant neuritic plaques and neurofibrillary tangles in his sections of the patient's brain. These features had been described before in patients with senile dementia, but Auguste D. was young for that diagnosis and her histopathologic findings were severe.

Alzheimer didn't think that this case represented a new disease, but the disease was called Alzheimer's disease by Emil Kraepelin in his textbook of psychiatry published in 1910. The reason for his decision is unknown, but possible contributing factors include that Alzheimer was well-liked and a respected researcher, Emil Kraepelin was his boss and there was the usual competitive atmosphere between the Institutes in Munich where Kraepelin and Alzheimer worked and the one in Prague where Arnold Pick (1851 – 1924) had described the dementia-causing disease that bears his name in 1892.

The significance of these characteristic histologic findings is still controversial and the subject of extensive research. For many years, Alzheimer's disease was distinguished from senile dementia, but following a series of papers published in the 1960s, it appeared that the distinction could no longer be made. Over the years various theories of AD etiology have been proposed including Aluminum toxicity, prion exposure, autoimmunity, a variant of a normal aging process and, recently, a response to bacterial infection. [6 – 8]

20.4 Laboratory medicine

20.4.1 Pseudomembranous colitis

The genus Clostridium comprises endospore-forming, anaerobic, catalase negative, Gram positive bacilli and includes the organisms responsible for botulism, tetanus, neutropenic enterocolitis, and enteritis necroticans. Clostridium difficile is common in soil, water, and household pets and it is carried asymptomatically by 3 – 8% of hospitalized adults, up to 70% of newborn infants, and 20% of hospitalized adults and nursing home residents. Stool specimens should be taken for the diagnosis of Clostridium difficile colitis. The specimen is cultured and tested for the presence of toxins A and B. Only liquid or unformed stools are processed to avoid treating patients with normal colonization by the bacteria. There are various enzyme-linked immunoassay tests available for the toxins. There is a similar test for the presence of a glutamate dehydrogenase that is relatively specific for C. difficile. Patients with a negative toxin test, but a positive culture may have a toxigenic culture test in which colonies of C. difficile are isolated on selective media and tested in vitro for toxin production. Tests using the polymerase chain reaction are available that detect the tcdA and tcdB toxin genes. A cultured strain may also be examined to identify the virulent NAP1 (North American pulsed-field type 1) type of C. difficile. Patient's with colonization by the NAP1 strain tend to have more severe disease with an increased risk for renal failure, toxic megacolon, and colonic perforation.

Patients for whom the clinical suspicion of the disease is high, but with negative tests, may have colonoscopy to confirm the presence of pseudomembranes and CT scan may be used in fulminant disease to detect toxic megacolon or perforation. [1,2,9,10]

20.5 Study questions

1. Why is the finding of colonic pseudomembranes on colonoscopy insufficient for a diagnosis of Clostridium difficile colitis?

2. Where can Clostridium difficile be found in the environment?

3. Name several causes of dementia.

4. Alzheimer didn't think that the case that he reported in 1906 was a new disease. How did it come to be considered one?

5. What problems might one encounter finding donors for fecal transplantation?

20.6 References

1. Lentino JR. Anaerobic bacteria. In: Porter RS, Kaplan JL, editors. The Merck Manual of Diagnosis and Therapy. Whitehouse Station, NJ: Merck Sharp & Dohmc Corp.; 2011. p. 1288 - 1289.
2. Aberra FN, Curry JA. Clostridium difficile colitis medication. BS Anand, editor. 2015. emedicine.medscape.com/article/186458-medication. Accessed 2016.
3. Rao K, Young VB. Fecal microbiota transplantation for the management of Clostridium difficile infection. Infect Dis Clin North Am. 2015;29:109-122.
4. Frosch MP, Anthony DC, De Girolami U. The Central Nervous System. In: Kumar V, Abbas AK, Aster JC, editors. Robbins and Cotran Pathological Basis of Disease. Philadelphia: Elsevier Saunders; 2015. p. 1287 - 1292.
5. Morris JH, Nagy Z. Alzheimer's disease. In: Esiri MM, Morris JH, Trojanowski JQ editors. The neuropathology of dementia. Cambridge: Cambridge University Press; 2004. p. 161 - 206.
6. Maurer K, Volk S, Gerbaldo H. Auguste D.: The history of Alois Alzheimer's first case. In: Whitehouse PJ, Maurer K, Ballenger JF, editors. Concepts of Alzheimer disease. Biological, clinical and cultural perspectives. Baltimore: The Johns Hopkins University Press; 2000. p. 5 - 29.
7. Berrios GE. Alzheimer's disease: A conceptual history. International J of Geriatric Psychiatry. 1990;5:335 - 365.
8. Kumar DKV, Choi SH, Washicosky KJ *et al.* Amyloid-ß peptide protects against microbial infection in mouse and worm models of Alzheimer's disease. Science Translational Medicine. 2016;8:340ra72.
9. Tille PM. Bailey & Scott's Diagnostic Microbiology. St. Louis: Elsevier Mosby; 2014
10. Delmée M. Laboratory diagnosis of clostridium difficile disease. Clin Microbiol Infect. 2001;7:411-416.

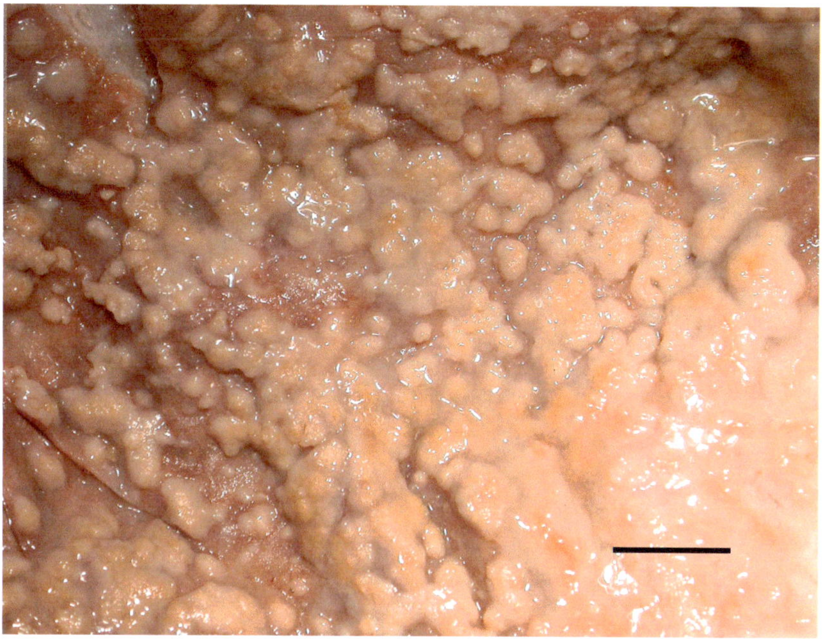

Figure 20.1 The patient's colonic mucosal surface had a geographic to confluent appearance with a tan pseudomembranous exudate. The black bar is 1 cm long.

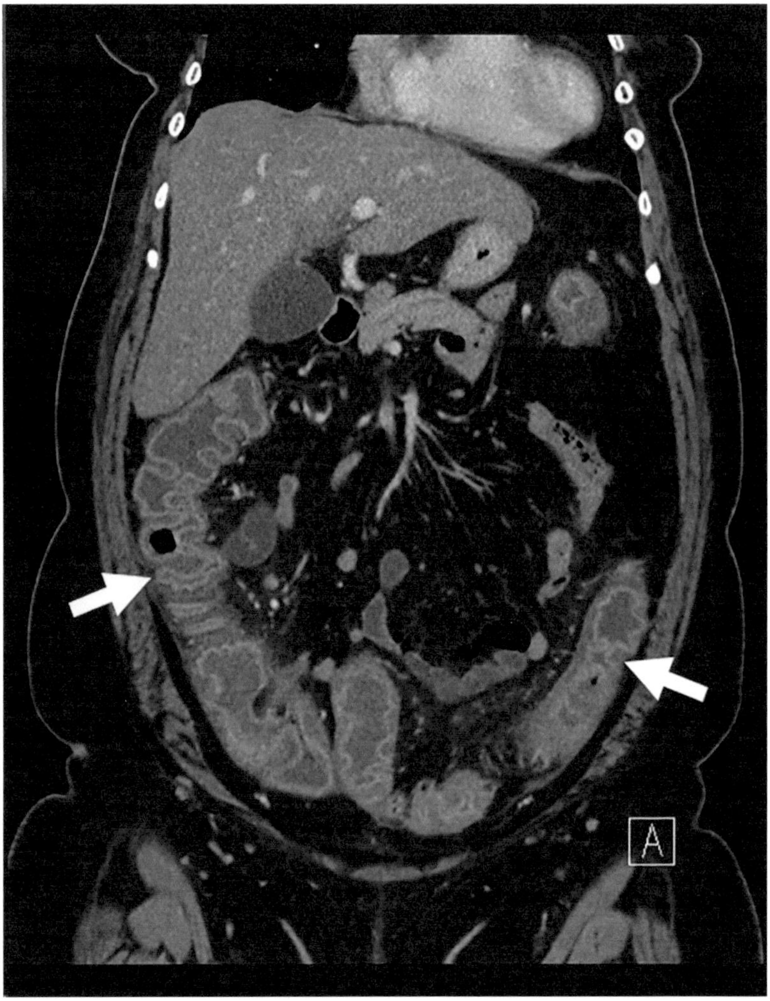

Figure 20.2 A coronal contrast enhanced CT of the abdomen from a different case shows diffuse wall thickening, mucosal enhancement and surrounding inflammation of the ascending colon, the descending colon and sigmoid colon (arrows). These findings are compatible with pseudomembranous colitis.

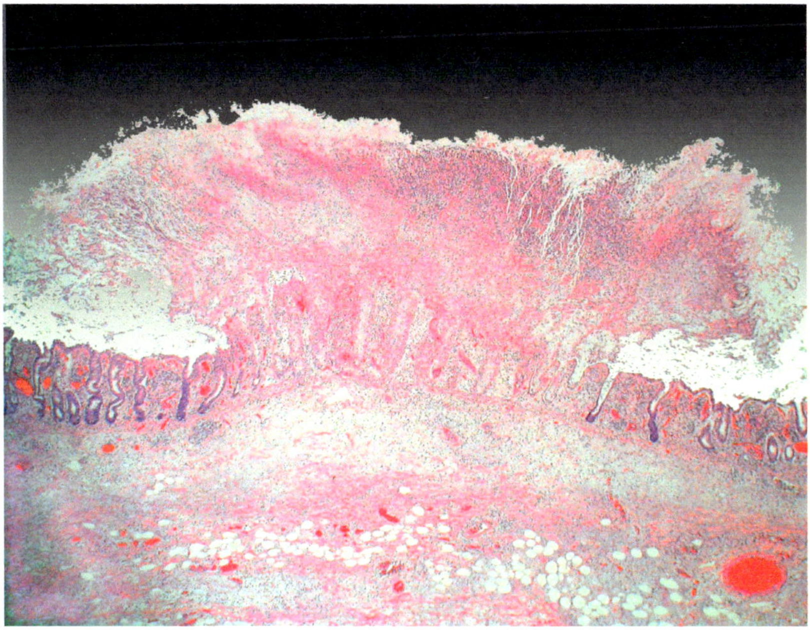

Figure 20.3 Histologic examination of the patient's colon showed the characteristic mushroom cloud-like surface exudate overlying mucosal ulceration. This appearance is typical for Clostridium difficile pseudomembranous colitis. (Original magnification 40x, H&E stain)

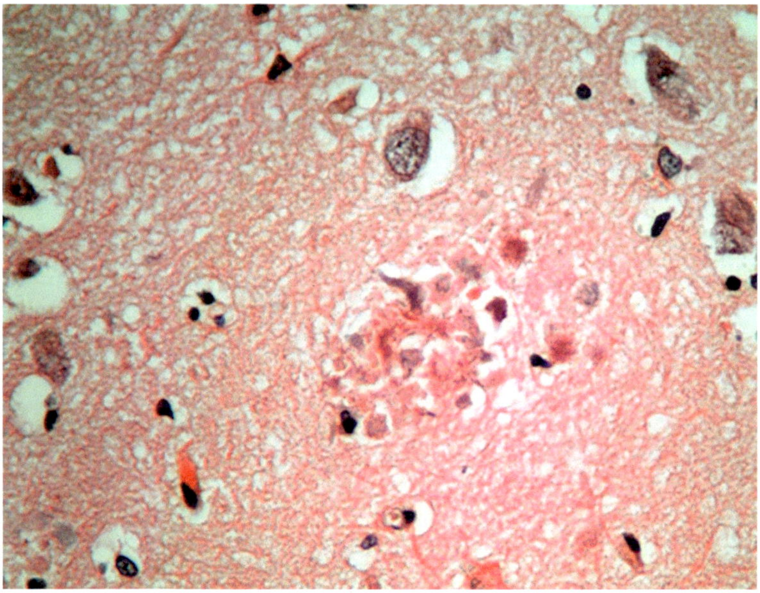

Figure 20.4 A histologic section from the left hippocampus shows a senile plaque with areas of central pink amyloid material. (Original magnification 400x, H&E stain)

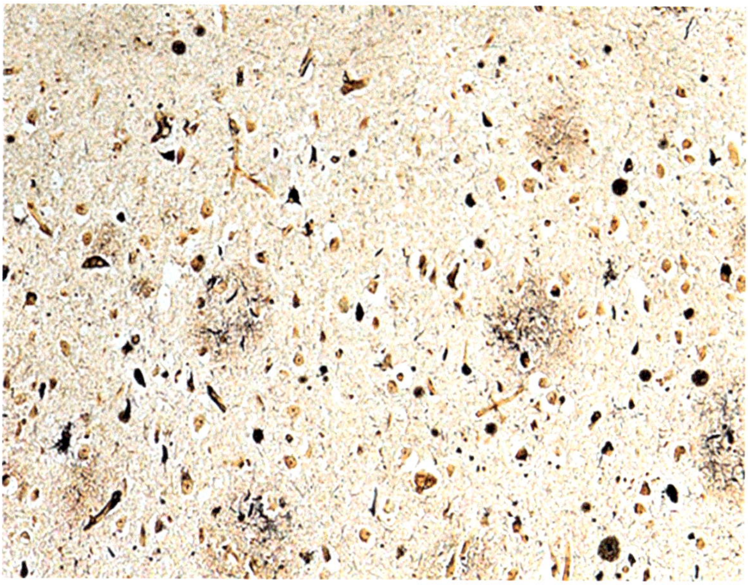

Figure 20.5 A low-power image showing multiple plaques resembling circular areas of increased density in the neuropil mostly between cell bodies using a silver impregnation stain. (Original magnification 100x, Bielschowsky stain)

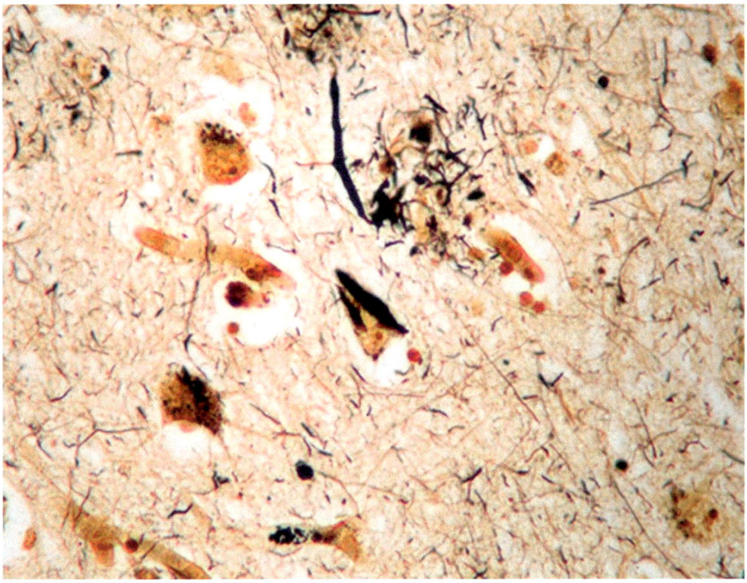

Figure 20.6 A neurofibrillary tangle is present in the central neuron and appears black and elongate on silver stain in this image. The images in figures 20.3, 20.4 and 20.5 are courtesy of Dr. Michael Kanzer at the Christiana Care Health Services and were taken from another similar case. (Original magnification 400x, Bielschowsky stain)

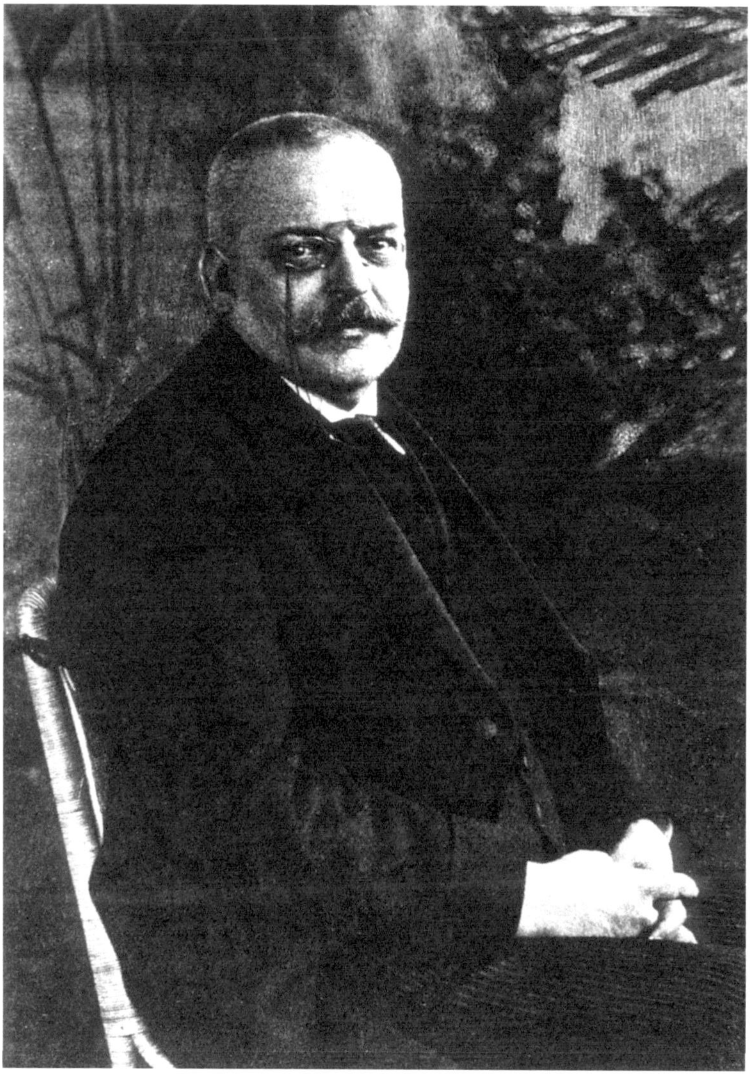

Figure 20.7 Alois Alzheimer (1864 – 1915). Courtesy of the National Library of Medicine.

CHAPTER 21

A stillborn female fetus at 27 weeks gestation with hepatosplenomegaly (uIndiCate, infectious, congenital)

"Cure the evils of Democracy by the evils of Fascism! Funny therapeutics! I've heard of their curing syphilis by giving the patient malaria, but I've never heard of their curing malaria by giving the patient syphilis." Sinclair Lewis (1885 – 1951)

21.1 The Autopsy

21.1.1 Case history

A G1P0 woman in her 20's presented to the hospital at about 27 weeks gestation with a one week history of loss of fetal movement. Ultrasonographic examination showed no fetal heart beat and a diagnosis of intrauterine fetal death was made. The woman had a history of a positive RPR (Rapid Plasma Reagin) test with a titer of 1:256. She had been treated with a dose of penicillin G the day before her presentation (i.e. several days after fetal movements stopped). She was Rubella immune, hepatitis B surface antigen negative, antibody screen negative, HIV negative and blood type O positive. A stillborn female fetus was delivered vaginally after induction with Cytotec (misoprostol, a synthetic prostaglandin analogue).

21.1.2 Postmortem findings

The fetus was female and weighed 780 grams. It was externally grossly normal except for slight abdominal enlargement and peeling skin on the hands, feet, face, back, abdomen, and legs (Peeling skin is a postmortem change.). There was a small amount of hemorrhagic fluid in the pericardial sac and in the abdomen. The liver and spleen were enlarged, and the brain to liver weight ratio was 2.5 (normal is about 3). The spleen was about four times normal weight. The placenta weighed 320 grams (normal = 226 ± 100g) and had some green discoloration of the fetal surface. The umbilical cord had red discoloration and edema. Histologic examination was remarkable for autolytic changes and hypocellularity of the spleen. A Steiner silver stain was negative for microorganisms on multiple visceral paraffin blocks, but an immunostain for spirochetes was positive on a block from the spleen. (figures 21.1, 21.2)

21.1.3 Case summary

The patient's mother was a young G1P0 woman who presented with intrauterine fetal death in the late second trimester and with a history of a positive RPR test. Postmortem examination of the stillborn female fetus showed organisms in the spleen that stained with an immunostain for spirochetes. I attributed the patient's death to congenital syphilis.

21.2 Discussion

21.2.1 Syphilis

Syphilis is a systemic sexually transmitted disease caused by the spirochete Treponema pallidum and characterized by three sequential clinical stages called primary, secondary, and tertiary syphilis. According to the Centers for Disease Control and Prevention there were about 24,000 cases of primary and secondary syphilis reported in the US in 2015. The stages of syphilis have many different clinical manifestations making diagnosis difficult and the disease has been called the "great imitator". Treponema pallidum enters the body through the mucous membranes or the skin, but reaches regional lymph nodes in a matter of hours. The risk of getting the disease is about 30% with a single sexual encounter with someone with primary syphilis. The risk of transplacental infection of a fetus is 60 – 80% if the mother has primary syphilis. Infection does not lead to acquired immunity. Treponema pallidum is sensitive to both drying and disinfectants.

The characteristic lesion of primary syphilis is the chancre, a painless ulcer in the area of sexual contact sometimes associated with regional lymphadenopathy. The chancre usually develops about 3 – 4 weeks after infection occurs.

Secondary syphilis occurs about 6 – 12 weeks after the chancre develops. It is characterized by lymphadenopathy and systemic symptoms such as fever, anorexia, nausea, and fatigue. More than 80% of these patients have mucocutaneous lesions. The classic lesions are a macular scaly rash on the palms and soles, and hypertrophic papular lesions developing in moist areas of skin called Condyloma lata. Symptoms of syphilis may disappear between the clinical stages of syphilis; this is called the latent period. These patients will still test positive with serological tests for syphilis.

About 30% of patients with syphilis who are not treated will progress to tertiary syphilis, often many years after their initial infection. Tertiary syphilis has many manifestations including the formation of soft inflammatory masses called gummas. These may occur in almost any organ and may cause symptoms due to local growth and tissue destruction. Another manifestation of tertiary syphilis is cardiovascular disease which usually occurs as ascending aortic aneurysm, aortic valve insufficiency, or coronary artery narrowing. The aortic aneurysm may erode into and through the chest wall. Some patients will develop neurological disease. Neurosyphilis has many manifestations including mild asymptomatic meningitis, a more severe meningovascular inflammation, general paresis due to destruction of the cortex of the brain, and tabes dorsalis. Tabes dorsalis is due to progressive destruction of the posterior columns of the spinal cord and nerve roots and is characterized by shooting pain in the back and legs, gait ataxia, paresthesias, urinary incontinence, and impotence. Syphilis may have many other manifestations including various lesions of the eyes, ears, skin and bones.

Other spirochetes, either classified as other species in the genus Treponema or as subspecies of Treponema pallidum are the causative agents for the related diseases, yaws, bejel, and pinta.

The mechanism of Treponema pallidum toxicity is uncertain. So, for example, why does the chancre resolve, and if it is due to a successful immune reaction, why does the disease progress? Why do some patients not progress to secondary syphilis, and why do 70% of patients with secondary syphilis not progress to tertiary syphilis? Trepenoma pallidum is often seen around arterioles histologically, it incites a strong plasma cell rich inflammatory reaction, and it may be associated with an endarteritis (figures 21.3 – 21.5). Some have suggested that ischemia associated with the endarteritis might be the cause of some tissue damage. The organism has fewer transmembrane proteins than other Gram-negative bacilli, and some of its transmembrane proteins are known to be highly antigenically variable.

Treponema pallidum does not reproduce in culture, and the diagnosis of syphilis following clinical suspicion is based on screening and confirmatory serological tests and observation of the causative organism by dark field microscopy on material from a chancre or lymph node aspirate or by silver impregnation stain on a tissue biopsy. Syphilis is treated with penicillin by intramuscular injection. The patient's sexual partners should also be evaluated and treated if necessary. Some patients with primary syphilis and more patients with secondary syphilis will have a systemic reaction following penicillin treatment by several hours. This is called the Jarisch-Herxheimer reaction and is usually self-limited and benign. [1 – 5]

21.2.2 Congenital Syphilis

Congenital syphilis occurs when Treponema pallidum crosses the placenta from mother to fetus. The risk of infection is 60 – 80% in a mother with primary or secondary syphilis. Tertiary syphilis is usually not transmissible. The probability of fetal infection is higher after 20 weeks gestational age. The features of syphilis in infants are divided into those that occur before 2 years of age, called early congenital disease, and those that occur after 2 years of age, called late congenital disease. Many patients with congenital syphilis are asymptomatic.

Infants with early congenital syphilis may have a vesiculobullous or copper colored rash on the palms and soles, hepatosplenomegaly, lymphadenopathy, and failure to thrive with a characteristic mucopurulent or blood-tinged nasal discharge called snuffles. Rarely, meningitis, hydrocephalus, and intellectual disability may occur. Long bone and costal osteochondritis may occur with a characteristic radiographic appearance.

Late congenital syphilis is typically marked by destructive gummas in the nose and nasal palate and periosteal bone growth causing frontal bossing and so-called saber shins. Acoustic nerve deafness can occur at any age. Characteristic, but unusual sequelae include abnormal secondary teeth (Hutchinson's incisors, screw driver incisors, turret and mulberry molars) and so-called bulldog facies from abnormal development of the jaw.

The diagnosis of congenital syphilis is usually suspected because the mother has positive serology. Pregnant women should be routinely given a serological screening test for syphilis. Newborns who are suspected of having the infection should have a serological test and dark field examination or fluorescent antibody staining of material from skin lesions and the placenta. Tests done on blood from the umbilical cord are relatively insensitive. Maternal IgG that has crossed the placenta may give a false positive test in the infant. A quantitative serology that is more than four times higher than the maternal titer suggests that the neonatal test is truly positive. Some studies have been done using an antibody for antitreponemal IgM, which does not cross the placenta. Children with suspected late congenital syphilis often have negative anti-reagin tests, but they usually are positive for the specific anti-treponemal antibody tests.

The first drug of choice in the treatment of congenital syphilis is also penicillin. [6]

21.3 Medical History

21.3.1 Syphilis

A pandemic of syphilis swept over Europe and into Africa and Asia beginning at the end of the 15th century. The disease resembled modern syphilis, but was much more virulent and with significant mortality. The disease had many names, usually blamed on a neighboring country, and was also called the great pox to distinguish it from small pox. Writing in 1546, Girolamo Fracastoro (1483 – 1553), an Italian polymath best known for his work on contagion and his description and naming of syphilis, said, "…our time has witnessed a new disease long unknown to our hemisphere….It invaded Italy…about the time the French under King Charles occupied the Kingdom of Naples about ten years before 1500…they say [the disease] is very common in certain regions which the Spanish navigators discovered — a new world where that contagion abounded to the widest extent, and was as well known a disease as Scabies is with us." [7] Prior to the germ theory of disease in the 19th century, the various sexually transmitted diseases were often confused with one another. This was aggravated by the surgeon and experimentalist John Hunter who, in 1767, inoculated someone with pus from a patient with gonorrhea. The patient developed a typical chancre and Dr. Hunter maintained that the diseases were the same. These two diseases were conclusively distinguished by Philippe Ricord (1800 – 1889) in 1838. The causative organism was identified in 1905 by Fritz Schaudinn (1871 – 1906) and Erich Hoffman (1868 – 1959) and first named Spirochaeta pallida.

Beginning early in the history of syphilis, it was treated with mercury, either with oral calomel, by injection, or with a salve. Mercury had long been used for the treatment of leprosy and it was known to be a diuretic and to increase salivation when given in large doses. It was thought that the agent responsible for syphilis could be eliminated in this way.

Paul Ehrlich (1854 – 1915, figure 21.6) was born in Strehlen in Upper Silesia. He studied at the University in Strasbourg, where he became interested in the chemistry of stains, and he graduated MD from Leipzig in 1878. He worked with the anatomist Wilhelm Waldeyer (1836 – 1921) and he stained and described mast cells in 1875. While working with Friedrich Theodor von Frerichs (1819 – 1885) in Berlin he discovered stains for blood cells, and in 1882 he developed a stain for Robert Koch's newly discovered tubercle bacillus. Ehrlich used his stain to diagnose his own tuberculosis and spent a year in Egypt recuperating. Ehrlich developed his famous side chain theory, that cells had side chains like those present, for example, on a benzene molecule, in 1897. He later changed the name from side chain to receptor. Ehrlich proposed that specific toxins would bind to the cell receptors and inactivate them. The cell would respond by secreting the receptor as an anti-toxin into the blood stream. We now know this theory to be incorrect, but it was an important step towards modern immunology, and Ehrlich won the Nobel Prize in Medicine in 1908. Although he initially doubted it, Ehrlich later decided that drugs might bind to specific receptors. He began a methodical search for a drug to treat syphilis using arsenical compounds. His assistant Sahachiro Hata (1873 – 1938) discovered that substance No. 606, arsphenamine, was active against syphilis. This lead to the production of the drug Salvarsan.

It had been noticed that patients with neurosyphilis had some amelioration of their symptoms when they were febrile. The psychiatrist Julius Wagner-Jauregg (1857 – 1940) received the Nobel Prize in 1927 for treating these patients with blood from patients with malaria. The patients were allowed to become febrile and then treated with quinine. One of the difficulties of the therapy was insuring that patients were given blood containing Plasmodium vivax and not the more virulent Plasmodium falciparum. These various therapies became obsolete in the 1940s after the discovery of penicillin by Alexander Fleming (1881 – 1955) and its later successful production.

There have been several hypotheses for the origin of syphilis including the Columbian (The disease came back with Columbus from the new world.), the Pre-Columbian (The disease was already present in the old world, but a new strain had broken out.), the Alternative (The disease came from baboon treponemes in Africa.), and the Unitarian (All treponemal diseases are caused by the same organism; the course and virulence is determined by environmental factors.). Evidence supporting the Columbian theory includes the absence of skeletal lesions of syphilis in Old World specimens from before 1492 and the written accounts of two physicians, Fernandez de Oviedo and Ruy Diaz de Isla, that claim that Columbus' pilot had returned with this disease and that it spread in Barcelona in 1493. Syphilis was called "Isla Española" or Hispaniola disease in Spain at the time. Some favored the Alternative theory, since exploration of Africa had also increased at that time, and there are continued occasional reports describing apparent syphilitic skeletal lesions in specimens from before 1492. Rothschild pointed out that single specimens would not be expected to have syphilitic changes, and that it is necessary to study many bone specimens from a community to determine if syphilis was present there. [8] Recent genomic studies have shown that the genomes of the various Treponemal species are different, eliminating the Unitarian theory from consideration. Treponema pertenue (the causative agent of yaws) has been shown to be similar to the treponeme found in African baboons, and the genetic diversity between Treponema pallidum and Treponema pertenue is most compatible with evolution over thousands of years. These findings are not completely consistent with any of the promulgated theories. Smajs et al. suggest that Treponema pallidum evolved from African baboon strains over thousands of years, yet still might have been brought to Europe by Columbus from the New World. [8 – 11]

21.4 Laboratory medicine

21.4.1 Syphilis

August von Wassermann (1866 – 1925, figure 21.7) was born in Bamberg, Germany the son of a banker. He graduated from Strasbourg in 1888 and became an assistant to Robert Koch. Wassermann was both a student of Koch and a follower of Paul Ehrlich. He was said to be a fine and humorous lecturer. He had many famous collaborators and didn't start research in his own laboratory until relatively late in life, beginning in 1913. In 1901 Bordet and Gengous developed the complement fixation test at the Pasteur Institute. Sheep red blood cells will lyse in the presence of antibodies to the red cells and complement. If one wants to know if a patient has a particular antibody, he or she combines the patient's serum with the antigen of interest – along with the sheep red blood cell system. If the antibody is present, it combines with the antigen and binds complement. In the absence of complement, the sheep red blood cells do not lyse. Wasserman wanted to use this system to detect antibody to Treponema pallidum which had just been discovered in 1905. He decided to use extracts from syphilitic lesions to obtain antigen, since Treponema pallidum cannot be cultured. His test worked and became the first serological test for infection with syphilis. It is interesting that none of Wassermann's controls were positive, since we now know that the Wassermann test is not specific for syphilis. Patients with a positive Wassermann test have an antibody to an antigen that was later identified as a component of the mitochondrial membrane called cardiolipin (first isolated from mammalian hearts). These antibodies are sometimes called reagin. False positive results may be seen in patients with leprosy, tuberculosis, chancroid, malaria, measles, chickenpox, hepatitis, pregnancy, recent immunization, drug addiction, autoimmune disease, aging, and in several other conditions. Over time the Wassermann test was replaced by the VDRL and RPR tests (Venereal Disease Research Lab and Rapid Plasma Reagin) that use lipid antigens from bovine heart to detect reagin.

The non-treponemal reagin tests may be reported qualitatively or quantitatively as a titer. Since they are sensitive but not specific for the detection of syphilis, they are used as screening tests. Confirmatory tests using anti-treponemal antibody include the fluorescent treponemal antibody absorption test (FTS-ABS), the microhemagglutination assay for treponemal antibodies (MHA-TP) and the Treponema pallidum hemagglutination assay (TPHA). Neither the reagin nor the treponemal tests are positive for 3 to 6 weeks after initial infection. The reagin tests become negative after treatment, but the treponemal tests are positive for decades.

Microscopically, Treponema pallidum (and the other Treponema species) are Gram negative, 8 to 10 microns long, and have 8 to 14 corkscrew-like spirals. They have a characteristic corkscrew-like motion. Material from a chancre can be placed on a glass slide and examined using a microscope set up for dark field examination. There are some anti-treponemal antibodies for direct observation of the organism using immunofluorescence or immunohistochemistry, but at the time of this writing, the latter are for research use only. [1, 11 – 13]

21.5 Study questions

1. What is the difference between a reagin and a treponemal test for syphilis?

2. What evidence is there to support the theory that syphilis first came to Europe with the return of Christopher Columbus?

3. Why did William Osler say, “He who knows syphilis knows medicine.”?

4. How often does congenital syphilis occur in the US?

5. Can you catch syphilis from a public toilet seat?

21.6 References

1. McCutchen JA. Sexually Transmitted Diseases. In: Porter RS, Kaplan JL, editors. The Merck manual of diagnosis and therapy. Whitehouse Station, NJ: Merck Sharpe & Dohme Corp.; 2011. p. 1475 - 1482.
2. Robinson ENJ, Hitchcock PJ, McGee ZA. Syphilis a disease with a history. In: Schaechter ME, NC Eisenstein, BI Medoff, G, editor. Mechanisms of microbial disease. Philadelphia: Lippincott, Williams & Wilkins; 1999. p. 243 - 250.
3. McAdam AJ, Miller DA, Sharpe AH. Infectious diseases. In: Kumar V, Abbas AK, Aster JC, editors. Robbins and Cotran Pathologic basis of disease. Philadelphia: Elsevier Saunders; 2015. p. 341 - 402.
4. Doolery JR, Binford CH. Treponematoses. In: Doolery JR, Binford CH, editors. Pathology of tropical and extraordinary diseases. Washington, D.C.: Armed Forces Institute of Pathology; 1976. p. 110 - 117.
5. Giacani L, Molini BJ, Kim EY *et al.* Antigenic variation in Treponema pallidum: TprK sequence diversity accumulates in response to immune pressure during experimental syphilis. J Immunol. 2010; 184:3822-3829.
6. Caserta MT. Infections in neonates. In: Porter RS, Kaplan JL, editors. The Merck manual of diagnosis and therapy. Whithouse Station, NJ: Merck Sharp & Dohme Corp.; 2011. p. 2821 - 2823.
7. Long ER. Selected readings in pathology. Springfield, Illinois: Charles C. Thomas; 1961
8. Rothschild BM. History of syphilis. Clin Infect Dis. 2005; 40:1454-1463.
9. Tampa M, Sarbu I, Matei C, Benea V, Georgescu SR. Brief history of syphilis. J Med Life. 2014; 7:4-10.
10. Smajs D, Norris SJ, Weinstock GM. Genetic diversity in Treponema pallidum: implications for pathogenesis, evolution and molecular diagnostics of syphilis and yaws. Infect Genet Evol. 2012; 12:191-202.
11. Talbott JH. A biographical history of medicine: excerpts and essays on the men and their work. New York: Grune & Stratton; 1970:1211.
12. Tille PM. Bailey & Scott's Diagnostic Microbiology. St. Louis: Elsevier Mosby; 2014
13. Bynum WF, Bynum HB. Dictionary of Medical Biography. Westport, Connecticut: Greenwood Press; 2007

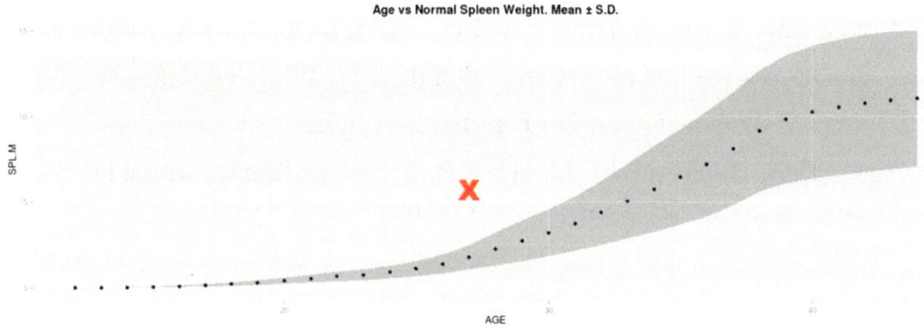

Figure 21.1. A graph of average fetal spleen weights and their standard deviations by gestational age. The case discussed in this chapter is represented by the red X. (Graph from https://markm2315-fw.shinyapps.io/Fetal_Growth_Curves/)

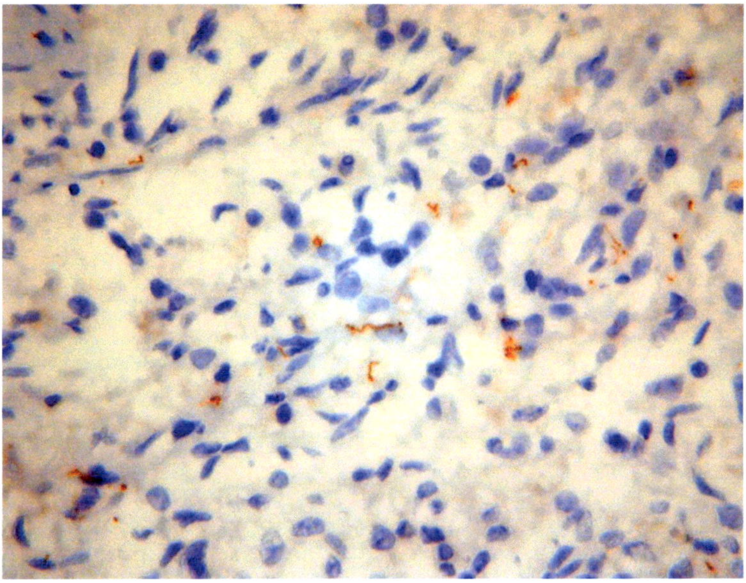

Figure 21.2. A section of the patient's spleen shows brown-stained spirochetes with an immunohistochemical stain. (Original magnification 400x, Anti-spirochete immunohistochemical stain)

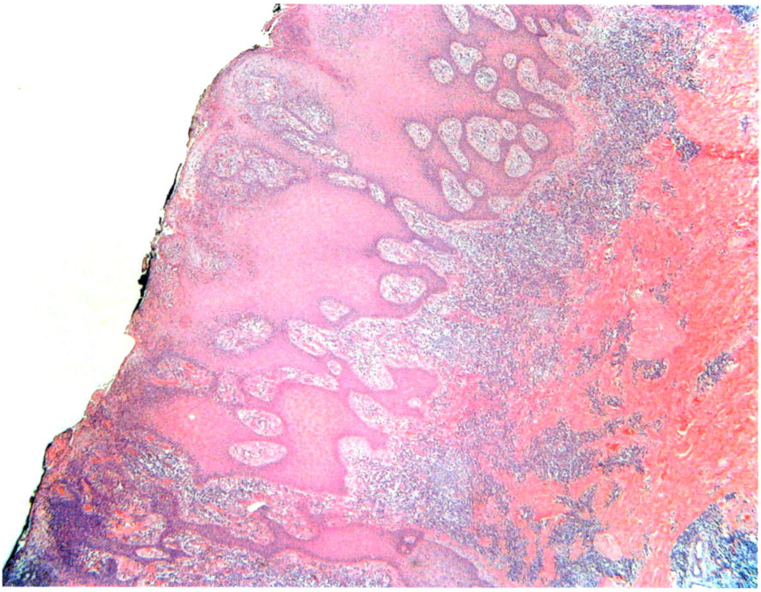

Figure 21.3. A histologic section from a different case of syphilis. This is a biopsy of a perianal lesion in an adult showing pseudoepitheliomatous squamous hyperplasia with a chronic inflammatory infiltrate. (Original magnification, x100. H&E stain)

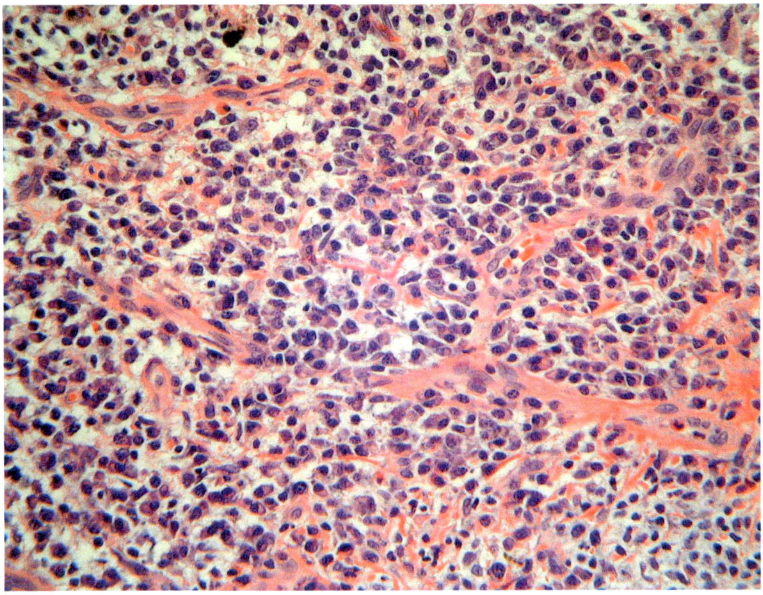

Figure 21.4. The inflammatory infiltrate in the lesion shown in Figure 21.3 is seen to be composed of many plasma cells. Plasma cells often have lilac-colored cytoplasm because of contained rough endoplasmic reticulum producing immunoglobulin. They also have a perinuclear clear zone from their Golgi apparatus and a characteristic eccentrically placed nucleus and coarse appearing chromatin. (Original magnification, x200. H&E stain)

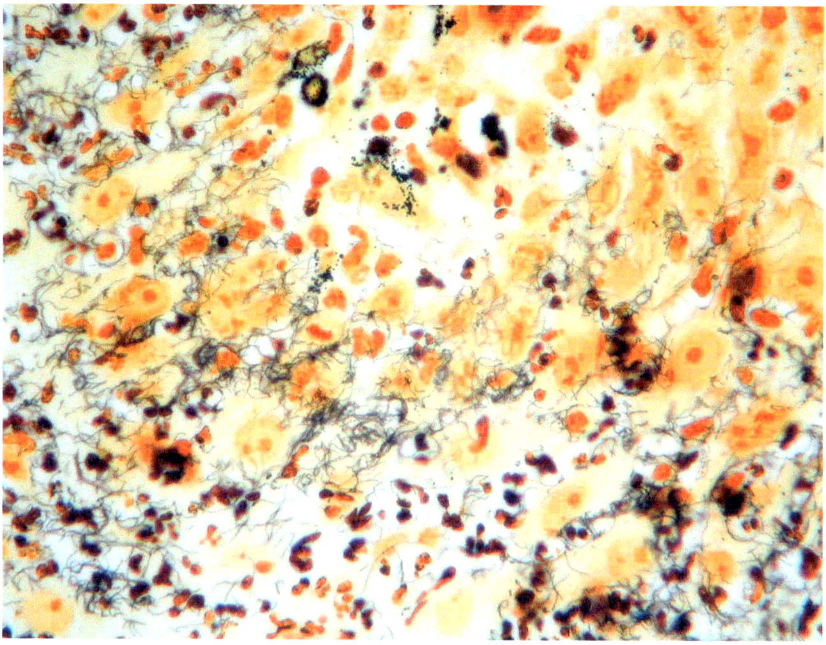

Figure 21.5. A Steiner silver impregnation stain on a section from the lesion shown in Figure 21.3 shows many thin black spirochetes. (Original magnification, x500. Steiner stain)

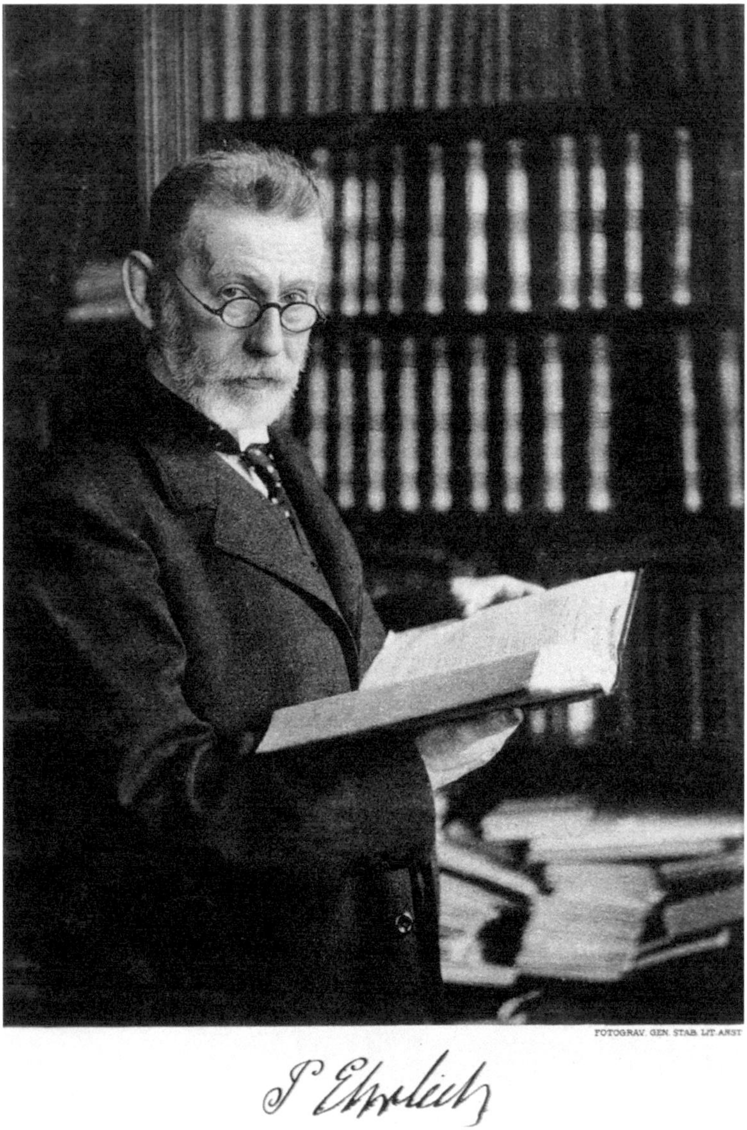

Figure 21.6. Paul Ehrlich (1854 – 1915). Courtesy of the National Library of Medicine.

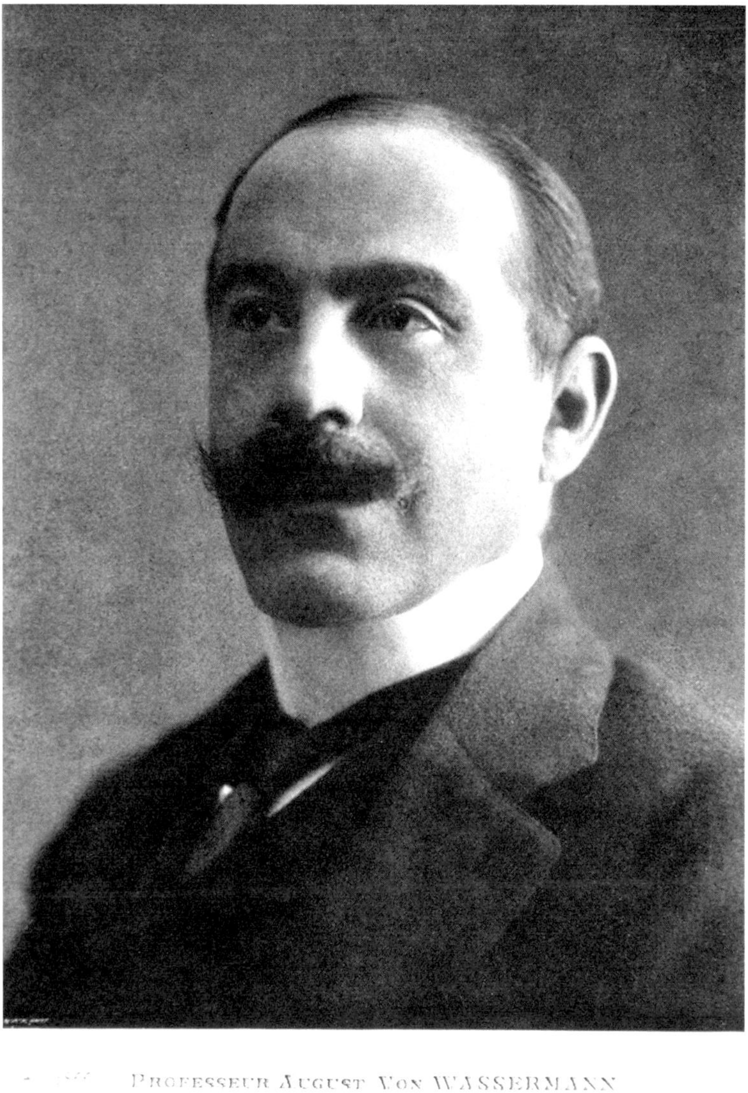

Figure 21.7. August von Wassermann (1866 – 1925) . Courtesy of the National Library of Medicine.

CHAPTER 22

An elderly man with left chest pain (viNdicaTe, neoplastic, toxic exposure)

"At dry dock, they'd gut all the asbestos insulation in the fire room then throw it into the bilges at the bottom of the ship. My job was to crawl on my belly in the ship's forward fire room bilges and sweep up the asbestos dust and debris. It was hot and poorly ventilated so breathing the asbestos dust was just part of the job." Navy boiler tender with mesothelioma. [1]

22.1 The Autopsy

22.1.1 Case history

The patient was an elderly man who had worked as a pipe fitter in the Philadelphia ship yards many years before. He developed left chest pain and he had left pleural thickening and a left pleural effusion on chest radiographs during the year prior to his death. A pleural biopsy and a left pleural fluid specimen had both been negative for malignancy seven months prior to his death, but the patient had a clinical diagnosis of malignant mesothelioma. The patient developed chest pain that was difficult to treat and he died while on hospice care.

22.1.2 Postmortem findings

The autopsy was limited to examination of the thoracic contents. There was obliteration of most of the pleural space on the left side and there was nodular tan-white thickening of the visceral pleura that was most prominent medially. The left pleura was up to 1.5 cm in thickness. A single 1 cm diameter nodule of tumor was present in the lung parenchyma grossly and the tumor penetrated into the mediastinum. The tumor appeared to surround and possibly penetrate lymph nodes in the mediastinum (figure 22.1 – 22.3). The patient had marked thoracic aorta atherosclerosis with complicated plaques and he had mild to moderate coronary artery atherosclerosis, but his heart was otherwise unremarkable. The right lung and esophagus appeared normal.

Histologic examination of the left pleura showed an extensive mixed epithelial and spindle cell type malignant neoplasm compatible with malignant mesothelioma. The tumor cells stained positively for epithelial membrane antigen, but were mucicarmine, carcinoembryonic antigen, and CD15 negative.

22.1.3 Case summary

The autopsy confirmed the presence of malignant mesothelioma and this was the cause of death. The patient's previous biopsies may have been negative because the tumor was most prominent medially.

22.2 Discussion

22.2.1 Asbestos

Asbestos is a naturally occurring fibrous mineral that can be woven like cloth. The mineral is a calcium, magnesium and/or iron silicate that is resistant to heat and fire, and is both sound damping and does not conduct electricity. It has been widely used as insulation, in construction and shipbuilding, in domestic products such as ironing boards and electric hair dryers, and in the manufacture of brakes, clutch linings, and gaskets. Asbestos was a component of Kent cigarette filters from 1952 to 1956 and it was used as artificial snow in Christmas decorations and in the motion picture industry (figure 22.4). Exposure to asbestos fibers is associated with pulmonary fibrosis, called asbestosis; pleural fibrosis; pleural effusions; carcinoma of the lung, larynx, ovary, and possibly the colon; and malignant mesothelioma of the pleura and of the peritoneum. The use of asbestos is currently tightly restricted or prohibited in many developed countries, but it is still widely used, sometimes with little protection, in developing countries.

Asbestos occurs in different mineral forms and is called white, blue, brown, or green asbestos when mined. The largest amounts of asbestos are in Canada and Russia, but it occurs widely. The various types of asbestos can be divided into serpentine and amphibole forms. About 90% of the asbestos that has been used is the serpentine form chrysotile. Serpentine asbestos is curled looking under the microscope and more water soluble than amphibole asbestos. It is thought to be more likely to be caught in the upper airways and removed by pulmonary macrophages. Amphibole asbestos, typical minerals being crocodilite and amosite, has straighter fibers that are less water soluble and which penetrate to the lower airways and out to the pleura. Both fiber types cause fibrosis of the lung and are carcinogenic, but amphibole asbestos is more likely to be associated with malignant mesothelioma. Asbestos exposure and cigarette smoking are more than additive risk factors for carcinoma of the lung. Patients with both pulmonary fibrosis from asbestos and who smoke cigarettes are many times more likely to get lung cancer than the general population.

Asbestos workers are at risk to get diffuse pulmonary interstitial fibrosis. Asbestosis starts in a subpleural location and is most prominent at the base of the lungs. Patients usually present with difficulty breathing 20 or 30 years after their asbestos exposure. The fibrosis is progressive and leads to pulmonary hypertension and right heart disease (cor pulmonale) like other forms of pulmonary fibrosis. Examination of lung tissue from patients with asbestosis usually shows small fibrous, often iron encrusted, bodies called asbestos bodies (figure 22.5). Exposure to asbestos also causes focal areas of benign fibrous thickening of the pleura called fibrous plaques. These lesions often calcify and are visible on chest radiographs. [2, 3]

22.2.2 Malignant Mesothelioma

Malignant mesothelioma is a rare malignancy of the pleura, peritoneum, pericardium, or tunica vaginalis arising from the lining mesothelial cells. The incidence in developed countries has ranged between 1 and 4 cases per 100,000 people in the last 20 years. Men are five times more likely than women to get mesothelioma, but this is due to the higher exposure in occupations where men are more likely to work. In occupations where women are more common, e.g. some asbestos factories where asbestos was woven by women, women have had the expected incidence of mesothelioma. The proportion of mesotheliomas that are asbestos related is controversial, but it is about 80 – 90% of cases. Mesothelioma has also been seen in patients who were exposed to Thorotrast (an old radiocontrast agent that was an alpha particle emitter) and in patients who had external beam irradiation for other malignancies, e.g. Hodgkin's lymphoma. There is some evidence of a genetic susceptibility to mesothelioma in families with mutations in the BRCA1 gene. The lifetime risk for getting mesothelioma in patients with heavy asbestos exposure is 7 – 10%. The tumor has a long latent period; patients present 25 to 45 years after their first asbestos exposure. Mesothelioma may be epithelioid, sarcomatoid, or mixed histologic type. These types occur in the ratio 3:1:1. The tumor is diffuse and pleural tumors can originate in either the visceral or parietal pleura. Patients present with chest pain and dyspnea. Only about 20% of them also have asbestosis. The median survival time is 12 months. Therapy may include any or all the usual modalities, depending on cancer stage and the patient's condition. Typical chemotherapy includes cisplatin and an antifolate drug like pemetrexed.

The diagnosis of mesothelioma may be difficult. In some cases, the clinicians and radiologists are quite certain that a patient has the disease, but the pathologist is unable to make a conclusive diagnosis by cytology or histopathology. This is because benign reactive mesothelial cells may appear very atypical cytologically and histologically, and because historically there have been no conclusive additional studies, e.g. immunohistochemical stains, to separate benign from malignant mesothelial cells. Pathologists often use multiple special stains on these cases to help exclude the diagnosis of a non-mesothelioma malignancy in the pleura, e.g. lung cancer, and to help exclude benign reactive mesothelial cells masquerading as a malignancy. The stains used have included mucicarmine, a pan-keratin antibody, calretinin, WT-1, D2-40, cytokeratin 5/6, CD-15, carcinoembryonic antigen, e-cadherin, TTF-1, and others. Recently, an antibody for BAP1 (BRCA1 associated protein) and fluorescent in situ hybridization (FISH) for p16 (CDKN2A) have been shown to be sensitive and specific for the detection of malignant mesothelioma. Both genes may be lost, or their expression diminished in many different malignancies, and it has been proposed that there might be a BAP1 cancer syndrome characterized by mesothelioma and melanoma.

The first poliovirus vaccines were prepared in rhesus monkey kidney cell cultures. In 1959 the DNA virus SV40 was discovered in these vaccines and was later shown to be oncogenic in rodents. Tumors in exposed rodents included mesothelioma, ependymoma, osteosarcoma, and non-Hodgkin's lymphoma. These vaccines were inactivated with formaldehyde, but some batches of vaccine contained infectious SV40. It is estimated that 30 - 100 million people in the US alone received potentially contaminated polio vaccine between 1955 and 1963. SV40 DNA sequences have been identified in human mesothelioma tumor cells, and it was proposed in the 1990s that SV40 and asbestos exposure might act synergistically to produce mesothelioma. Other studies have questioned these results, and epidemiological studies have shown no link between SV40 and mesothelioma.

Man-made carbon nanotubules are beginning to be widely used as structural materials and in Medicine for bone grafting, dental implants, targeted drug delivery, and imaging diagnostics. Little is known about their toxicity, but there is evidence that they persist in the body as fibers with possible carcinogenic potential. In mice, these nano-fibers migrate to the pleura and induce inflammation after a single inhalation. The pleural changes have been described as resembling the changes seen after exposure to asbestos. Detected changes have included gene expression profiles that resemble those seen in human lung cancer risk and progression. Recall that malignancy may follow asbestos exposure only after several decades have passed. The US National

Institute for Occupational Safety and Health (NIOSH) recommended an exposure limit for carbon nanotubules of 1 microgram/cubic meter elemental carbon as a respirable mass in 2013. [3 – 8]

22.3 Medical History

22.3.1 Asbestos and Malignant Mesothelioma

Asbestos was known to the ancient Greeks and Romans, and it was mentioned and named by the Roman historian Pliny the Elder. Marco Polo said that he saw it mined on his travels. Røe and Stella show a picture of asbestos bowls used for cooking food in Norway from the bronze age up to about 575 C.E. Large scale mining and production of asbestos started in the mid 19th century. There were some reports of adverse health effects of exposure to asbestos as early as 1899. William Cooke (1881 – 1939) of the Wigan Infirmary Department of Pathology published a case report of a 33-year-old woman who had worked in the spinning room of Turner Brothers Asbestos in Rochdale since she was 13. She died of pulmonary fibrosis and tuberculosis, and the case suggested the possibility of a relationship of her lung disease and her asbestos exposure. Following a similar case report in Glasgow, Edward Merewether (1892 – 1970), a 36-year-old medical inspector was asked to investigate. In his 1929 report he stated that asbestos workers were at increased risk for pulmonary fibrosis leading to complete disablement and death. The British Asbestos Industry Regulations were enacted in 1931 requiring the suppression of dust in asbestos factories and leading to a subsequent reduction in the incidence of asbestosis. There was little regulation in the United States prior to the 1970 act creating the Occupational Safety and Health Administration.

Pleural tumors were described prior to the 20th century. The French physician Joseph Lieutand (1703 – 1780) described a case of a pleural tumor in 1767, but prior to significant production of asbestos, malignant mesothelioma was so rare that many physicians were not familiar with it. One of the first good descriptions of mesothelioma was by Klemperer and Rabin in 1931. Some thought that the incidence of lung cancer was also increased in these workers, and in 1955 Richard Doll (1912 – 2005) at Central Middlesex Hospital published the results of a case control study that seemed to confirm an increased incidence of carcinoma of the lung in patients exposed to asbestos. In 1960 J. C. Wagner, C. A. Sleggs, and P. Marchand reported that South African miners working with crocodilite asbestos had an increased incidence of malignant mesothelioma. The idea that asbestos exposure was linked to mesothelioma became well established in the 1960s, and reports by Irving Selikoff (1915 – 1992) at Mt. Sinai Medical Center in New York also indicated that there was some increased risk for those who worked with asbestos products, not just in asbestos miners and factory workers.

Law suits seeking compensation for asbestos related disease started in 1969 in the United States and ultimately became the longest running mass tort in US history. Famous criminal cases included those against the Adamo Wrecking Company in Detroit in 1973 and W. R. Grace and Company in Libby, Montana in 2005. The mass tort case led to the bankruptcy of the Johns Manville Corporation in the 1980s. The US Environmental Protection Agency only began to require that manufacturers mention if their products contained asbestos in 1988. A permitted exposure limitation to 0.1 ff/mL of respired air was introduced in the US in 1994. It is estimated that 1000 tons of asbestos were released when the World Trade Center was destroyed on September 11, 2001. Currently the use of asbestos is banned in the European Union, Australia, New Zealand, Japan, and Hong Kong. Asbestos is still used for some construction purposes in the United States. [4, 5, 9]

22.4 Laboratory medicine

22.4.1 Malignant Mesothelioma

Laboratory tests don't currently play a large role in the diagnosis of malignant mesothelioma, but many possible biomarkers have been tested, and some FDA approved tests are available. The mesothelin gene encodes a 69 kDa precursor protein that is cleaved into two pieces, a soluble portion called Megakaryocyte potentiating factor, and a membrane-bound glycoprotein called

Mesothelin. Tests for the detection of both moieties have been devised. Mesothelin is present in normal mesothelial cells, but it is increased in epithelioid mesothelioma cells, ovarian cancer and in carcinoma of the pancreas. Its sensitivity for the detection of mesothelioma has been quite variable in different laboratories. The gene ERC, first isolated from renal cell carcinoma cells in the rat, is a homologue of the human mesothelin gene. An ELISA test for the N-terminal fragment that is cleaved from the mesothelin precursor protein has been sensitive and moderately specific for the detection of mesothelioma. Other potential biomarkers have included fibulin-3 and osteopontin.

A relatively new assay using slow off-rate modified aptamers (SOMAmers) to bind and detect small amounts of proteins in patient's blood has been used to identify a 13-protein signature that appears to be characteristic for malignant mesothelioma. It has been tested for use for early detection and measurement of progression in mesothelioma. Similarly, work has been done with the use of microRNA miR-625-3p in patient's plasma for the detection of mesothelioma.

Years ago, it was common to take a portion of lung from autopsy or surgical specimens from patients who were suspected of having asbestos exposure and to digest it in bleach. The digested material was washed and concentrated on a slide by centrifugation or with a filter and the slide was examined by light microscopy for asbestos bodies. The test results were often used in legal testimony as proof of asbestos exposure, but since patients without a history of any significant asbestos exposure may have some asbestos bodies in this type of concentrated specimen, and since a quantitative normal range for the number of bodies found was never established, the test was discontinued (figure 22.5). [5, 10 – 12]

22.5 Study questions

1. Why did it take so long to determine that asbestos exposure was a risk factor for malignant mesothelioma?

2. Are men more susceptible to getting mesothelioma than women?

3. Why did the Johns Manville Corporation file for bankruptcy in 1982 and what is the Manville Trust?

4. What is the relative risk for getting lung cancer between white males who neither smoke nor are exposed to asbestos and white males who both smoke and are exposed to asbestos?

5. What would be the clinical usefulness of a blood test that was moderately sensitive but highly specific for mesothelioma, and what would be the usefulness of a test that was highly sensitive but only moderately specific for mesothelioma?

22.6 References

1. Anonymous. Quotes from those whose lives have been affected by asbestos disease. http://www.mesotheliomaweb.org/quotes.htm. Accessed 2017.
2. Husain AN. The Lung. In: Kumar V, Abbas AK, Aster JC, editors. Robbins and Cotran Pathological Basis of Disease. Philadelphia: Elsevier Saunders; 2015. p. 690 - 692.
3. Husain AN. The Lung. In: Kumar V, Abbas AK, Aster JC, editors. Robbins and Cotran Pathologic Basis of Disease. Philadelphia: Elsevier Saunders; 2015. p. 723 - 724.
4. Bartrip PWJ. History of asbestos related disease. Postgrad Med J. 2004; 80:72 - 76.
5. Røe OD, Stell GM. Malignant pleural mesothelioma: history, controversy and future of manmade epidemic. Eur Respir rev. 2015; 24:115 - 131.
6. Cigognetti M, Lonardi S, Fisogni S *et al.* BAP1 (BRCA1-associated protein 1) is a highly specific marker for diferentiating mesothelioma from reactive mesothelial proliferations. Mod Pathol. 2015; 28:1043-1057.
7. Anonymous. NIOSH: Occupational exposure to carbon nanotubles and fibers. https://www.nano.gov/node/1007. 2013.
8. Hwang HC, Sheffield BS, Rodriguez S *et al.* Utility of BAP1 immunohistochemistry and p16 (CDKN2A) FISH in the diagnosis of malignant mesothelioma in effusion cytology specimens. Am J Surg Pathol. 2016; 40:120-126.

9. Anonymous. Asbestos and the Law. https://en.wikipedia.org/wiki/Asbestos_and_the_law. Accessed 2017.
10. Ostroff RM, Mehan MR, Stewart A *et al.* Early detection of malignant pleural mesothelioma in asbestos-exposed individuals with a non-invasive proteomics-based surveillance tool. PLoS One. 2012; 7:e46091.
11. Sato T, Suzuki Y, Takanori M *et al.* Newly established ELISA for N-ERC/mesothelin improves diagnostic accuracy in patients with suspected pleural mesothelioma. Cancer Medicine. 2014; 3:1377 - 1384.
12. Hollevoet K, Reitsma JB, Creaney J *et al.* Serum mesothelin for diagnosing malignant pleural mesothelioma: an individual patient data meta-analysis. J Clin Oncol. 2012; 30:1541 - 1549.

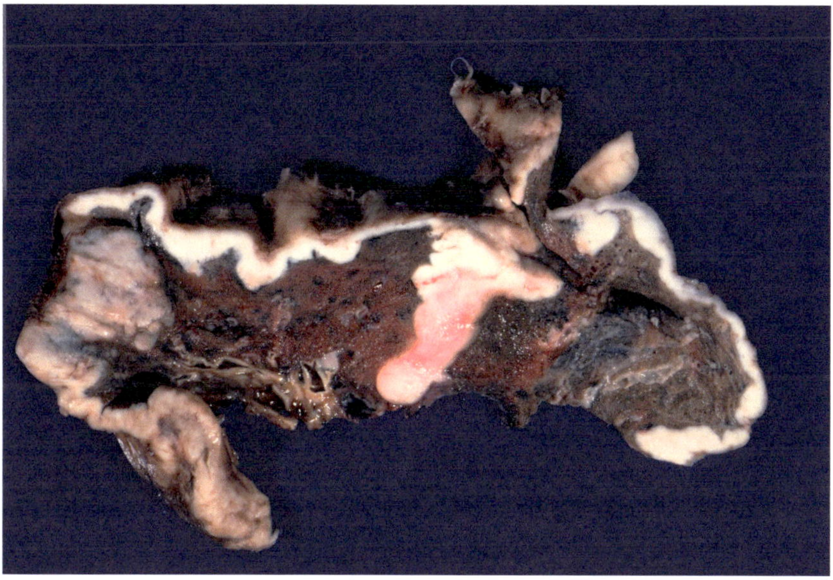

Figure 22.1 A specimen from a different case of malignant mesothelioma. The tumor forms a white rind around the dark collapsed lung.

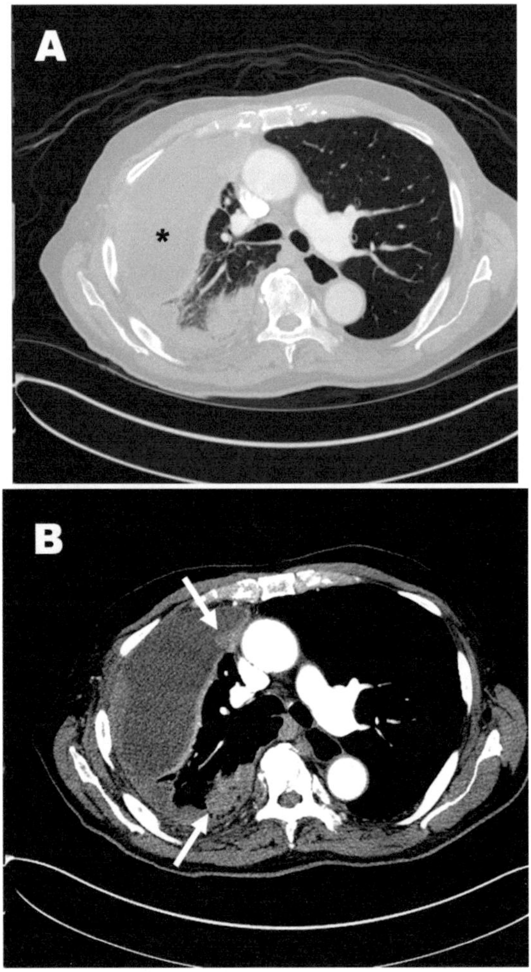

Figure 22.2.A An axial contrast enhanced CT of the chest in lung windows from a different patient shows a large loculated right pleural effusion (black asterisk).

Figure 22.2.B The axial contrast enhanced CT of the chest in soft tissue windows shows a large loculated right pleural effusion with nodular tissue along the pleural surface (arrows) concerning for malignant mesothelioma. Some smooth non-nodular thickening is atelectasis from the pleural effusion.

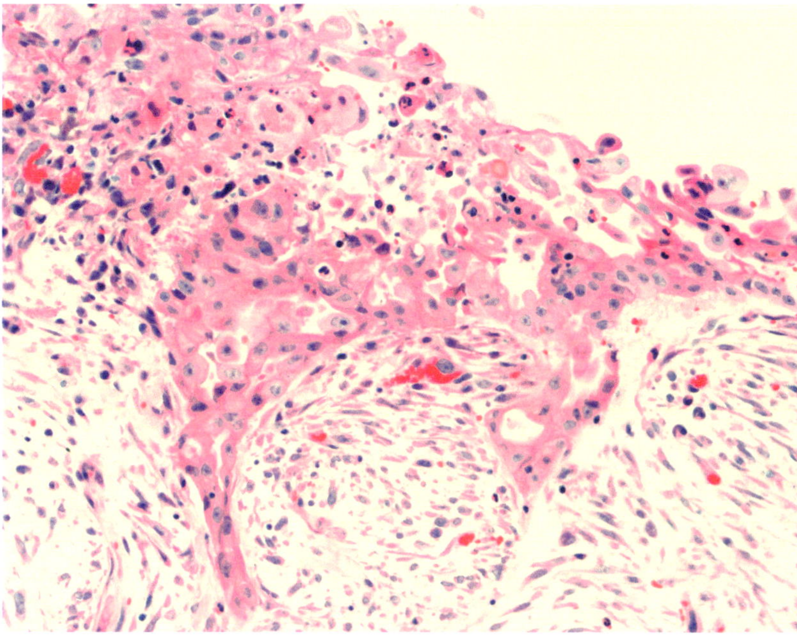

Figure 22.3 A histologic section from a different case of malignant mesothelioma. The tumor is biphasic with atypical epithelioid cells on the pleural surface and atypical spindle cells in the underlying stroma. Although this is a case of malignant mesothelioma, benign reactive mesothelioma cells may sometimes have a similar appearance. (Original magnification, x200. H&E stain)

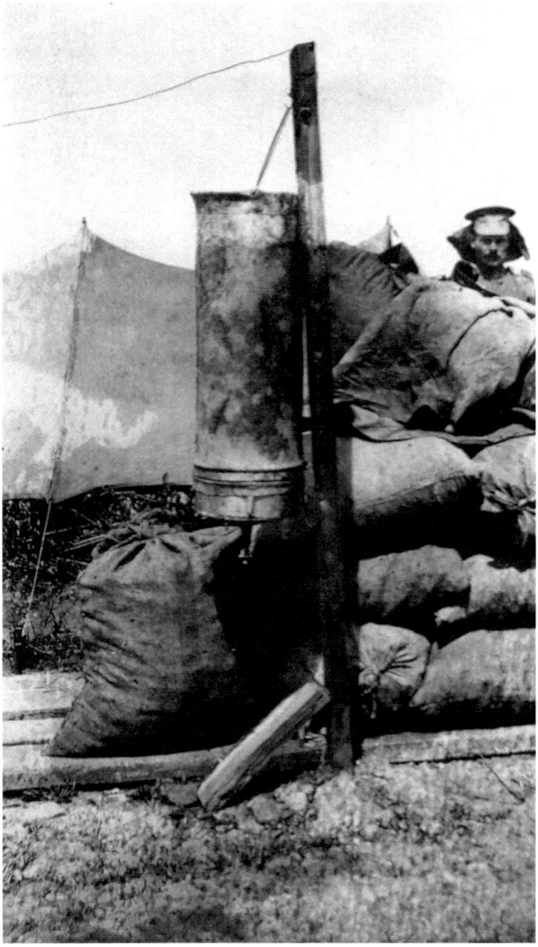

Figure 22.4 A water filter used in the Russo-Japanese war of 1904 - 1905. The filter is a linen bag filled with asbestos. Courtesy of the National Library of Medicine.

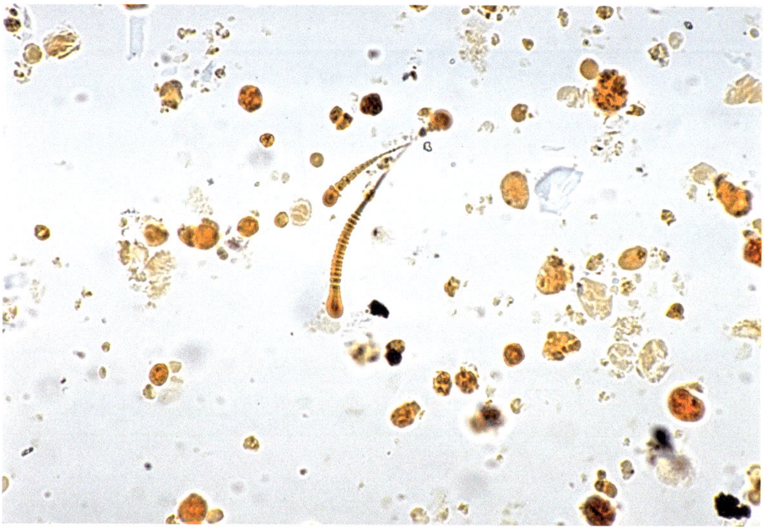

Figure 22.5 Asbestos bodies from a digested portion of the patient's lung. Asbestos bodies have a central transparent or translucent fiber that is surrounded by nodular accreted material that contains iron giving it a golden-brown color. (Original magnification, x500. No stain used)

CHAPTER 23

An elderly man with cough and weight loss (viNDicate, neoplastic, drug)

"Now I'm being blamed not only for anorexia but for lung cancer". - On being a social smoker. Kate Moss (1974 –)

23.1 The Autopsy

23.1.1 Case history

The patient was a man in late middle-age with generalized weakness and a 50-pound (23 Kg) weight loss in 3 months. He also had been hoarse, with difficulty swallowing, a nonproductive cough, and left posterior chest pain over the same period. The patient had a smoking history and a recent chest radiograph had shown "a new process" in the right upper lung lobe with fullness in the right pulmonary hilum. The patient had a history of non-insulin dependent diabetes mellitus and a previous coronary artery bypass graft procedure for coronary artery atherosclerosis. At the time of admission to the hospital the patient had a serum lactate dehydrogenase of 434 (normal = 60 - 160 U/L), an aspartate aminotransferase, AST, of 167 (normal = 0 - 35 U/L), a hemoglobin of 10.1 (normal = 14 - 17 g/dL) and a slightly elevated urea nitrogen, BUN, with normal serum creatinine. His medications were listed as Ascriptin (aspirin, possibly as an anti-platelet aggregation drug), Capoten (captopril, an angiotensin converting enzyme inhibitor for high blood pressure and congestive heart failure), Tylenol (acetaminophen, for pain relief), Codeine (a narcotic, for pain relief), Tagamet (cimetidine, to decrease gastric acidity), Digoxin (a natural alkaloid from the digitalis plant, for heart failure), Xanax (alprazolam, a benzodiazepine for anxiety), Darvocet (acetaminophen and propoxyphene (a narcotic), for pain relief, no longer available in the US), Tylenol #3 (acetaminophen and codeine, for pain relief), and Percocet (acetaminophen and oxycodone, for pain relief). The list almost certainly included the drugs he had taken over some time, since the patient could not take all of these narcotics and acetaminophen containing drugs at one time. CT scan of the chest showed an infiltrate in the left lung base with air bronchograms (i.e. there was some consolidation of the lung and the air in the contained bronchi showed up as an area of decreased density on the radiograph), a right pleural effusion, and evidence of metastatic disease in the liver. CT scan of the head was normal. The patient had a generalized seizure on the 16th hospital day followed by cardiac arrest and death.

23.1.2 Postmortem findings

At autopsy the patient had a 3-cm maximum diameter subpleural tumor in his right upper lung lobe. Histologic examination was compatible with small cell undifferentiated carcinoma of the lung. Metastases were present in right pulmonary hilar lymph nodes, the left visceral pleura, the liver, and in bone marrow (figures 23.1 – 23.5). The patient had bilateral small to moderate pleural effusions, an enlarged spleen, 680 grams (normal = 150 grams), and organizing regional alveolar damage in the left lower lung lobe. The patient's liver weighed 3630 grams (normal = 1500 grams). The patient had marked coronary artery atherosclerosis with three patent vein grafts. He had extensive scarring of the lower third of his left cardiac ventricle compatible with old myocardial infarcts, and he had biventricular hypertrophy with a heart weighing 619 grams (normal = 350 grams).

The patient's stomach contained 50 - 60 white only partially degenerated tablets. The tablets were roughly elliptical with a central score mark. They had no other marking on them. An additional 40 - 50 tablets were present in the patient's intestines (figure 23.6). I provided a sample of these tablets and of the patient's liver to the Medical Examiner for toxicological examination. The case fell into the Medical Examiner's purview since I now suspected an unnatural manner of death. Throughout most of my career, the hospitals where my autopsies were performed did not have elaborate toxicology laboratories. They were designed to perform screening tests on blood and urine, and to refer more complicated specimens to outside laboratories, since those analyses are expensive and unusual. But at the time and place that this autopsy was done, the clinical chemistry laboratory had a gas-liquid chromatograph. I gave a tablet to the laboratory and the technologists informed me that their analysis had not turned up any of the approximately 150 drugs that they could detect. I asked if there were any common drugs that GLC could not detect. They said, yes, aspirin and acetaminophen, and that these were detected by simple thin layer chromatography. A methanol extract of one of the tablets was positive for acetaminophen. I informed the Medical Examiner's laboratory that my laboratory had found acetaminophen, and they confirmed this later.

23.1.3 Case summary

This case appeared to be a relatively straight forward case of stage IV small cell undifferentiated carcinoma of the lung in a patient who also had marked coronary artery atherosclerosis, but when the gastrointestinal tract was opened at the end of the autopsy, I was surprised to find about 100 tablets. Obviously, patients are not prescribed 100 of the same tablets at one time, and the findings were compatible with suicide from acetaminophen overdose. The patient had obtained a 100-count bottle of acetaminophen and taken its entire contents. The minimum lethal dose of acetaminophen in an adult is 25 grams. The patient had probably ingested three times that much in a short period of time, and the patient had abundant metastatic carcinoma in his liver and some degree of cancer associated cachexia. There was no clinical information to indicate that anyone on the medical staff was aware that this had happened, and there was never any comment from the patient's family about the autopsy report.

23.2 Discussion

23.2.1 Carcinoma of the Lung

Carcinoma of the lung is second behind breast cancer in incidence in the US, but it is first in cancer-related deaths. There were only 18,000 new cases of lung cancer in 1950, but there were 226,160 in 2012. Lung cancer was responsible for 28% of all cancer related deaths in 2012 in the US. Breast cancer was the leading cause of cancer-related death in women from about 1947 until 1987, but since then lung cancer deaths have been more common.

About 85% of lung cancer cases are caused by cigarettes, and about 11% of heavy smokers develop lung cancer. The cause of the other 15% of cases is unknown. Possible causes include radon gas, EGFR mutations, exposure to other people's exhaled cigarette smoke (so-called second-hand smoking), asbestos, radiation, arsenic, nickel and chromates. The risk of lung cancer is increased in patients with pulmonary fibrosis. Patients who smoke have the accumulation of somatic mutations in their bronchial epithelium over time. These mutations may cause increased cell growth (K-RAS and MYC), abnormal growth factor receptor signaling (EGFR, ALK, HER-2), decreased apoptosis (BCL-2), or inhibit tumor suppressor genes (p53, APC). There are several different histologic types of malignant lung tumors. The main categories of lung cancer are squamous cell carcinoma, adenocarcinoma, small cell undifferentiated carcinoma and poorly differentiated non-small cell or large cell carcinoma. Cigarette smokers may get any of these types, but squamous cell carcinoma and small cell undifferentiated carcinoma have the closest linkage to cigarette smoking. Common presenting symptoms are cough, chest pain, and dyspnea. Hemoptysis (blood in the sputum) may occur, but is uncommon. About 25% of cases have no symptoms and the tumor is detected incidentally by radiography. The prognosis of lung cancer is closely related to the patient's tumor stage. Lung carcinoma stages correspond to patients with local disease, those with relatively local metastases only or regional disease, and those with distant metastases. About 60% of patients have metastatic disease at the time of initial diagnosis. The five-year survival for all lung cancer patients with low stage disease that is confined to the lung is about 54% with treatment, and it is only about 4% for patients with distant metastases.

Small cell carcinoma is more aggressive than the non-small cell types of carcinoma. It is usually staged as either limited or high stage (extensive) disease. Less than one third of patients present in limited stage. The five-year survival for small cell undifferentiated carcinoma with treatment is 20% in limited stage and less than 1% in patients with extensive disease. Small cell carcinoma may arise centrally or peripherally in the lung. The tumor cells have a high nucleus to cytoplasm ratio and are often relatively small compared to other tumor cell types. They may resemble oats histologically, and the tumor has been called oat cell carcinoma (figures 23.4, 23.5). The tumor appears to arise from the normal neuroendocrine cells of the lung and the tumor cells often stain positively with immunohistochemical stains for neuroendocrine markers like chromogranin, synaptophysin and CD57.

Carcinoma of the lung may be treated with radiation, surgical resection, chemotherapy, or some combination of these. Some tumor types may also be treated with biological drugs that target specific tumor cell receptors, when other therapies have failed. The diagnosis of lung cancer is usually made radiographically and then confirmed by either bronchoscopic biopsy or fine-needle aspiration biopsy. The diagnosis of carcinoma may also be made cytologically from the patient's sputum, from a sample of pleural fluid, or from a biopsy of a metastatic site. [1 – 3]

23.2.2 Acetaminophen

Acetaminophen is available without a prescription and is widely used by itself and in combination with other drugs as an analgesic (pain relieving) and anti-pyretic (fever lowering) alternative to aspirin. Unlike aspirin, acetaminophen has only weak anti-inflammatory activity, has few gastrointestinal side effects, does not affect platelet function, and does not cause acid-base abnormalities. Patients with aspirin allergy only rarely react to acetaminophen, but rare patients are allergic to acetaminophen. The drug is usually well tolerated, but an acute overdose can cause severe liver damage and death. Acetaminophen is a common cause of drug overdose in the US. In 2009, the FDA recommended that the maximum daily dose of acetaminophen be lowered in adults and children, especially since so many combination drugs contain acetaminophen and the patient may unknowingly take a toxic dose.

Acetaminophen has a peak plasma concentration 30 - 60 minutes after an oral therapeutic dose and a plasma half-life of about 2 hours. Between 90 and 100% of the drug is excreted in the urine in one day following hepatic conjugation of the drug. A small amount of acetaminophen forms a highly reactive intermediate metabolite called N-acetyl-p-benzoquinone-imine, NAPQI. Normally, NAPQI is inactivated by glutathione unless the dose is so large that the amount of glutathione available is inadequate.

Acute ingestion of more than 7.5 grams of acetaminophen or repeated exposure to high doses can cause toxicity. The most serious side effect is liver necrosis. Renal tubular necrosis and hypoglycemic coma may also occur. In cases of toxic overdose, the patient's hepatic glutathione stores are depleted and the metabolite NAPQI binds to cell macromolecules disrupting normal cell metabolism. Reduction of glutathione by itself renders the hepatocytes more susceptible to oxidative stress. Doses of 20 - 25 grams are potentially fatal. Susceptibility of acetaminophen is increased in patients with low glutathione, e.g. patients who are fasting, malnourished, or alcoholic. After acute poisoning, patients may have deceptively mild symptoms for the first 48 hours with anorexia, nausea and abdominal pain. Plasma transaminases become elevated about 12 - 36 hours after ingestion. In 48 - 96 hours the patient will start to have signs and symptoms referable to the liver including jaundice, tender hepatomegaly, and coagulopathy. Liver enzymes will also peak in this time interval. The prognosis is poor if hepatic encephalopathy or worsening coagulopathy ensue after the fourth day after ingestion. Liver biopsy done at this time would show centrilobular necrosis with preservation of the periportal area (liver zone 1). The hepatic necrosis is reversible if the patient survives.

Acetaminophen overdose is a medical emergency. The patient's risk of liver injury can be seen on the Rumack-Matthew nomogram which relates acetaminophen plasma level and time after ingestion to the risk. So, for example, 90% of patients with an acetaminophen level > 300 micrograms/mL at 4 hours after ingestion are likely to have severe liver injury. About 10% of patients who don't receive treatment will develop severe liver injury and about 10% of those patients will eventually die of liver failure. Standard treatment consists of early use of activated charcoal and early use of N-acetylcysteine (Mucomyst or Acetadote). N-acetylcysteine replenishes liver glutathione and may bind directly with NAPQI to inactivate it. Aggressive supportive care may also be necessary. Some patients with severe hepatonecrosis may require liver transplantation. [4, 5]

23.3 Medical History

23.3.1 Carcinoma of the Lung

Except possibly among certain miners, lung cancer was a rare disease in the 19th century. Malignant lung tumors only comprised 1% of all cancers in 1878 in autopsies done at the Institute of Pathology of the University of Dresden. Miners in the area of Schneeberg, Saxony were known to have a disease called Schneeberg lung disease as early as the 16th century. Drs. Hartung and Hesse showed in 1879 that about 75% of these miners died from carcinoma of the lung. In the 20th century it was shown that the air in these mines had a high content of radon gas. The surgeon Alton Ochsner (1896 – 1981) told the story that while he was a student at Washington University Medical School his entire junior class was called to see an autopsy on a lung cancer patient, and that George Dock (1860 – 1951), then their chief of medicine, said that the group might not see another case in their lifetimes. Ochsner did not see another case of lung cancer for 17 years, but he then saw eight cases in six months among patients who had started smoking during their service in World War I.

Inhalation of the smoke from burning tobacco leaves was a widespread practice among North and South American Indians, and some cultivation sites are thought to be as old as 3400 years. Tobacco was brought to Europe in the 16th century. Tobacco contains the alkaloid stimulant nicotine and its use is addictive. Tobacco smoke contains many other toxic substances, including carbon monoxide, cyanide and various carcinogens. In the 19th century tobacco cigarettes were relatively expensive because they were hand made. In 1876, the cigarette manufacturer Allen & Ginter offered a prize for an invention to help produce cigarettes and James Albert Bonsack (1859 – 1924) invented a machine that could make 200 cigarettes in one minute; a skilled cigarette roller could make 200 cigarettes in an hour. This reduced the price of cigarettes by 50%. Allen & Ginter were reluctant to use the machine because they did not believe there was a market for this volume of uniformly made cigarettes. James Buchanan Duke (1856 – 1925) leased two of the machines and had great commercial success; in 1889, he became president of the new American Tobacco Company formed by the combination of many different tobacco companies. The Sherman Anti-Trust Act was passed in 1890 and The American Tobacco Company was broken up in 1907 – 1911. Cigarettes were popularized during the First World War and became even more popular among civilian men, women, and adolescents in the 1920's.

In 1929, the German physician Fritz Lickint (1898 – 1960) published a paper that showed that lung cancer patients were likely to be cigarette smokers, and he then started an anti-smoking campaign in Germany. F. H. Müller published a case control study in 1940 and stated, "the extraordinary rise in tobacco use was the single most important cause of the rising incidence of lung cancer".

On April 5, 1933 Evarts A. Graham (1883 – 1957) performed the first one stage pneumonectomy for lung cancer in which the patient survived the procedure. The patient, Dr. James Gilmore, a 48-year-old gynecologist, lived until 1963, but Dr. Graham himself, a cigarette smoker, died of lung cancer in 1957. Alton Ochsner and his student, Michael DeBakey (1908 – 2008) the great future cardiac surgeon, published a study in 1939 in which they hypothesized that cigarette smoking was "probably a responsible factor" for an increase in lung cancers. The idea of the association of lung cancer with cigarette smoking was ridiculed by some. Dr. Evarts Graham himself reportedly told Ochsner that, "Yes, there is a parallel between the sale of cigarettes and the incidence of cancer of the lung, but there is also a parallel between the sale of nylon stockings and the incidence of lung cancer." In the first edition of Lauren

Ackerman's textbook of surgical pathology in 1953, Dr. Ackerman (1905 – 1993) wrote, "Carcinoma of the lung has become increasingly important during the past fifteen years. This is apparently due not only to increased recognition and better radiologic and bronchoscopic diagnoses, but also to a definite true increase .... the incidence of carcinoma of the lung is still less than carcinoma of the stomach. There has been much speculation as to the cause of this increase .... Tobacco may be one of the factors, but there probably remain multiple other causes."

Additional studies linking tobacco use to lung cancer were published in the 1950's by Richard Doll (1912 – 2005) and Bradford Hill (1897 – 1991) in the UK and E. Cuyler Hammond (1912 – 1986) and Ernst Wynder (1922 – 1999) in the US. Since cigarette smoking was widely popular, tobacco growth and cigarette production were an important industry, and cigarette smoking is addictive, there was an underlying opposition to accepting these findings, but in 1962 a committee of the Royal College of Physicians reported that cigarette smoking was associated with lung cancer and chronic bronchitis. The report of the Advisory Committee to the Surgeon General of the United States was published in 1964 and concluded after a two-year study analyzing 7000 publications that smoking was, among other things, a cause of lung cancer with a 10 to 20-fold increase in the occurrence of lung cancer among smokers. This led to legislation in 1965 and 1969 that required warning labels on packages of cigarettes and eliminated cigarette advertisements on television in the US. The ubiquity of those advertisements is supported by this author's tenacious memory of several and perhaps a score of cigarette advertisements and their jingles from the 1950s and 60s. [6 – 9]

23.3.2 Acetaminophen

Josef von Mering (1849 – 1908, figure 23.7) was born in Cologne and graduated from Strasbourg in 1873. He had an appointment in the department of medicine at Halle, but Mering had unusually wide interests. He was an assistant to the psychiatrist Krafft-Ebing, worked with Frerichs in the medical clinic in Berlin, studied the absorption of sugar with Ludwig in Leipzig, physiology with Goltz in Strasbourg, and became a professor of Forensic Medicine in 1886. He is probably most famous for his 1889 studies with Oskar Minkowski (1858 – 1931) in which they resected the pancreas from dogs causing diabetes mellitus closely resembling the human disease. The further significance of these experiments, i.e. that the pancreas makes insulin, wasn't determined until the 20th century. Mering helped discover the barbiturates in his work with Emil Fischer (1852 - 1919) which led to the marketing of diethylmalonylurea as the drug Veronal. The aniline drug acetanilide was discovered to be an analgesic and an antipyretic in the late 19th century. It was sold as the drug Antifebrin beginning in 1886. Acetanilide had some toxic side effects including cyanosis from methemoglobinemia (see note below). In 1877, Harmon Northrop Morse (1848 – 1920) synthesized acetaminophen (also called paracetamol) at Johns Hopkins, but Josef von Mering was the first to give the drug to humans in 1887. Von Mering wrote that unlike the newly discovered phenacetin, acetaminophen caused some degree of methemoglobinemia just as acetanilide did. This led to the abandonment of acetaminophen and the popularization of phenacetin for the next seventy years.

In the late 1940s it was reconfirmed that acetaminophen was a major metabolite of acetanilide and of phenacetin, it was shown that acetaminophen does not cause methemoglobinemia, and it was hypothesized that sixty years earlier von Mering had used a specimen that was contaminated with acetanilide. Acetaminophen began to be marketed in the 1950s as Tylenol in the US and Panadol in the UK at first with the emphasis on it having much lower gastrointestinal irritation than aspirin. Over the next thirty years acetaminophen became more popular because of the association of aspirin with Reye's syndrome in children, and with the linkage of phenacetin with cases of autoimmune hemolytic anemia, renal papillary necrosis, hemolysis associated with G6PD deficiency, and urothelial cell carcinoma. The FDA banned phenacetin in 1987.

Note: Recall that hemoglobin has four ferrous iron atoms in each molecule. Methemoglobinemia occurs when hemoglobin contains one or more ferric iron atoms. Oxygen binds more weakly to ferric than to ferrous iron, and when hemoglobin has one ferric iron the remaining ferrous iron binding sites bind oxygen more strongly. This leads to less oxygen delivery to the peripheral tissues.

Relatively normal patients may tolerate methemoglobin up to 15% without symptoms, but patients with other medical problems, such as ischemic heart disease, anemia, sepsis, lung disease, or sickle cell anemia and infants are especially susceptible to methemoglobinemia. Methemoglobinemia is treated with oxygen and with intravenous methylene blue which acts as a reducing agent to replenish the normal mechanisms that maintain hemoglobin iron in the ferrous state. [10,11]

23.4 Laboratory medicine

23.4.1 Carcinoma of the Lung

The diagnosis of lung cancer is usually made radiographically and confirmed with some form of biopsy. Blood tests are not currently used for the diagnosis of lung cancer, but there has been work done using new technologies to either make the diagnosis of lung cancer outright, or to help find a group of patients who will benefit from more traditional screening methods. Previous studies had shown that screening smokers for lung cancer by plain chest radiograph did not work since detecting lung tumors earlier did not affect patient mortality. More recently, because of the evolution of chest radiography and of lung cancer therapy, The National Lung Screening Trial (NLST) screened 53,000 patients between the ages of 55 and 74 with at least a 30 pack-year smoking history using low radiation dose spiral CT. Participants who received CT screening had a 20% reduction in lung cancer mortality compared to those who did not and 24.2% of study participants had a positive finding on CT scan. The vast majority of positive findings (96.4%) were false positive findings, e.g. a scar from old pneumonia, but cost effectiveness analyses have shown a clear benefit in the group of patients resembling those who were studied. Cost effectiveness studies often report their findings as a ratio of costs and quality adjusted life years (QALYs) with and without the test, called the incremental cost-effectiveness ratio (ICER). The ICER for the NLST and similar studies is between $28,000 and $169,000/QALY. The US Preventative Services Task Force has recommended the use of low dose CT scan for screening for lung cancer in these patients. They determined that 50% of lung cancers would be detected at stage I or II and there would be a reduction of lung cancer mortality between 8.2 and 23.5%.

A biomarker blood test (Paula's test, Gensys Biolabs) is available that purports to filter the patient population into a group with a higher pre-CT probability of lung cancer. The test first recommends that the patient be 50 years of age or older, have a 20 pack-year smoking history, and not currently be being examined by CT scan for screening for lung cancer. It uses a panel of three tumor antigens and one tumor auto-antibody, and is used to detect non-small cell carcinoma. The vendors claim a sensitivity of 74% and a specificity of 80%, but the predictive value of a positive result is only 8.4%, so, just like CT scanning alone, there is a high false positive rate.

Work has also been done measuring volatile substances in the patient's breath or in the air over tumor cell cultures. Many substances have been identified that are associated with lung cancer, but no clinical test has been developed. Theoretically, this technology could lead to a simple point of care breath test for lung cancer. [12 – 18]

23.5 Study questions

1. Why don't all cigarette smokers get carcinoma of the lung?

2. Is cigarette smoking associated with any carcinomas besides lung cancer?

3. Why were people reluctant to believe that cigarette smoking caused lung cancer? Can you think of any other relatively well-proven scientific theories that people are reluctant to believe?

4. Make a table showing the advantages and disadvantages of acetaminophen, aspirin, and phenacetin.

5. What problems can you imagine in the development of a point of care breath analyzer for the diagnosis of lung cancer?

23.6 References

1. Hong WK, Tsao AS. Tumors of the Lungs. In: Porter RS, Kaplan JL, editors. The Merck Manual of Diagnosis and Therapy. Whitehouse Station, NJ: Merck Sharp & Dohme Corp; 2011. p. 2004 - 2014.
2. Husain AN. The Lung. In: Kumar V, Abbas AK, Aster JC, editors. Robbins and Cotran Pathological Basis of Disease. Philadelphia: Elsevier Saunders; 2015. p. 712 - 719.
3. Anonymous. Cancer Stat Facts: Lung and Bronchus Cancer. https://seer.cancer.gov/statfacts/html/lungb.html. Accessed 2017.
4. Grosser T, Smyth E, FitzGerald GA. Anti-inflammatory, antipyretic, and analgesic agents; Pharmacotherapy of gout. In: Brunton LL, Chabner BA, Knolmann BC, editors. Goodman & Gilman's The Pharmacological Basis of Therapeutics. New York: McGraw Hill Medical; 2011. p. 982- 984.
5. Bird SR. Acetaminophen. In: Linden CH, Rippe JM, Irwin RS, editors. Manual of Overdoses and Poisonings. Philadelphia: Lippincott Williams & Wilkins; 2006. p. 14 - 18.
6. Ackerman LV. Respiratory Tract. In: Surgical Pathology. St. Louis: The C. V. Mosby Company; 1953. p. 133 - 189.
7. Horn L, Johnson DH. Evarts A. Graham and the first pneumonectomy for lung cancer. J Clin Oncol. 2008; 26:3268.
8. Robison RF. Schneeburg Lung Disease. Mining and Selling Uranium. New York: Springer; 2014. p. 219 - 222.
9. Witschi H. Profiles in toxicology. A short history of lung cancer. Toxicological Sciences. 2001; 64:4 - 6.
10. Talbott JH. A biographical history of medicine: excerpts and essays on the men and their work. New York: Grune & Stratton; 1970:1211.
11. Anonymous. Paracetamol. https://en.wikipedia.org/wiki/Paracetamol. Accessed 2017.
12. Team NLSTR. Reduced lung-cancer mortality with low-dose computed tomographic screening. N Engl J Med. 2011; 365:395 - 409.
13. de Koning HJ, Meza R, Plevritis SK *et al.* Benefits and harms of computed tomography lung cancer screening strategies: a comparative modeling study

for the U.S. Preventive Services Task Force. Ann Intern Med. 2014; 160:311-320.

14. Moyer VA, Force USPST. Screening for lung cancer: U.S. Preventive Services Task Force recommendation statement. Ann Intern Med. 2014; 160:330-338.

15. Black WC. Computed tomography screening for lung cancer in the National Lung Screening Trial: a cost-effectiveness analysis. J Thorac Imaging. 2015; 30:79-87.

16. Curl PK, Kahn JG, Ordovas KG, Elicker BM, Naeger DM. Understanding cost-effectiveness analyses: An explanation using three different analyses of lung cancer screening. AJR. 2015; 205:344 - 347.

17. Schmidt K, Podmore I. Current challenges in volatile organic compounds analysis as potential biomarkers of cancer. J Biomark. 2015; 2015:981458.

18. Schallschmidt K, Becker R, Jung C *et al.* Comparison of volatile organic compounds from lung cancer patients and healthy controls-challenges and limitations of an observational study. J Breath Res. 2016; 10:046007.

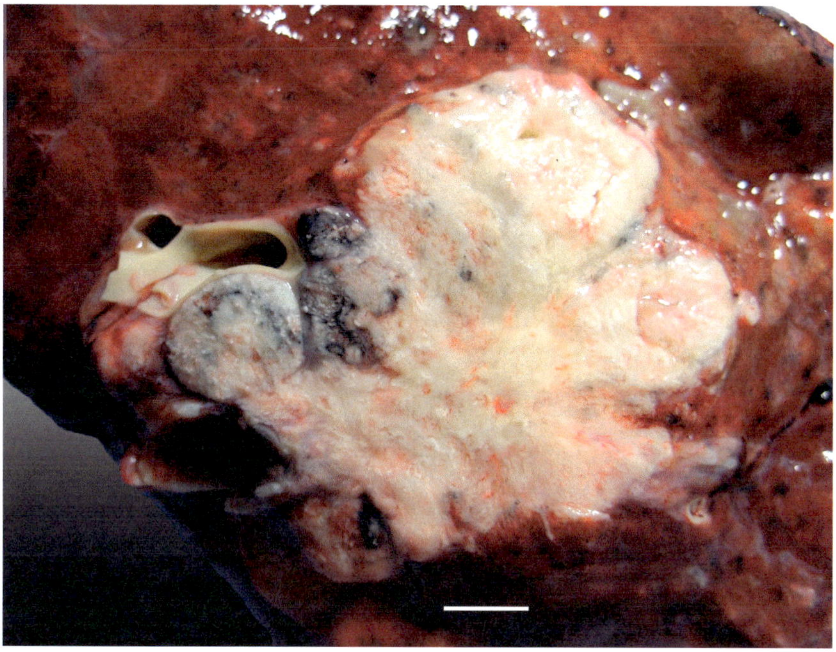

Figure 23.1. A lung specimen from a different case of small cell undifferentiated carcinoma. The tumor is invading adjacent lymph nodes that are partially discolored by black anthracotic pigment (the pigment is a normal finding in lymph nodes that drain the lung). The white bar is 1 cm long.

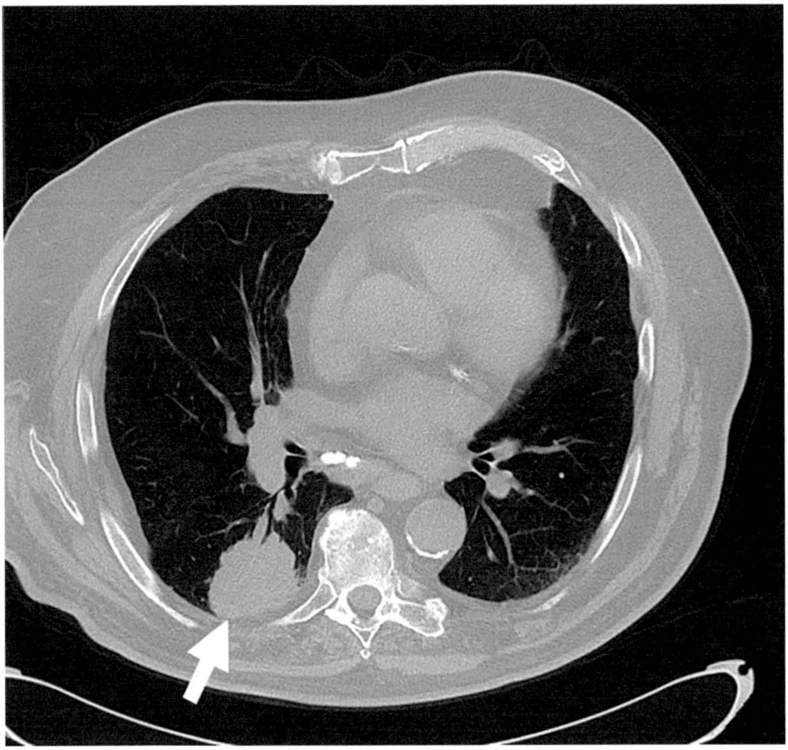

Figure 23.2 An axial non-contrast CT in lung window from a different case shows a round peripheral lobular mass (arrow) in the right lower lobe concerning for lung cancer.

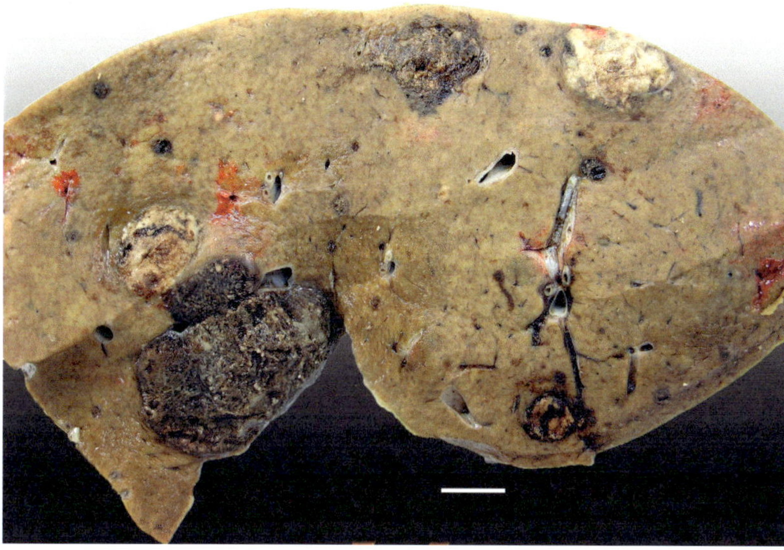

Figure 23.3. A liver specimen from a different case of metastatic small cell undifferentiated carcinoma of the lung. The metastases are white and roughly spherical. The metastases are red where there has been hemorrhage into the tumor. The patient in the case described in this chapter had a much larger volume of metastatic carcinoma. The white bar is 1 cm long.

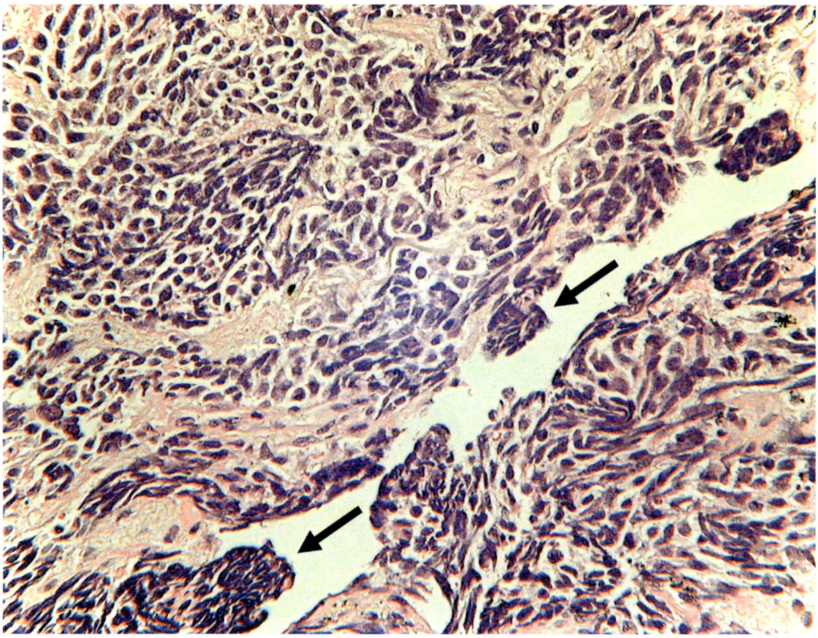

Figure 23.4 Small cell undifferentiated carcinoma of the lung. The tumor cells are relatively small with a high nucleus to cytoplasm ratio. The tumor cells are fragile and show areas of crush artifact (arrows). (Original magnification, x200. H&E stain)

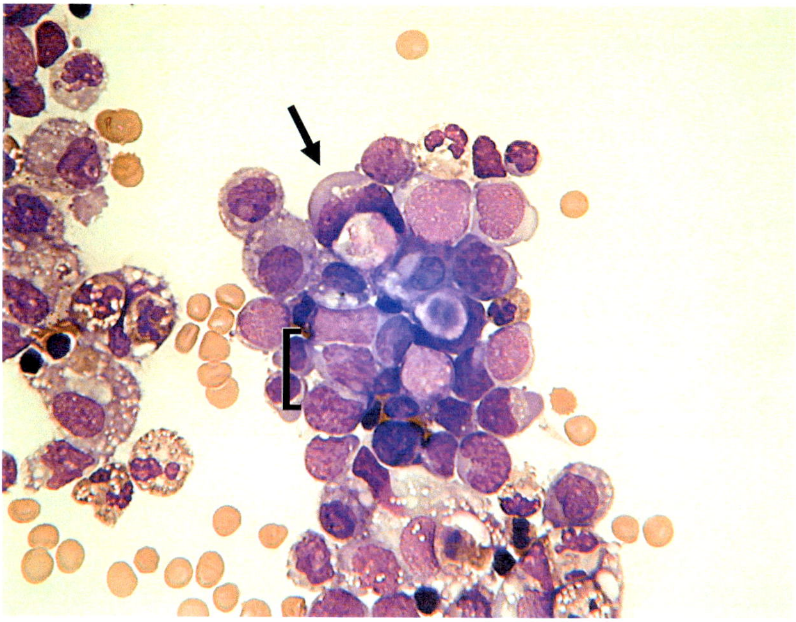

Figure 23.5 Small cell undifferentiated carcinoma of the lung in an air-dried cytologic preparation. In addition to benign red blood cells, neutrophils, mesothelial cells, and lymphoid cells, the central group has a vertical row of tumor cells. The tumor cell at the top (arrow) is larger than the others and has a cell within cell configuration possibly containing a mitotic figure. The tumor cells by the bracket appear to be molded together, a characteristic feature of this tumor. (Original magnification, x400. Wright-Giemsa stain)

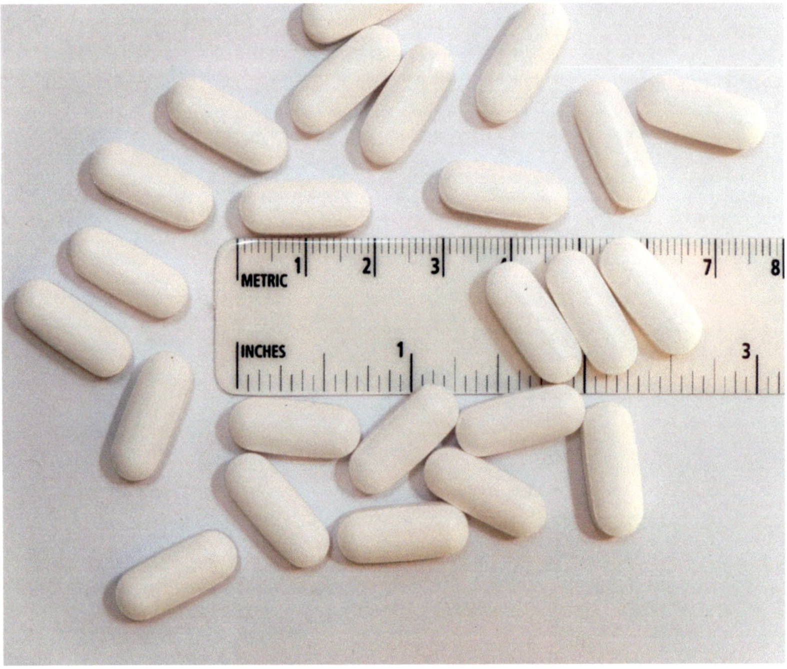

Figure 23.6 I don't have a good picture of the tablets found in the patient's gastrointestinal tract. These are extra strength Tylenol tablets that I bought at the pharmacy. They are similar, but they are not scored and they are slightly smaller.

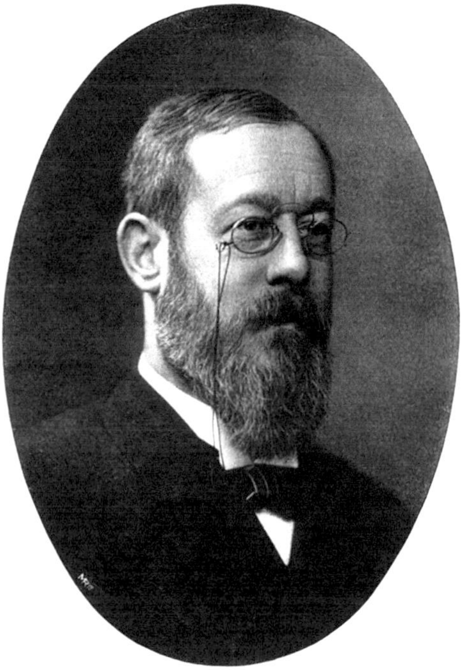

Figure 23.7 Josef von Mering (1849 – 1908). Courtesy of the National Library of Medicine.

CHAPTER 24

An elderly man with chronic lymphocytic leukemia, peptic ulcer disease and Pneumocystis jirovecii pneumonia (vINdicate, infectious, neoplastic)

"Never forget that it is not a pneumonia, but a pneumonic man who is your patient." William Gull (1816 – 1890)

24.1 The Autopsy

24.1.1 Case history

The patient was an elderly man with chronic obstructive lung disease and hypertension. About three months earlier he had a diagnosis of chronic lymphocytic leukemia (CLL) made when he was found to have a peripheral white blood cell count of 170,000 (normal = 4000 – 10,700 cells/μL) and a hemoglobin of 6 (normal = 14 – 17 g/dL). At that time, a diagnosis of hemolytic anemia was made. He was treated with transfusion, Cytoxan and prednisone. Two weeks prior to hospital admission the patient developed cough, right pleuritic chest pain, and fever. Chest radiograph showed left lower lobe pneumonia and he was treated with erythromycin. The patient was admitted at another hospital with respiratory distress, nausea, vomiting, and diarrhea. He was transferred to our hospital, his chest radiograph showed bilateral pneumonia, and he was treated empirically with amikacin, ampicillin, and trimethoprim-sulfamethoxazole. A cytologic specimen from bronchoscopy showed Pneumocystis jirovecii and the patient's trimethoprim-sulfamethoxazole was continued. The patient developed nausea, diarrhea, and dyspnea and required mechanical ventilation. Two days prior to his death the patient vomited about 250 mL of clotted blood and complained of left upper quadrant abdominal pain. He had slight prolongation of his protime and his partial thromboplastin time. The patient died on the 14th hospital day following a hypotensive episode.

24.1.2 Postmortem findings

The patient's lungs were grossly normal except for centrilobular emphysema, but histologic sections of the lungs showed organizing Pneumocystis jirovecii pneumonia bilaterally and increased intravascular lymphocytes (figures 24.1, 24.3, 24.4). The patient's bone marrow was moderately hypercellular for an elderly man and had hyperplasia of immature and mature myeloid cells. A 3 x 0.5 cm acute ulcer was present on the posterior wall of the duodenum 2 cm superior to the Ampulla of Vater. Histologic examination showed that the ulcer had eroded into two underlying arteries. A postmortem blood culture was negative. Other findings included hypertensive heart disease and a pancreatic duct calculus with atrophy of the tail of the pancreas.

24.1.3 Case summary

The patient was an elderly man with CLL and hemolytic anemia who had received chemotherapy including prednisone. He developed signs and symptoms of pneumonia and gastrointestinal symptoms and was treated with antibiotics. Pneumocystis jirovecii was found in a bronchoscopy specimen and the patient was treated with trimethoprim-sulfamethoxazole. He developed respiratory failure and hematemesis and died. Postmortem examination confirmed the presence of Pneumocystis pneumonia and showed that the patient had an acute duodenal ulcer that had eroded into underlying arteries.

24.2 Discussion

24.2.1 Chronic lymphocytic leukemia

Chronic lymphocytic leukemia (CLL) is the most common leukemia in the Western world and is characterized by the proliferation of cytologically mature-appearing, but neoplastic, B lymphocytes. CLL-type small lymphocytic lymphoma is essentially the same disease, but presenting in lymph nodes and to a much lesser degree in the peripheral blood. As a lymphoma, the disease is uncommon and only accounts for 4% of non-Hodgkin lymphomas. Tumor cells may also be present in the bone marrow and spleen. The incidence of CLL increases with age and it typically occurs in patients who are 60 years-old or older. Men with CLL outnumber women by 2 to 1. The diagnosis is made by examination of the patient's peripheral blood smear, lymph node biopsy, and/or bone marrow biopsy. CLL is a rare disease in China and Japan, and it is also rare in Americans of Japanese ancestry. Patients with CLL are often asymptomatic and they may be identified incidentally on examination of a routine blood smear. When symptomatic, CLL patients usually present with nonspecific findings such as weight loss, anorexia and fatigue. About half of symptomatic patients have lymphadenopathy and hepatosplenomegaly. Hypogammaglobulinemia is common and these patients are at increased risk for infection. CLL appears to originate either from a naive B-cell or a postgerminal center B memory cell, since the immunoglobulin genes of some cases are somatically hypermutated, but others are not. The cases that resemble naive B-cells behave more aggressively. Unlike most other lymphoid malignancies, CLL does not usually have a chromosomal translocation. Certain chromosomal deletions and trisomy 12q are the most common genetic abnormalities. Some models of CLL suggest that the tumor cells are dependent on signals from membrane bound immunoglobulin for survival. These signals require a cascade of kinases including Bruton tyrosine kinase (BTK). Several BTK inhibitors are in clinical trials and preliminary studies suggest that treatment may inhibit CLL in human patients.

Treatment is delayed until symptoms are present in CLL. Therapy may include prednisone and various chemotherapeutic agents. Alemtuzumab (anti-CD52, present on mature lymphocytes, but not on stem cells) and rituximab are also used. Rituximab (anti-CD20) has a partial response rate of 10 - 15% in CLL. In previously untreated patients the response rate is 75% with 20% of patients having a complete remission. Alemtuzumab has the side effect of immunosuppression with activation of CMV being especially common.

Median survival is about 5 years, but some patients with small tumor burdens may live 10 or more years. About 5 - 10% of patients with CLL may eventually have their tumor transform into a more aggressive tumor. The most common transformation is into a diffuse large B-cell lymphoma, so-called Richter syndrome. These patients usually survive less than 1 year. [1, 2]

24.2.2 Pneumocystis jirovecii

Pneumocystis jirovecii is an atypical fungus with a world-wide distribution that is commonly present in the human pulmonary alveolus in very small numbers. As many as 85% of infants have developed antibody to Pneumocystis by age 20 months. Pneumocystis was, for many years, considered to be a protozoan since it does not form hyphae, it does not form budding yeast, and it responds to anti-protozoal drugs, but not to antifungal drugs. Examination of its genome has shown it to be an unusual fungus. The organism has three morphologic forms in its life cycle, still called the trophozoite, the precyst, and the cyst; names which originated when the organism was thought to be a protozoan. Infection with Pneumocystis occurs in a sporadic and an epidemic form. The epidemic form usually occurs in infants. The sporadic form occurs in immunosuppressed patients. The disease was rare, but became more common when the AIDS epidemic began in the 1980s. Pneumocystis is extracellular in the alveolus. Its proliferation leads to the formation of a characteristic eosinophilic exudate (figure 24.3) and is associated with an interstitial chronic inflammatory infiltrate. The disease was formerly called interstitial plasma cell pneumonia, especially in infants. Some patients with HIV infection may have Pneumocystis in bone marrow, spleen, or lymph nodes. Patients usually have a non-productive cough, low grade fever, dyspnea, and night sweats. The diagnosis is usually made in the appropriate clinical setting with a characteristic ground-glass appearing chest radiograph (i.e. opacification that does not obscure the underlying pulmonary architecture, figure 24.2) and by identifying the organism in a bronchoalveolar lavage specimen. Sputum specimens usually do not contain identifiable organisms. Several different staining methods are available, but cysts in cytologic and tissue specimens are usually examined with the Gomori methenamine silver (GMS) stain (figure 24.4). Pneumocystis pneumonia is usually treated with trimethoprim-sulfamethoxazole or pentamidine. Other drugs and prednisone may be used in patients with severe disease. [3, 4]

24.2.3 Peptic ulcer disease

Recall that about 80% of the stomach has a lining mucosa that contains oxyntic glands that secrete hydrochloric acid, pepsinogen, intrinsic factor and mucus. One of the constituent cells of these glands is the oxyntic or parietal cell. Hydrochloric acid is formed at villous projections into intracytoplasmic canaliculi in these cells. This yields a solution with a pH of 0.8 and hydrogen ion concentration that is 3 million times higher than that found in arterial blood. The hydrogen ions are actively secreted in exchange for potassium ions using the proton pump enzyme $H^{+}K^{+}$-ATPase, and secretion of hydrogen ions is stimulated via cell membrane receptors by both gastrin and histamine. Two classes of drugs used to reduce gastric acidity are H2 receptor antagonists and proton pump inhibitors.

Helicobacter pylori is a species of helically shaped Gram-negative bacteria that can survive in the acidic environment of the stomach. About 50% of 60-year-old patients in the US are infected with H. pylori. H. pylori in the gastric antrum increases gastrin secretion and results in increased gastric acidity. Most patients with H. pylori infection are asymptomatic, but infection with H. pylori, especially with strains whose genome contains a collection of about 20 genes called the cag pathogenicity island, is the most common cause of chronic gastritis. Patients with H. pylori chronic gastritis are at increased risk for peptic ulcer disease, gastric carcinoma, and low-grade gastric lymphoma.

A peptic ulcer is a defect in the gastric or proximal duodenal mucosa that penetrates through the muscularis mucosae (a band of smooth muscle at the base of the musosa). Nearly all are caused by infection with Helicobacter pylori or the use of non-steroidal anti-inflammatory drugs (NSAIDs). Ulcers may occur at any age, but they are usually seen in middle-aged adults. They range in size from a few millimeters to several centimeters (figure 24.4). H. pylori is present in 50 - 70% of patients with duodenal ulcers and 30 - 50% of patients with gastric ulcers. Ulcers recur in 10% of patients who have their H. pylori eradicated, but in 70% of patients who are treated with acid suppression alone. Symptoms depend on the location of the ulcer and the patient's age. Elderly patients often have no symptoms. The typical symptom is burning or gnawing epigastric pain that is relieved by food or antacids. Ulcers in the pyloric channel may cause symptoms of obstruction including nausea and vomiting. Patients with duodenal ulcers may be awakened at night by their pain. Pain is more common in duodenal than in gastric ulcers; it is often absent when the patient awakens in the morning but appears in mid-morning. The diagnosis of a gastric or duodenal ulcer is usually made by endoscopy. Biopsies and cytologic specimens may be collected to exclude the possibility of an ulcer in a gastric carcinoma and to identify H. pylori (figure 24.5). Stomach cancer is usually suspected clinically in patients with severe or refractory symptoms and weight loss. These findings may also be found in patients with the Zollinger-Ellison syndrome in which gastric ulcers form because the patient has a gastrin secreting tumor. Those patients often have multiple ulcers. If the diagnosis of Z-E syndrome is suspected, serum gastrin is measured. Possible complications of peptic ulcer include hemorrhage, perforation, and gastric outlet obstruction. The risk of subsequent carcinoma of the stomach is increased 3 to 6-fold in patients with H. pylori associated ulcers. Treatment of peptic ulcer disease includes antibiotic therapy to eradicate H. pylori and acid-suppressive drugs.

Cessation of smoking and reduction of alcohol consumption are also helpful. Surgery is usually reserved for patients with perforation, obstruction, or uncontrolled hemorrhage, and rarely for patients who are refractory to medical treatment. [5 – 7]

24.3 Medical History

24.3.1 Leukemia

Like most concepts, the idea of leukemia as a neoplastic proliferation of white blood cells developed over time. Key figures included Alfred Armand Louis Marie Velpeau (1795 – 1867) and Alfred François Donné (1801 – 1878).

Alfred Armand Louis Marie Velpeau (figure 24.7) was born in the small French village of Breche. His father was a blacksmith, and, as was apparently not uncommon, his father also served as the local veterinarian. Velpeau did not attend any formal school until he was about 20 years old. He received some lessons from a local priest and a school teacher and he read some of his father's veterinary texts. Velpeau had an early interest in medicine and he treated some patients in his village. People in the area were impressed with his intelligence and he tutored the children of a wealthy neighbor. In 1816, a physician arranged for him to train to be the community health officer in Tours. He continued his medical studies supporting himself as an anatomical assistant. Velpeau received his medical degree in 1824 when he completed his thesis, in Latin, on intermittent and chronic fevers. He was appointed surgeon at the Pitié Hospital in 1828 and became chief of surgery at the University of Paris in 1833 and remained there until his death in 1867. During his career, and despite having no formal primary education, Velpeau had 340 publications. His publications included a two volume Treatise of Surgical Anatomy in 1825, a two volume Elementary Treatise on the Art of Midwifery in 1829, and the three volume New Elements of Operative Surgery in 1832. A bandage designed to support the arm in cases of fracture of the clavicle is named for him. In his 1854 book on breast disease Velpeau distinguished benign from malignant tumors (which were inoperable) and he suggested that some patients might have a constitutional predisposition to cancer. Velpeau was resistant to early attempts to use anesthesia, but he did eventually use ether in surgery and in obstetrics. Similarly, he felt that his clinical experience made him a better diagnostician than those who had taken up microscopy, but he did submit his resected tumors for microscopic examination.

In 1827, Velpeau reported the case of a 63-year-old man who had urinary stones, abdominal swelling, fever, and weakness. The patient had been ill since age 54. His fever was treated with an antipyretic agent. He had two tumors on the left side of his abdomen and he died on the second hospital day. Velpeau performed an autopsy and found marked enlargement of the liver and spleen. The blood was altered so that it resembled pus-filled blood. Velpeau thought that the blood alteration could occur without prior inflammation and he suspected that the disease was related to the circulatory system. This is the first known description of leukemia at postmortem examination. [8 – 10]

Alfred François Donné was born in Noyon. He graduated MD in 1831. Donné was an early user of microscopy in the study of disease. He began teaching a course in medical microscopy in 1837 at a time when the microscope was not widely used in medicine. In 1844 and 1845 Donné published *Cours de microscopie complémentaire des études médicales*, the first medical atlas illustrated with photomicrographs. These images were taken by Donné's student Léon Foucault (the future physicist) and used a technique to create engravings from the one of a kind metal plate daguerreotypes. The images included pictures of platelets, Trichomonas vaginalis, and leukemic leukocytes, all first described by Donné.

Donné reported the case of a 44-year-old woman with splenomegaly who had died at hospital Hotel Dieu in Paris in 1839. He examined the patient's blood under the microscope and noted that half of the corpuscles in her blood resembled mucous globules. He thought that the patient's physicians had mistakenly identified her circulating mucous/purulent globules (leukocytes) as pus. Donné hypothesized that the accumulation of these globules was due to the arrest of differentiation of the leukocytes. He did not describe the associated symptoms in leukemic patients, but his atlas illustrated leukemic cell morphology. His studies were before the discovery of the stains that are now used to differentiate these cells; at the time, the nucleus of the leukocytes was made more visible by treatment with acetic acid. Donné said, "There are conditions in which white cells seem to be in excess in the blood. I found this fact so many times, it is so evident in certain patients, that I cannot conceive the slightest doubt in this regard. One can find in some patients such a great number of these cells that even the least experienced observer is greatly impressed. I had an opportunity of seeing these in a patient under Dr. Rayer at the Hôpital de la Charité.... The blood of this patient showed such a number of white cells that I thought his blood was mixed with pus, but in the end, I was able to observe a clear-cut difference between these cells, and the white cells . . . " This abnormality was associated with typical symptoms and recognized as a new blood disease by John Hughes Bennett (1812 – 1875, a former student of Donné) and by Rudolf Virchow (1821 – 1902). [10 – 12]

24.3.2 Pneumocystis jirovecii

Pneumocystis was first described by Carlos Chagas (1879 – 1934) and Antonio Carini (1872 – 1950) in Sao Paulo, Brazil in 1909 – 1910 in rats infected by Trypanosoma cruzi and T. lewisi. They believed that the organism was a part of the Trypanosome's life cycle. Dr. Chagas placed the organism in a new genus called Schizotrypanum. In 1912 Delanoë and Delanoë at the Pasteur Institute identified the organism in rats and guinea pigs that were not infected with trypanosomes and they named it Pneumocystis carinii. A similar organism was found in other animals and it was described in three human patients in 1942. In 1952 Otto Jirovec (1907 – 1972) and M. Vanek described it again in premature infants associated with the histologic features that had been called interstitial plasma cell pneumonia. The name Pneumocystis jiroveci was proposed in 1976 by J. K. Frenkel when it was demonstrated that P. jiroveccii in humans and P. carinii in rats were different species. There has been some controversy concerning the name change, and some workers have felt that if the name were changed it should honor workers who they thought had precedence over Dr. Jirovec. [13 – 15]

24.3.3 Peptic ulcer disease

In the 19th century, peptic ulcers were only diagnosed clinically and at autopsy, consequently, patients with dyspepsia were labeled with a host of different diagnoses that are no longer made, many of them with a presumed neurological or psychiatric etiology. Since the modern rediscovery of H. pylori, many of these diagnoses have been replaced by our current concept of Helicobacter pylori gastritis and its consequences.

From the late 19th to the late 20th century gastric and duodenal ulcers were often treated surgically. The first partial gastrectomy was described in 1879 by Pean. In 1901, B. G. A. Moynihan (1865 – 1936) reviewed 51 cases of gastric ulcer that were operated on in Europe between 1888 and 1901. Only 8 patients survived the procedure. The main competing therapy was described by Bertram W. Sippy (1866 – 1924) in 1915. Sippy developed a medical treatment characterized by small feedings alternating with antacids throughout the day. The diet started with milk and cream and gradually expanded its content. Diets of this type were a mainstay of medical treatment at least until the coming of the H2-receptor antagonist drugs.

Gastric bacteria were identified by German researchers as early as 1875, but the organisms were not successfully cultured. Walery Jaworski (1849 – 1924) described organisms compatible with Helicobacter pylori in gastric lavage specimens in 1899 and Giulio Bizzozero (1846 – 1901) had seen similar organisms in the dog stomach in 1893. Jaworski called the organisms Vibrio rugula and suggested that they might play a role in gastric pathology, but these observations were published in Polish and were essentially lost or ignored. Occasional subsequent observations described gastric mucosal spirochetes, but a large study by E. D. Palmer in 1954 failed to show any organisms in 1180 gastric biopsies. Drs. Robin J. Warren (1937 –) and Barry J. Marshall (1951 –) observed helical organisms in 1979 and 1981 in association with gastric inflammation. They successfully cultured these organisms, initially naming them Campylobacter pyloridis. Dr. Marshall drank cultured organisms and succeeded in giving himself gastritis, thus dramatically fulfilling Koch's postulates. Over the next ten years, multiple researchers duplicated the observation of the organism now called Helicobacter pylori and older notions of the etiology of peptic ulcer disease including diet and stress, were replaced. Drs. Warren and Marshall won the Noble prize in Medicine in 2005 for this work.

Carcinoma of the stomach was the most common visceral malignancy in the US from the late 19th century until carcinoma of the lung overtook it after the second world war. Similarly, carcinoma of the stomach has been the most common visceral malignancy in China and Japan, but its incidence began to decline in the last decades of the 20th century. It has been hypothesized that the time of infection, extent of infection, and gastric distribution of infection with Helicobacter pylori changed at these times with changes in the refrigeration of food, the availability of fresh fruits and vegetables out of season, and general sanitation and hygiene. These changes are thought to have also led to a decrease in the incidence of gastric ulcer and carcinoma and an increase in the incidence of duodenal ulcer. [16 – 19]

24.4 Laboratory medicine

24.4.1 Chronic lymphocytic leukemia

Patients with CLL have more than 5000 lymphocytes per microliter in their peripheral blood. The neoplastic nature of this proliferation is usually confirmed by flow cytometry to detect clonality. The tumor cells in CLL have the pan-B-cell antigens CD19 and CD20 on their surface. They also usually have surface immunoglobulin light chain, CD20, and CD79b, but these antigens are present in a lesser amount than usually seen on normal B-cells. CLL cells express CD5 (a T-cell marker, but also present on normal naive B-cell and post-germinal center B memory cells) and CD24. Mantle cell lymphoma in leukemic phase may simulate CLL, but those cells are usually CD24 negative, and the cases that do express CD24 are usually cyclin-D1 negative. Rare cases of marginal zone lymphoma and lymphoplasmacytic lymphoma may have some markers in common with CLL, and a small proportion of normal people have a population of B-cells that have the surface antigen features of CLL cells.

About 80% of patients with CLL have a cytogenetic abnormality by FISH. Unlike other leukemias and lymphomas, CLL does not have a characteristic chromosomal translocation. Abnormalities may include various chromosomal deletions and trisomy 12.

Other laboratory findings in patients with CLL may include hypogammaglobulinemia, anemia (sometimes hemolytic), or thrombocytopenia. [1, 2, 20]

24.4.2 Pneumocystis jirovecii

The best diagnostic specimens for the detection of Pneumocystis are bronchoalveolar lavage specimens. Sputum specimens have a high false negative rate. Pneumocystis cysts may be detected with calcofluor white, Gomori methenamine silver, and by immunofluorescent stain. The cysts are spherical to concave, 4 - 7 microns in size, do not bud, and contain an intracystic body (figure 24.4). Giemsa stain may be used to identify trophozoites. The immunofluorescent method, compared to the other stains, has higher sensitivity, but the negative predictive value is smaller. There are real-time PCR tests being developed for the detection of Pneumocystis. Some commercial kits using monoclonal antibodies against Pneumocystis jirovecii are available.

Serology is of limited value because antibody levels only increase 2 - 3 weeks after infection and may not occur in immunocompromised patients. [3, 4]

24.4.3 Helicobacter pylori

The diagnosis of H. pylori infection is usually made with a serological test for the presence of H. pylori antibodies. The test has a sensitivity and specificity greater than 85%. Since serum antibodies may persist for years after treatment, they cannot be used to determine if the patient has been cured. Tests to assess cure include the urea breath test and a stool antigen test. Both have sensitivity and specificity greater than 90%. The urea test is done by giving the patient an oral dose of urea that is tagged with radioactive carbon and measuring exhaled carbon dioxide to detect C14 from bacterial metabolism. Some patients may also have endoscopy and biopsied tissue can be stained for the organism, or used in a rapid urease detection test. Helicobacter pylori can be seen using silver impregnation stains or with an immunohistochemical stain (figure 24.6). [6]

24.5 Study questions

1. Which is correct, Pneumocystis jerovici or Pneumocystis jerovicii? Why do some workers still call the organism Pneumocystis carinii f. hominis?

2. Is Pneumocystis jirovicii part of normal human flora?

3. What is the most commonly occurring leukemia in adults in the Western world?

4. Why is treatment of CLL delayed until the patient is symptomatic?

5. At what stage in human evolution did we acquire gastric Helicobacter pylori?

24.6 References

1. Freireich EJ. Leukemias. In: Porter RS, Kaplan JL, editors. The Merck manual of diagnosis and therapy. Whitehouse Station, NJ: Merck Sharp & Dohme Corp.; 2011. p. 1010 - 1012.
2. Kumar V, Abbas AK, Aster JC. Diseases of white blood cells, lymph nodes, spleen, and thymus. In: Kumar V, Abbas AK, Aster JC, editors. Robbins and Cotran Pathologic basis of disease. Philadelphia: Elsevier Saunders; 2015. p. 592 - 594.
3. Tille PM. Opportunistic atypical fungus: Pneumocystis jirovecii. In: Tille PM, editor. Bailey & Scott's Diagnostic microbiology. St. Louis: Elsevier Mosby; 2007. p. 768 - 770.
4. Krogstad DJ, Englebert NC. Blood and tissue protozoa. In: Schaechter ME, NC Eisenstein, BI, Medoff G, editors. Mechanisms of microbial disease. Philadelphia: Lippincott Williams & Wilkins; 1999. p. 456 - 458.

5. Guyton AC, Hall JE. Secretory functions of the alimentary tract. Textbook of medical physiology. Philadelphia: Elsevier Saunders; 2006. p. 797 - 799.
6. Cohen S. Gastritis and peptic ulcer disease. In: Porter RS, Kaplan JL, editors. The Merck manual of diagnosis and therapy. Whitehouse Station, NJ: Merck Sharp & Dohme Corp.; 2011. p. 133 - 138.
7. Szabo IL, Cseko K, Czimmer J, Mozsik G. Diagnosis of gastritis - Review from early pathological evaluation to present day management. In: Mozsik G, editor. Current Topics in Gastritis - 2012. Intech; 2012. p. 1 - 19.
8. Talbott JH. A biographical history of medicine: excerpts and essays on the men and their work. New York: Grune & Stratton; 1970:1211.
9. Bynum WF, Bynum HB. Dictionary of Medical Biography. Westport, Connecticut: Greenwood Press; 2007
10. Kampen KR. The discovery and early understanding of leukemia. Leuk Res. 2012;36:6-13.
11. Diamantis A, Magiorkinis E, Androutsos G. Alfred Francois Donné (1801-78): a pioneer of microscopy, microbiology and haematology. J Med Biogr. 2009;17:81-87.
12. Anonymous. Foundation of Microphotography; Landmark in Hematology, Oncology, and Pathology (1844 – 1845). http://www.historyofinformation.com/expanded.php?id=3219. Accessed 2017.
13. Frenkel JK. Pneumocystosis. In: Binford CH, Connor DH, editors. Pathology of tropical and extraordinary diseases. Washington, D.C.: Armed Forces Institute of Pathology; 1976. p. 303 - 307.
14. Anonymous. Pneumocystis jirovecii. https://en.wikipedia.org/wiki/Pneumocystis_jirovecii. Accessed 2017.
15. Hughes WT. Pneumocystis carinii vs Pneumocystis jiroveci: Another misnomer (Response to Stringer et al.) [letter]. Emerg Infect Dis 2003;9(2):276 - 277.
16. Graham DY. History of Helicobacter pylori, duodenal ulcer, gastric ulcer and gastric cancer. World J Gastroenterol. 2014; 20:5191 - 5204.
17. Konturek SJ, Konturek PC, Brzozowski T, Konturek JW, Pawlik WW. From nerves and hormones to bacteria in the stomach; Nobel prize for achievements in gastrology during last century. J Physiol Pharmacol. 2005; 56:507 - 530.

18. Konturek JW. Discovery by Jaworski of Helicobacter pylori and its pathogenetic role in gastritis, peptic ulcer and gastric cancer. J Physiol Pharmacol. 2003; 54:23 - 41.

19. Anonymous. Helicobacter pylori. https://en.wikipedia.org/wiki/Helicobacter_pylori. Accessed 2017.

20. Ioachim HL, Medeiros LJ. Chronic lymphocytic leukemia / Small lymphocytic lymphoma. Ioachim's Lymph Node Pathology. Philadelphia: Wolters Kluwer/Lipincott Williams & Wilkins; 2009. p. 352 - 362.

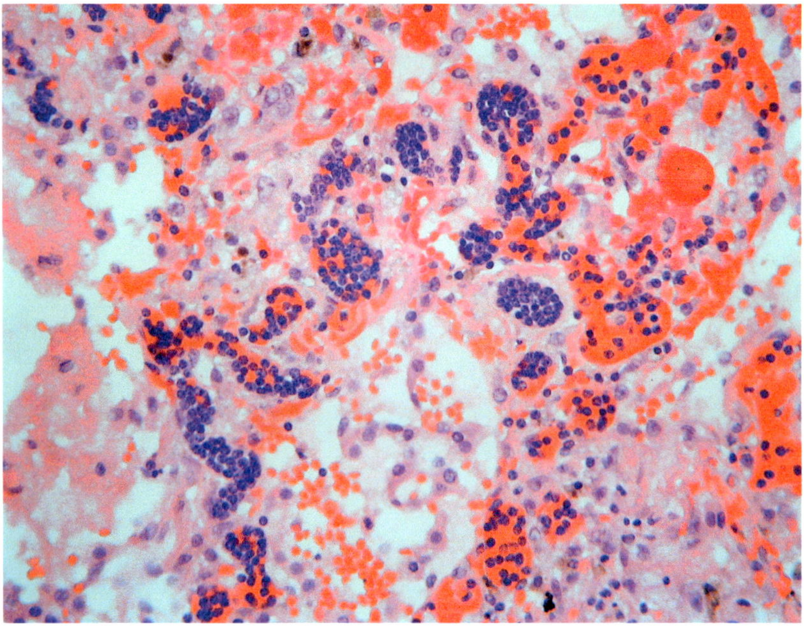

Figure 24.1 A histologic section of lung showing abundant mature appearing lymphocytes in alveolar capillaries in a patient with Chronic Lymphocytic Leukemia. (Original magnification, x200. H&E stain)

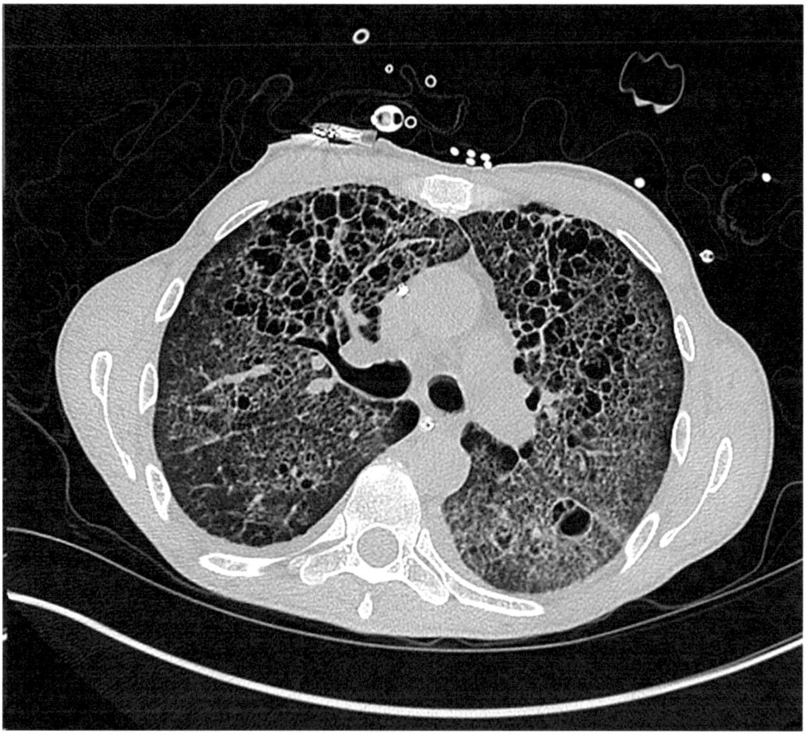

Figure 24.2 An axial contrast enhanced CT in lung window from a different patient shows diffuse bilateral hazy ground glass opacities and multiple lung cysts in both lungs. These findings have a limited differential, although if given the history of HIV, then Pneumocystis pneumonia is on the top of the differential list.

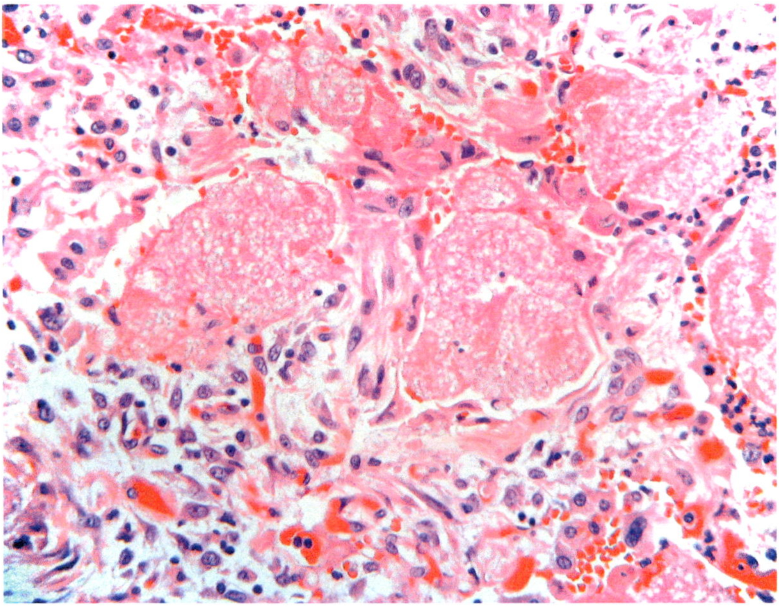

Figure 24.3 A section of lung shows abundant frothy appearing pink exudate in alveolar spaces. Some of the spaces in the exudate are caused by the presence of Pneumocystis cysts. (Original magnification, x200. H&E stain)

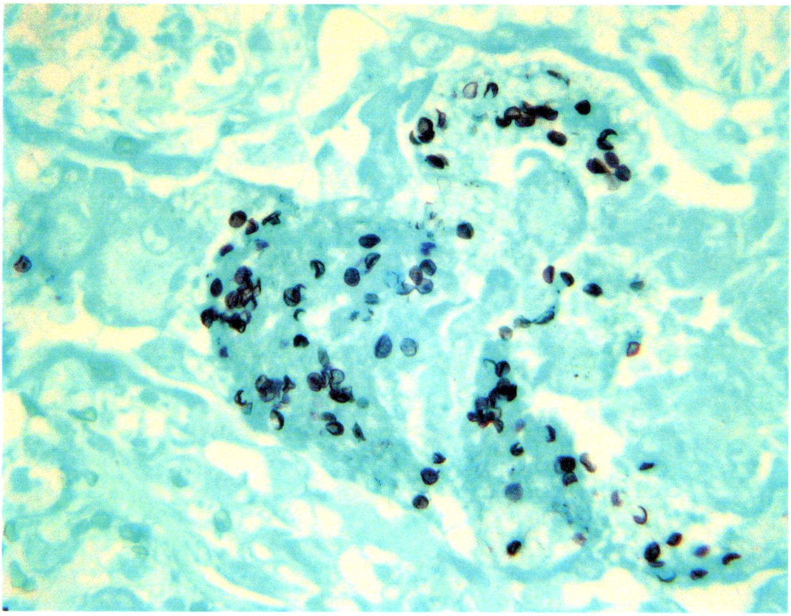

Figure 24.4 A silver stain of lung shows abundant Pneumocystis cysts in the alveolar exudate. Some cysts have a collapsed beach ball appearance and some contain a central inclusion. (Original magnification, x400. GMS stain)

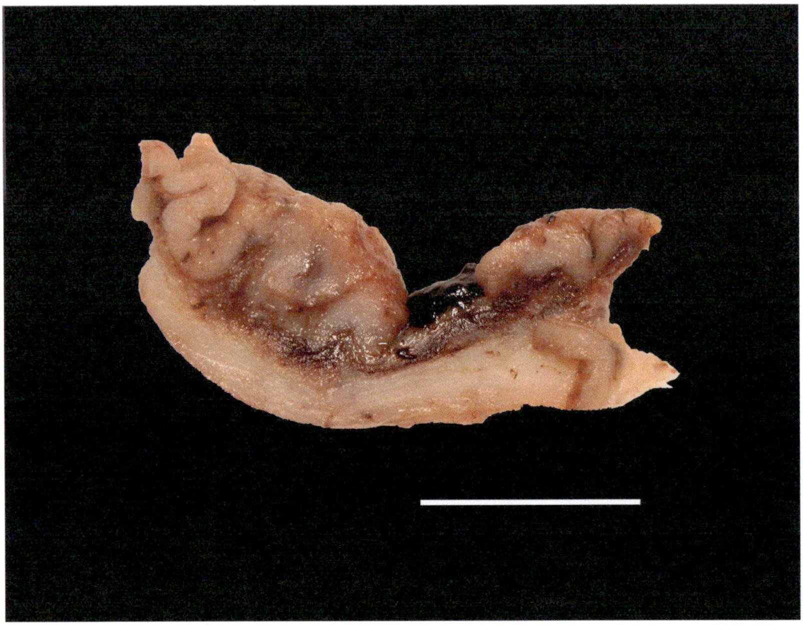

Figure 24.5 A portion of gastric wall from a different patient showing a central ulcer with some hemorrhagic gastric contents on the ulcer base. The white line is 1 cm long.

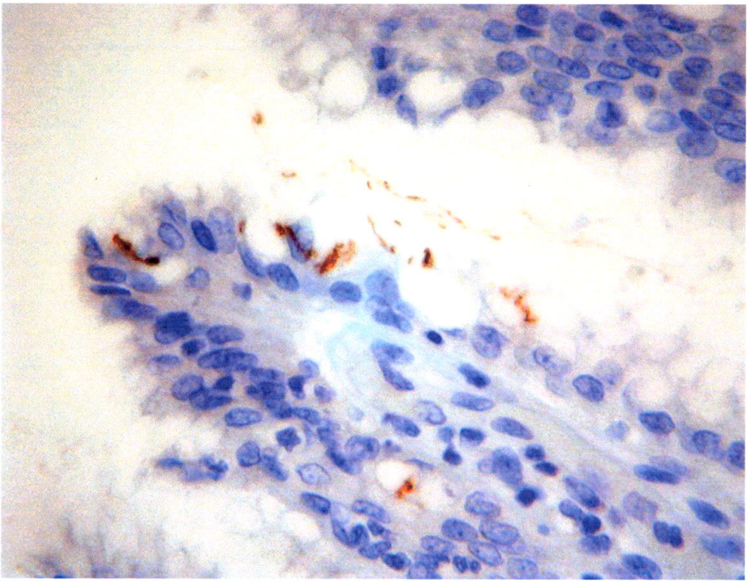

Figure 24.6 A section of the surface of the gastric mucosa. Helicobacter pylori organisms stain brown with an immunohistochemical stain. (Original magnification, x500. Anti-Helicobacter pylori immunohistochemical stain)

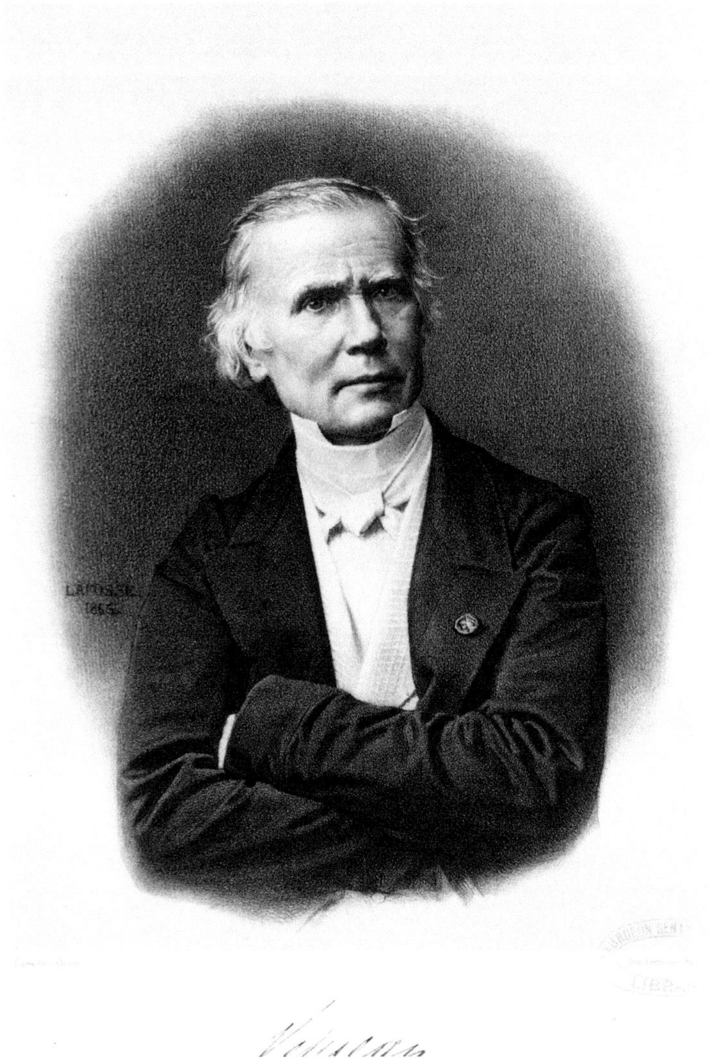

Figure 24.7 Alfred Velpeau (1795 – 1867). Courtesy of the National Library of Medicine.

Chapter 25

Statistical review of the autopsy database

"The importance of precise measurements in research is inarguable. Yet, one must guard against the delusions of precision that can result from such information." Edwin R. Fisher (1923 – 2008)

The autopsies that I've described here were selected from 971 cases that I performed between 1979 and 2014 at Strong Memorial Hospital in Rochester, New York, a University hospital, or at the Christiana Hospital in Christiana, Delaware, a not for profit private teaching hospital. Of the 971 cases, 633 (65.2%) were adults, 92 (9.5%) were children and 246 (25.3%) were stillborn infants. The median age of the adults was 64 years with a range of 20 – 98 years. The median age of the stillborn infants was 23 months gestation with a range of 14 – 42 months.

Decedents were 46% female and 54% male. The sex was indeterminate in 2 stillborn cases.

I tried to summarize the cause of death in each autopsy using a brief diagnostic code. About 80% of the cases could be summarized with a single word or abbreviation such as AMI for acute myocardial infarct. The remaining 20% had too much going on and required two or three words or abbreviations. Figures 25.1 and 25.2 are a currently popular type of statistical graphic called a word cloud made from the diagnostic codes for the adult and stillborn patients. [1,2] The size of the printed code word in the word clouds is proportional to the frequency of its occurrence. So, among the adult patients, acute myocardial infarct, stage IV carcinoma and bacterial sepsis were the most common causes of death. Among the stillborn infants, a congenital anomaly, acute chorioamnionitis and unknown were the most common causes of death. Note that some diseases might be rare, but they could be a common reason for requesting an autopsy. A congenital anomaly in a stillborn infant is an example of this phenomenon.

25.1 References

1. R Core Team. R: A language and environment for statistical computing. 2014. http://www.R-project.org/. Accessed 2015
2. Fellows I. wordcloud:Word Clouds. R package version 2.5. 2014. http://CRAN.R-project.org/package=wordcloud. Accessed 2015

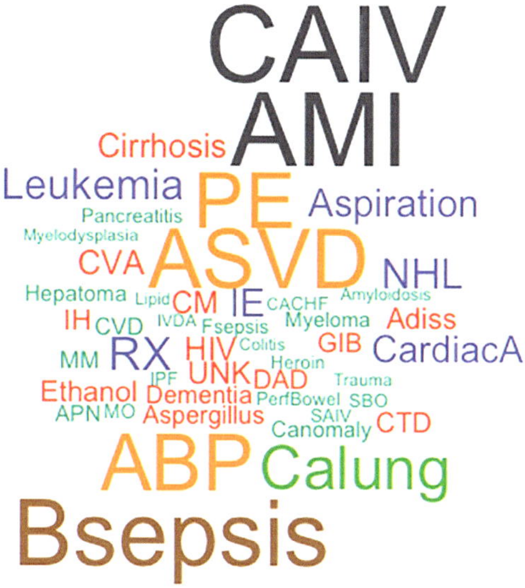

Figure 25.1 Word cloud of diagnostic codes associated with patient death in adult decedents. The size of the word is proportional to the frequency of the diagnostic code. **Stage IV carcinoma, acute myocardial infarct and bacterial sepsis were the three most common codes among adult decedents.** CAIV = stage IV carcinoma, AMI = acute myocardial infarct, Bsepsis = bacterial sepsis, ABP = acute bronchopneumonia, ASVD = atherosclerotic vascular disease, PE = pulmonary thromboembolus, CAlung = carcinoma of the lung (the only primary site that I have labeled specifically), Rx = a therapeutic or diagnostic procedure effect, NHL = non-Hodgkin's lymphoma, CardiacA = cardiac arrhythmia, IE = infective endocarditis, CVA = stroke, CM = cardiomyopathy, UNK = unknown, Adiss = aortic dissection, GIB = gastrointestinal hemorrhage, CVD = cardiac valve disease, IH = internal hemorrhage, DAD = diffuse alveolar damage (adult respiratory distress syndrome), CTD =

connective tissue disease, MM = malignant mesothelioma, MO = morbid obesity, APN = acute pyelonephritis, Fsepsis = fungal sepsis, SAIV = stage IV sarcoma, IPF = interstitial pulmonary fibrosis. Word clouds were made with the R package, "wordcloud". [1,2]

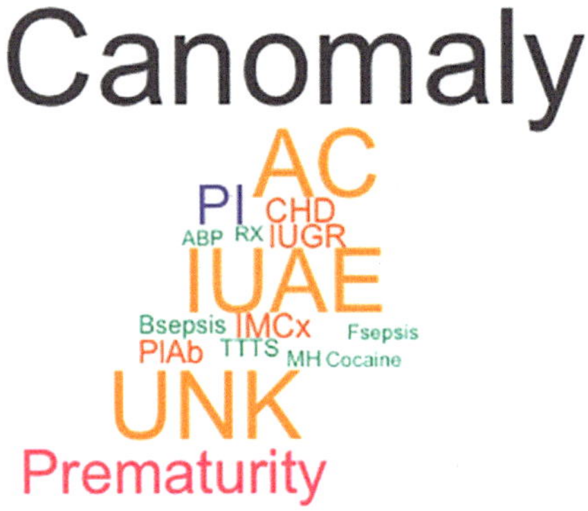

Figure 25.2 Word cloud of diagnostic codes associated with patient death in fetal and child decedents. The size of the word is proportional to the frequency of the diagnostic code. **Congenital anomaly, unknown and acute chorioamnionitis were the three most common codes among fetal and child decedents.** Canomaly = congenital anomaly, UNK = unknown, AC = acute chorioamnionitis, IUAE = intrauterine asphyxial event, PI = placental insufficiency, IMCx = incompetent maternal cervix, PlAb = placental abruption, IUGR = intrauterine growth retardation, MH = maternal hypertension,

CHD = congenital heart disease, TTTS = twin-twin transfusion syndrome, Fsepsis = fungal sepsis, ABP = acute bronchopneumonia, RX = therapy. Word clouds were made with the R package, "wordcloud". [1,2]

Index

An index of discussion topics, personal names, and figures. Pages for figures are bold face and pages for quotations at the beginning of chapters are italicized.

A

B

C

D

E

F

G

H

O

P

R

S

T

About the Authors

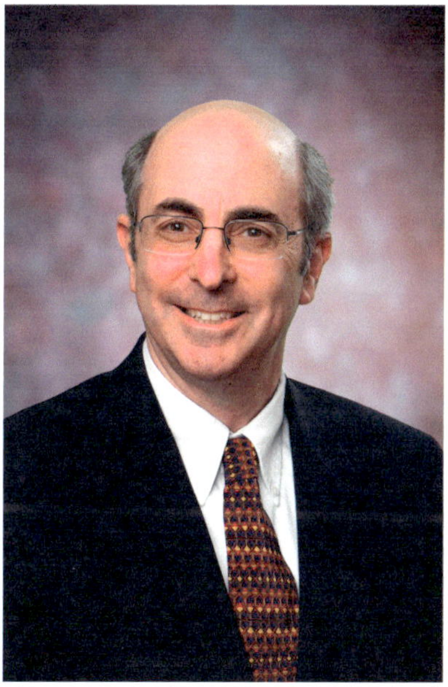

Mark L. Mitchell is a retired Anatomic Pathologist, the former Medical Director of the Department of Medical Laboratory Science in the College of Health Sciences at the University of Delaware, and the former Section Chief of Surgical Pathology and the Autopsy Service at Christiana Care Health Services in Newark, Delaware.

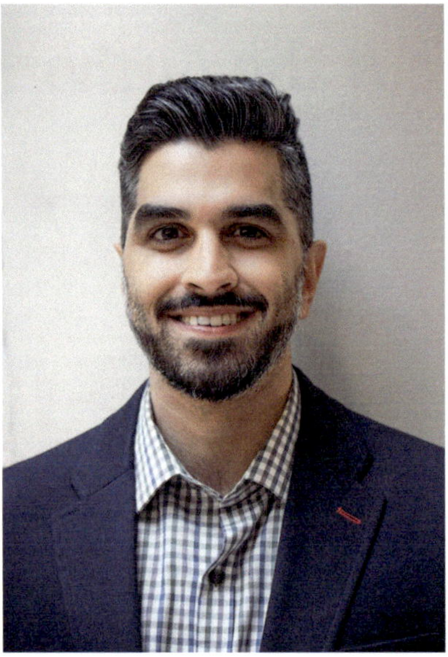

Omar Zahid Chohan is a graduate of Drexel University and Lake Erie College of Osteopathic Medicine. He is currently the Chief Resident in the Department of Radiology at Christiana Care Health Services, in Newark, Delaware, and will be a Fellow in Interventional Radiology in 2018. He enjoys teaching and hopes this book provides valuable information to anyone seeking to learn more about medicine.

Made in United States
Troutdale, OR
11/11/2026

57125325R00243